At a time when disinformation and misinformation about gender-affirming care are rampant, this book is a much needed scientifically based resource for mental health providers to better understand and appropriately work with trans and nonbinary people. This second edition not only includes more recent research but also expands on how mental health professionals can and must support and advocate for trans and nonbinary communities in the face of bad science and hostile governments.

—**Genny Beemyn, PhD,** Trans Scholar and Director of the Stonewall Center, University of Massachusetts Amherst

The new edition of this book is a timely update on an important community at a time when professional support and accurate knowledge are especially crucial. The authors share cutting-edge information and are established experts in their respected areas. This text would be among my top choices for teaching and training in clinical psychology and other mental health fields.

—**Lauren Mizock, PhD,** Core Faculty, Clinical Psychology PhD Program, Fielding Graduate University, Santa Barbara, CA

AFFIRMATIVE COUNSELING AND PSYCHOLOGICAL PRACTICE WITH *TRANS* AND *NONBINARY* CLIENTS

Perspectives on Sexual Orientation and Gender Diversity

David P. Rivera, Series Editor

Affirmative Counseling and Psychological Practice With Trans and Nonbinary Clients, Second Edition
  Edited by Anneliese Singh and Rafe McCullough

Affirmative Counseling and Psychological Practice With Transgender and Gender Nonconforming Clients
  Edited by Anneliese Singh and lore m. dickey

Affirming LGBTQ+ Students in Higher Education
  Edited by David P. Rivera, Roberto L. Abreu, and Kirsten A. Gonzalez

Dismantling Everyday Discrimination: Microaggressions Toward LGBTQ People, Second Edition
  Kevin Leo Yabut Nadal

The Gender Affirmative Model: An Interdisciplinary Approach to Supporting Transgender and Gender Expansive Children
  Edited by Colt Keo-Meier and Diane Ehrensaft

HIV+ Sex: The Psychological and Interpersonal Dynamics of HIV-Seropositive Gay and Bisexual Men's Relationships
  Edited by Perry N. Halkitis, Cynthia A. Gómez, and Richard J. Wolitski

Lesbian and Gay Parents and Their Children: Research on the Family Life Cycle
  Abbie E. Goldberg

LGBTQ Mental Health: International Perspectives and Experiences
  Edited by Nadine Nakamura and Carmen H. Logie

Supporting Gender Identity and Sexual Orientation Diversity in K–12 Schools
  Edited by Megan C. Lytle and Richard A. Sprott

Teaching LGBTQ Psychology: Queering Innovative Pedagogy and Practice
  Edited by Theodore R. Burnes and Jeanne L. Stanley

That's So Gay! Microaggressions and the Lesbian, Gay, Bisexual, and Transgender Community
  Kevin L. Nadal

AFFIRMATIVE COUNSELING AND PSYCHOLOGICAL PRACTICE WITH *TRANS* AND *NONBINARY* CLIENTS

SECOND EDITION

EDITORS
ANNELIESE SINGH
AND
RAFE McCULLOUGH

AMERICAN PSYCHOLOGICAL ASSOCIATION

Copyright © 2026 by the American Psychological Association. All rights, including for text and data mining, AI training, and similar technologies, are reserved. Except as permitted under the United States Copyright Act of 1976, no part of this publication may be reproduced or distributed in any form or by any means, including, but not limited to, the process of scanning and digitization, or stored in a database or retrieval system, without the prior written permission of the publisher.

The opinions and statements published are those of the Authors, and do not necessarily represent the policies of the American Psychological Association. The information contained in this work does not constitute personalized therapeutic advice. Users seeking medical advice, diagnoses, or treatment should consult a medical professional or health care provider. The Authors have worked to ensure that all information in this book is accurate at the time of publication and consistent with general mental health care standards.

Published by
American Psychological Association
750 First Street, NE
Washington, DC 20002
https://www.apa.org

Order Department
https://www.apa.org/pubs/books
order@apa.org

Typeset in Charter and Intrastate by TIPS Publishing Services, Carrboro, NC

Printer: Gasch Printing, Odenton, MD
Cover Designer: Gwen J. Grafft, Minneapolis, MN

Library of Congress Cataloging-in-Publication Data

Names: Singh, Anneliese A. editor | McCullough, Rafe editor
Title: Affirmative counseling and psychological practice with trans and nonbinary clients / edited by Anneliese Singh and Rafe McCullough.
Description: Second edition. | Washington, DC : American Psychological Association, [2026] | Series: Perspectives on sexual orientation and gender diversity series | Includes bibliographical references and index.
Identifiers: LCCN 2025018034 (print) | LCCN 2025018035 (ebook) | ISBN 9781433843228 paperback | ISBN 9781433843235 ebook
Subjects: LCSH: Transgender people--Mental health | Transgender people--Counseling of | Psychiatry, Transcultural | Cross-cultural counseling
Classification: LCC RC451.4.G39 A335 2026 (print) | LCC RC451.4.G39 (ebook) | DDC 616.890086/6--dc23/eng/20250806
LC record available at https://lccn.loc.gov/2025018034
LC ebook record available at https://lccn.loc.gov/2025018035

9781433849725 (pdf)

https://doi.org/10.1037/0000471-000

Printed in the United States of America

10 9 8 7 6 5 4 3 2 1

To the trans and nonbinary (TNB) organizers in the Deep South and transcestors of color who have labored to remind us of the power of our identities and communities—and ultimately liberation—in our experiences of healing, joy, and thriving; and to my always-and-forever-beloved, Lauren Lukkarila.
—ANNELIESE SINGH

To the TNB youth bravely fighting for their right to exist in perilous and uncertain times, the TNB mentors and elders who continue to light their way as they have always done, and to Kitt Kling, who modeled community care and illuminated his path with hope and optimism.
—RAFE McCULLOUGH

Contents

Contributors ix
Acknowledgments xvii

Introduction: Helping Trans and Nonbinary People Thrive 3
Anneliese Singh and Rafe McCullough

I. FOUNDATIONS OF TRANS AND NONBINARY-AFFIRMING CARE 17

1. Gender Diversity Within Trans and Nonbinary Communities 19
   Rafe McCullough, Anneliese Singh, and Heidi Breaux

2. Addressing Legal and Ethical Issues in Mental Health Care for Trans and Nonbinary Clients 31
   Cort M. Dorn-Medeiros, Sarah E. Burgamy, and Linda F. Campbell

3. Integrating Advocacy Into Gender-Affirming Care With Trans and Nonbinary Clients 57
   Robin M. Mathy

4. Affirmative Interdisciplinary Collaborative Care With Trans and Nonbinary Clients 77
   Kelly Ducheny, Michael L. Hendricks, G. Nic Rider, and Colt M. St. Amand

5. Debunking Bad Science With Trans and Nonbinary Communities 103
   Douglas Knutson, Bek Urban, and Aaron S. Breslow

II. WORKING WITH DIVERSE CLIENT IDENTITIES AND LIFE STAGES — 131

6. **Trans and Nonbinary People and Communities of Color: Resilience, Resistance, and Liberation** — 133
   Anneliese Singh, Sel J. Hwahng, Tochukwu Awachie, Aléx Bassi, Trae Brown, and Heidi Breaux

7. **Working With Nonbinary Communities** — 163
   Em Matsuno, Jay Bettergarcia, and Nat L. Bricker

8. **Affirmative Practice With Trans and Nonbinary Parents and Caregivers** — 189
   Daniel Walinsky, Julie M. Koch, and Anneliese Singh

9. **Affirmative Counseling With Trans and Nonbinary Children** — 211
   Aidan Key and Rafe McCullough

10. **Gender-Affirming Care With Trans and Nonbinary Adolescents** — 237
    Lisa Griffin

11. **Affirmative Care With Trans and Nonbinary Older Adults** — 269
    Kyle L. Bower and Mary Chase Mize

III. CLINICAL SKILLS AND INTERVENTIONS — 291

12. **Gender-Affirming Assessment and Treatment of Trauma With Trans and Nonbinary Clients** — 293
    Theodore R. Burnes, Jan E. Estrellado, and Anneliese Singh

13. **Trans and Nonbinary Suicidality and Suicide Risk Management** — 317
    Jayme Peta and Aspen Thomson

14. **Trans and Nonbinary Experiences of Religion, Spirituality, and Faith** — 345
    Ruben Hopwood and Jack Bruno

15. **Trans and Nonbinary Participation in Physical Activities, Competitive Sports, and Physical Education Classes** — 373
    John Gleaves, Matt Englar-Carlson, and Max Usman

Index — 395
About the Editors — 415

Contributors

Tochukwu Awachie (they/them), is a queer and trans genderfluid child of Nigerian immigrants who grew up on land stolen from Mvskoke and Aniyvwiyaʔi nations (Atlanta, GA). In personal and professional life, they are invested in the dynamic resistance, survival, and wellness practices that Black Diasporans have cultivated for generations. Their love for their communities is channeled through work in culturally informed psychology services, interdisciplinary research, educational programming, and spiritual care.

Aléx Bassi, MSEd (they/them), has a master's degree in school counseling and is currently working on getting their master's in professional mental health counseling. They have a passion for working with Black, Indigenous, and people of color (BIPOC) and youth populations, as well as discussing and exploring intersectionality. Aléx is a first-generation child of two immigrant parents, nonbinary, and transmasculine.

Jay Bettergarcia, PhD (they/them), is an associate professor in psychology and child development at California Polytechnic State University, San Luis Obispo. Their research explores queer- and trans-affirming care, trans resilience and resistance, and interventions centering radical healing and joy in the lives of queer and trans people of color. They are a Latiné, mixed race, transmasculine, and nonbinary counseling psychologist.

Kyle L. Bower, PhD (she/her), is the administrative director of the Youth Development Institute at the University of Georgia. She studies the life course and intergenerational family systems using qualitative methodology enhanced through digital technologies. As an ATLAS.ti professional trainer and proficient user of qualitative data analysis software (QDAS), she uses QDAS to engage reflexively throughout her research process, emphasizing the experiences of socially minoritized older adults and their social networks. She is a White, cisgender female of Jewish heritage.

Heidi Breaux, DSW, LCSW-BACS-R (she/they), is an assistant professor of professional practice at the Louisiana State University School of Social Work. They have worked in the LGBTQ+ community for over 15 years and taught graduate students for over a decade. Heidi is a White, queer, nonbinary activist originally from New York, now living in the Deep South.

Aaron S. Breslow, PhD (he/him), is an assistant professor with the Prime Center for Health Equity and the Einstein-Rockefeller-CUNY Center for AIDS Research at Albert Einstein College of Medicine. As a licensed psychologist, he received his PhD from Teachers College, Columbia University and runs a gender-affirming clinical service for trans and nonbinary adults at Montefiore Medical Center in the Bronx, NY. Dr. Breslow is a queer, White scholar whose research aims to measure and mitigate mental health disparities for trans, nonbinary, and intersex people, as well as those affected by human immunodeficiency virus criminalization.

Nat L. Bricker, MS (they/them), is a White, nonbinary, queer, clinical psychology PhD candidate at Palo Alto University. They are completing their degree with an emphasis in LGBTQ+ psychology, and their research and clinical work focuses on working with trans, nonbinary, queer, alterhuman, and neurodivergent communities. Their work is rooted in values of liberation, empowerment, and challenging oppressive systems through research and advocacy that centers the voices of minoritized individuals.

Trae Brown (they/them), is a graduate student in the school psychology doctoral program at Tulane University. Their research explores the ways Black, Indigenous, and people of color (BIPOC) adolescents navigate systems and cope, with a particular focus on how gender-nonconforming queer and transgender BIPOC (QTBIPOC) adolescents cultivate and leverage resilience, build community, and create meaning. Trae is a Black, queer, nonbinary person and has extensive experience working directly with BIPOC youth, providing support for their emotional well-being while also being involved as a grassroots community organizer and advocate.

Jack Bruno, LCSW (he/him), works to serve community members as a therapist with Transhealth and is a consulting faculty member with the Northwest Portland Area Indian Health Board. His writing, training, and learning has focused on Two-Spirit and Indigiqueer history, community, wellness, and embodiment, as well as topics of care in rural settings, sexual expression, and health care provider education. He is an Indigenous (Citizen Potawatomi Nation/Shishibéni), multiracial, Two-Spirit, transmasculine person who has been working to braid together themes of Indigeneity, queerness, and belongingness for almost 2 decades.

Sarah E. Burgamy, PsyD (she/her), is a White, genderqueer, androgynous woman with nearly 20 years of clinical practice expertise working with children, adolescents, and adults. The primary foci of her clinical work, professional trainings, and speaking engagements are gender and sexual orientation diversity across the lifespan. She has previously served as an adjunct faculty member in both masters and doctor of psychology (PsyD) programs as well as helping cofound a multidisciplinary pediatric gender clinic in Colorado.

Theodore R. Burnes, MSEd, PhD (he/him), is a professor of clinical education at the University of Southern California and a licensed mental health practitioner on the traditional land of the Tongva people (known today by colonists as Los Angeles). His work explores sexual well-being with special attention to consensually nonmonogamous people and sex workers. He is a cisgender, White, queer person expressing diverse genders who has worked with trans and nonbinary communities as a healer for over 20 years.

Linda F. Campbell, PhD (she/her), is a professor in the Counseling Psychology Program at the University of Georgia and director of the Center for Counseling Training Clinic. Her teaching, publications, and professional service are in the areas of ethics, supervision, and research on effectiveness in providing services to those living in poverty. Dr. Campbell is chair of the American Psychological Association (APA) Task Force on Revision of the Ethics Code and president of the Georgia State Board of Examiners of Psychologists.

Cort M. Dorn-Medeiros, PhD, LPC, CADC III (he/him), is an associate professor and department chair at Lewis & Clark College. His research focuses on mental health and addiction issues in LGBTQ+ communities, and both the training and supervision of counseling students working with LGBTQ+ people. He is a White, queer, trans man who has instructed a variety of courses in counselor education over the past decade, including content on ethical practice with trans and nonbinary communities.

Kelly Ducheny, PsyD (she/her), is a health psychologist and the senior advisor for education and clinical practice at Howard Brown Health, an LGBTQ+ federally qualified health center in Chicago, Illinois. She specializes in integrated care and community-based participatory research in trans and nonbinary (TNB) health, which centers TNB voices and priorities while also being heavily involved in the development of TNB standards of care and guideline development work groups in the APA and World Professional Association for Transgender Health (WPATH). She is a White, straight, cisgender woman who has worked with TNB communities as a clinician, coresearcher, and advocate for over 20 years.

Matt Englar-Carlson, PhD (he/him), is a professor and department chair in counseling at California State University, Fullerton, where he also directs the Center for Boys and Men. He is a cisgender, White male whose scholarship emphasizing healthy boyhood impacts education in schools and community settings.

Jan E. Estrellado, PhD, is an associate professor in the PsyD program at the California School of Professional Psychology, Alliant International University, San Diego campus. Dr. Estrellado's research areas examine race, ethnicity, sexual orientation, and gender identity in trauma therapy. Dr. Estrellado's scholarly interests connect multicultural psychology and trauma psychology, with the goal of providing quantitative and qualitative evidence for effective, culturally informed supervision and training of graduate students. Dr. Estrellado runs a private practice dedicated to trauma recovery and is also a consultant to the Avellaka Program, a federally funded antiviolence program serving the La Jolla Band of Luiseño Indians.

John Gleaves, PhD (he/him), is a codirector of the Center for Sociocultural Sport and Olympic Research at California State University, Fullerton and a professor of kinesiology. Gleaves's primary research interest focuses on cultural issues at the intersection of sport, science, and society, including performance enhancing drugs and policies for TNB inclusion in sports and physical activity. Gleaves has authored and edited numerous influential books and articles on the subject.

Lisa Griffin, PhD (she/her), is a licensed clinical psychologist who has been in practice for 30 years, specializing in care for gender-diverse children and teens. A White, Jewish, queer mother, she has spoken nationally and internationally on issues pertaining to TNB care, particularly in the areas of youth, cultural literacy, and professional ethics. She has attended engagements ranging from organizational trainings to conferences to serve as an expert witness. She serves on the Board of Directors of the United States Association for Transgender Health (USPATH) and she practices under the Psychology Interjurisdictional Compact (PSYPACT), providing care via telehealth to youth and their families in PSYPACT states across the country.

Michael L. Hendricks, PhD, ABPP (he/him), is a clinical and forensic psychologist in private practice in Washington, DC, and a clinical professor in the Department of Psychology and Brain Sciences at The George Washington University. He is the first author on the seminal article on the minority stress model for trans individuals, for which he earned an APA Presidential Citation. He has served in governance in APA and in its divisions, where he has been an advocate for a broad array of diversity issues—specifically including sexual and gender minority—for more than 30 years.

Ruben Hopwood, MDiv, PhD, LP (he/him), is a licensed psychologist, consultant, author, and visiting researcher with the Danielsen Institute at Boston University. His work centers on healing wounded relationships with the self, others, and whatever is sacred or spiritual in people's lives. His work focuses on trans and gender-diverse people, sexual minorities, and people struggling with the effects of cultural masculinity in their lives. He is a White, male, and queer-identified person who has worked in trans and gender-diverse health care and education for 20 years, and in spiritual leadership, care, and advocacy in the larger LGBTQ+ community for over 40 years.

Sel J. Hwahng, ScM, PhD (they/them), is an assistant professor in the Department of Women's and Gender Studies, Health and Sexuality track, at Towson University and recently completed a master of science in cardiovascular epidemiology at Johns Hopkins University, Bloomberg School of Public Health. Dr. Hwahng's current research focuses on women of color and LGBTQ nutritional and cardiometabolic health disparities utilizing social, behavioral, and epidemiological methods. This research has been funded by the National Institute on Drug Abuse, National Institutes of Health, American Public Health Association, International AIDS Society, Association for Women in Psychology, and the American Heart Association. Publications include over 30 sole-, first-, and co-authored articles and book chapters in peer-reviewed journals and edited volumes. Dr. Hwahng is also coauthor and coeditor of *Global LGBTQ Health: Research, Policy, Practice, and Pathways*, was recently accepted into the Delta Omega Honorary Society in Public Health, and leads an ontological-based leadership course at higher education institutions.

Aidan Key (he/him), is the author of *Trans Children in Today's Schools* (Oxford University Press), and is the founder and director of Gender Diversity, an organization that offers trainings and educational curriculum for educators in K–12 schools. Key is also the founder of TransFamilies.org, a national organization offering crucial support for families of gender-diverse children. His award-winning work and media appearances have spanned over 25 years.

Douglas Knutson, PhD, LHSP, ABPP (he/him), holds the Myron Ledbetter and Bob Lemon Counseling Psychology Diversity Associate Professorship and is the director of clinical training for the Counseling Psychology Program at Oklahoma State University. He serves as director of the Health, Education, and Rural Empowerment Lab, a research and advocacy group focused on health, resilience, and resistance in LGBTQ+ people with an emphasis on gender-diverse and rural populations. He is a White, neurodivergent, gay, cisgender man, board certified in counseling psychology.

Julie M. Koch, PhD, LHSP (she/they), is a professor of counseling psychology at the University of Iowa. Her research interests include multicultural counseling, microaffirmations, and the interaction of nature and mental health. They identify as a White, cisgender, queer woman and have a small private practice serving LGBTQ+ people in rural areas.

Robin M. Mathy, MSW, MSc, MSt, MA (she/her), is pursuing her doctor of social work at Tulane University and works as a clinical social worker and administrator in California. Her research interests include LGBT mental health and the relationship between childhood cross-gender behavior and adult gender identity and sexual orientation. She is of Oneida and Belgian heritage and lives productively with mental and physical impairments, despite attitudinal and structural barriers. She identifies as a woman assigned male at birth. She is committed to using evidence-based research and education to promote social justice for sexual and gender minorities, and engages in interpersonal and social activism to confront discrimination and oppression against marginalized people.

Em Matsuno, PhD (they/them), is an assistant professor in counseling and counseling psychology at Arizona State University. Their research focuses on minority stress and resilience among TNB people, with special attention to the unique experiences of nonbinary people and TNB BIPOC. They are a mixed race, Japanese American, queer, trans, and nonbinary person who aims to empower and liberate trans and nonbinary communities through community-centered research, clinical training, and advocacy.

Mary Chase Mize, PhD, LPC, ACS (she/her), is an assistant professor of clinical mental health counseling at Agnes Scott College in Decatur, GA. Her research is focused on gerontological counseling, community-based suicide prevention, and preparing mental health counselors to work with older adults. She hopes she is lucky enough to become an older person and strives to leverage her power and resources to support the lives of trans and nonbinary older adults through clinical work, advocacy, and research.

Jayme Peta, PhD (he/they), is a licensed psychologist and the director of practicum training at the Wright Institute's clinical psychology program. Their research and clinical background focuses on LGBTQ wellness and the intersection of suicidality, psychiatric crisis, and serious mental illness for LGBTQ+ clients. They are White, nonbinary, trans-identified, and have been advocating for improved mental health care for trans and nonbinary youth for 25 years. Jayme is also a coauthor of *The Trans and Gender Diverse Teen Resilience Guide: Essential Skills for Building Community, Well-Being and Mental Health*.

G. Nic Rider, PhD (they/them), is an associate professor, a licensed psychologist, and the gender services program coordinator at the Institute for Sexual and Gender Health and director of the National Center for Gender Health, both within the University of Minnesota Medical School. Their work focuses on social and structural factors impacting the lived experiences of marginalized communities, as well as the resilience and strengths identified by these same communities. Their professional interests include intersectionality, health equity, sexual health and pleasure, decolonizing healing justice, systemic change, and social justice advocacy.

Colt M. St. Amand, MD, PhD (he/they), is a licensed psychologist and board-certified family medicine physician with expertise in gender and sexuality. He began this work in 2009. He is an openly trans, genderqueer, Two-Spirit man who works with LGBTQ+ children, teens, adults, and their loved ones. Colt mentors and learns from trans and gender-diverse clinicians in providing gender care and provides consultation and programming.

Aspen Thomson, MA (she/her), is a student at Lewis and Clark College pursuing a master of arts in mental health counseling. She is a White, disabled, trans, and queer therapist who has done crisis counseling services, research, and activism. Her work focuses on trans, nonbinary, and queer people of all ages and backgrounds, towards the goal of collective and intersectional liberation.

Bek Urban, MA (they/them), is a PhD candidate in counseling psychology at Oklahoma State University. Their research focuses on queer health and eating disorders with an emphasis on improving care for trans and genderqueer individuals with eating disorders. Bek is a White, (gender) queer, neurodivergent person who grew up in the rural, southern United States and uses their experiences with rurality and queerness to inform their research and clinical practice.

Max Usman, BA (they/them), is a graduate student in Lewis & Clark College's Graduate School of Education and Counseling, Professional Mental Health Counseling program. Their research explores the perception of racial passing, the educational use of live-action role-playing, and the parallels between tabletop role-playing games and therapy. They are a Middle Eastern, mixed race, nonbinary femme who has worked with queer communities of color in a participatory and research-oriented role throughout their life.

Daniel Walinsky, PhD (he/him), is a licensed psychologist and adjunct faculty member at Temple University. He is a cisgender, White male. His clinical work and scholarship have focused on supporting LGBTQ+ people in community, academic, and practice spaces in both rural and urban settings.

Acknowledgments

We want to offer deep gratitude to you for reading this text—it has truly been a labor of love and accountability to organize the second edition of this book! We also want to express profound thanks to the 34 incredible chapter authors who demonstrated so much care and compassion as they reviewed the science and practice to describe essential aspects of gender-affirming care for trans and nonbinary (TNB) communities.

There are many additional people we would like to thank—starting with lore m. dickey, who coedited the first edition of this text (as well as coauthored numerous chapters within it) with Anneliese. A beloved friend of both Anneliese and Rafe, lore's passion and commitment to gender-affirming mental health care ran through our hearts and minds through each step of this book's organization and completion. We love you, lore! We are also very appreciative of Christopher Kelaher at the American Psychological Association, who believed in and supported this text from the beginning to this second edition, as well as David Becker, Ann Butler, and Emily Ekle who helped with production. Thanks also to Robert Kern and Claire Cin, who managed the copy editing, proofreading, composition, and indexing. Anneliese would also like to thank their partner, Lauren Lukkarila, whose love and support makes life so much sweeter and a grand adventure! Special thanks as well to their soul siblings—Anki Sinha, Theo Burnes, SJ McNulty, Tommy Le, and Narin Hassan—and to the Trans Resilience Project and Project ATL AFFIRM research team members and community advisory board members, Tochukwu Awachie, Heidi Breaux, Bekah Estevez, Robin Mathy, Nat Truszczynski, Tori Cooper, Jamie Roberts, and Evelyn Olansky. Additionally, Rafe would like to thank his dad for showing him what humble, steadfast, and unassuming support and advocacy looks like. Gratitude for Manivong J. Ratts, whose nearly 20-year mentorship led him to this place. Rafe would also like to express special appreciation for his trans siblings, Kai, Jackal, and Gauge; for the countless trans women who made it possible for him to find his people; and for his beloved professional community, Tameeka Hunter, Alexia de León, Heather Hadraba, Nori Valdez Gruber, Lana Kim, and Lina Darwich, who see him clearly. Finally, Rafe would like to thank Scott Lavis for more than 20 years of patience and support.

It is our greatest wish that this second edition supports you in deepening your ability to provide gender-affirming care with TNB clients from a wide variety of cultural backgrounds and lived experiences—and reminds you of the important progress we have made and the work we still have ahead of us to building TNB-affirming counseling and psychological settings.

AFFIRMATIVE COUNSELING AND PSYCHOLOGICAL PRACTICE WITH *TRANS* AND *NONBINARY* CLIENTS

INTRODUCTION

Helping Trans and Nonbinary People Thrive

ANNELIESE SINGH AND RAFE McCULLOUGH

Welcome to the second edition of this book! We are grateful you have found this text, and we are excited for you to read the work of the incredible authors who shaped this edition. One of the main reasons we are excited about the book is that you will be able to see how the landscape of trans and nonbinary (TNB) mental health is changing—in many ways for the better. This is not to say there are not significant, enduring challenges we face in providing TNB-affirming care. For instance, since 2022 we have seen the field of TNB-affirming care face emboldened legislative attacks at the state and federal levels. However, as you will read in this text, we have a larger body of specific supportive interventions that uplift and affirm the TNB clients with whom we work. When we compiled the first edition of this text, there was a strong focus on the harmful impact of societal anti-TNB bias on mental health (Singh & dickey, 2017). While these challenges have, in some ways, become even more merciless, this edition also highlights the resilience and resistance of TNB communities in pushing back against transprejudice and other intersectional oppressive systems. Additionally, we explore how mental health providers (MHPs) are expanding and evolving TNB-affirming care, both within the counseling office and in broader support systems.

---

https://doi.org/10.1037/0000471-001
Affirmative Counseling and Psychological Practice With Trans and Nonbinary Clients, Second Edition, A. Singh and R. McCullough (Editors)
Copyright © 2026 by the American Psychological Association. All rights reserved.

As coeditors of this text, we have thought deeply about the topics that you will read about in this book. Do we include a chapter specifically exploring affirming mental health care for nonbinary communities? Yes. Do we call in new chapters exploring the harm of bad science that has been used to drive anti-TNB legislation and the attack on TNB communities in the sports and recreation world? Yes. We are at a time in trans and nonbinary where the field is rapidly changing (for the better, we hope). At the same time, we know the continued attacks on TNB communities are escalating and becoming more vicious. Therefore, MHPs have even more opportunities to identify, value, and support the immense diversity and unique needs within TNB communities, centering intersectionality within TNB-affirming care. In addition, we take a lifespan and development approach by distinguishing between children and adolescents, and dedicate a chapter to the experiences of older TNB clients. Throughout, we maintain a focus on TNB-affirming care that prioritizes, not only support, but also joy, liberation, and the thriving of TNB communities.

In addition to these recurring themes throughout the chapters, we encourage you to embrace an expansive and inclusive approach as MHPs. Whether we spend our time primarily in practice, teaching, research, advocacy, or a mix of each of these, providing TNB-affirming counseling and psychological practices calls us each to broaden our perspectives and commit to training and retraining in what creating healthy counseling spaces for TNB people actually entails. Whether we are TNB or cisgender, the field of TNB-affirming care will continue to evolve in new directions. As MHPs, we must remain flexible and open to expanding our awareness, knowledge, skills, and actions (Ratts et al., 2015) to cultivate truly TNB-affirming counseling environments.

One of the important contributions of the first edition was grounding the rapidly expanding field of TNB care in general in a definition of what affirming care entailed. In the first edition, we defined TNB-affirming psychological practice as

> counseling that is culturally relevant and responsive to [TNB] clients and their multiple social identities, addresses the influence of social inequities on the lives of [TNB] clients, enhances [TNB] client resilience and coping, advocates to reduce systemic barriers to [TNB] mental and physical health, and leverages [TNB] client strengths. (Singh & dickey, 2017, p. 4)

We also described theoretical and competency frameworks that undergirded this definition. For instance, the minority stress model (Meyer, 2003; Testa & Hendricks, 2012) and resilience theory (Masten, 2001; Singh et al., 2011) shaped this definition so MHPs could learn and understand how distal and proximal stressors drive the need for TNB-affirming care, and how to cultivate the resilience needed from TNB individuals and communities to navigate these stressors. Simultaneously, multicultural and social justice counseling competency (Ratts et al., 2016) is foundational to TNB-affirming care, meaning MHP interventions are culturally responsive in terms of the MHP's awareness, knowledge, skills, and actions that they would need to engage in TNB-affirming practice, while also addressing biased institutional systems and societal attitudes toward TNB communities.

In this second edition, we update the definition of TNB-affirming counseling and psychological practice to the following: practice that is culturally responsive to TNB clients and their multiple social identities, ensures that TNB clients are aware of the long lineage and history of TNB communities, demystifies counseling and psychological practice, addresses the influence of interlocking oppressions (e.g., racism, ableism) and resulting social inequities on the well-being of TNB clients, enhances TNB client resilience and thriving, leverages TNB client strengths to cultivate self-autonomy and joy, and advocates to reduce systemic barriers (e.g., gatekeeping in health care, anti-TNB societal beliefs, anti-TNB legislation and policies) to TNB mental and physical health.

With this new definition, you will notice a shift in terminology (from "transgender and gender-nonconforming" to "trans and nonbinary"). As language is constantly evolving, we strive to use terminology that is most affirming for TNB people. As TNB communities continue to develop, linguistic expansion is inevitable. At the time of writing, many TNB people have adopted the term "trans," perhaps as a more concise and inclusive way to capture an umbrella term representing many diverse gender identities. *Trans* may encapsulate identities such as, transgender, transsexual, genderqueer, genderfluid, Two-Spirit (Indigenous people), nonbinary, and many more. Since the term "trans" holds significant meaning for TNB communities, we use it because we believe it aligns with what is most affirming from the perspectives of TNB people currently.

Since the first edition's publication, many TNB people have embraced the term *nonbinary* to describe those whose gender exists outside the male and female categories or who experience a sense of being both or neither (Matsuno & Budge, 2017). Some individuals use *nonbinary* or *gender-nonconforming* to describe expressions of gender that do not align with traditional gender binary norms ("woman" or "man"). However, "nonbinary" seems to more specifically refer to those whose identity represents a distinct gender. It is important to recognize that TNB communities are dynamic and diverse, with individuals using a wide range of terms to describe themselves. (See Chapter 7 for a deeper discussion on working with nonbinary communities.) We believe this new definition highlights for MHPs the importance of centering TNB autonomy while emphasizing that TNB joy, liberation, and thriving must be central to our work. This approach remains essential, especially in the face of persistent societal anti-TNB prejudice and discrimination. In doing so, we draw from liberation psychology (Martín-Baró, 1994; see also Chapter 2 in this volume for further discussion of liberation psychology tenets) applied to TNB counseling and psychology (Singh, 2016; Singh & Awachie, 2025; Singh et al., 2020), such as the principles of recovering historical memory of TNB people's existence over time, continents and cultures, and demystifying psychology. Intersectionality (Crenshaw, 1991) and critical race theory (Delgado & Stefancic, 2005) tenets help us clarify that gender-affirming care must recognize that the societal inequities TNB communities experience exist alongside systemic interlocking oppressions that amplify these inequities for clients with multiple minoritized social identities (e.g., TNB people of color, young TNB people, disabled TNB people).

ADDRESSING THE CHALLENGES

We know we just referenced the importance of uplifting TNB joy, liberation, and thriving. We stand by the importance of this. At the same time, it is also vital to note that as we go to press, there are over 500 bills that have been proposed in nearly all states that block or reduce rights for TNB people. In 2024, we saw more bills that eliminate TNB rights than any other year on record. Out of the 674 bills proposed across states, 50 passed, mostly targeting education, health care, and sports (Trans Legislation Tracker, 2025). This is on the heels of a 2023 legislative year, where 86 anti-TNB bills passed in 24 states restricting TNB rights in education, sports, civil rights, bathrooms, health care, birth certificates, incarceration, and military settings; 14 were vetoed. Overall, the Biden administration was TNB-friendly, asserting Title IX to provide protections to TNB children and adolescents in schools (though 26 Republican-led states sued the federal government in opposition).

Since the writing of this book began, the political climate has swiftly shifted in a precarious and unsafe direction for TNB people. Since Donald Trump won the presidential election and took office in January 2025, his presidential administration has enacted several executive orders and "Dear Colleague" letters from the Department of Education that threaten the health and safety of TNB people. One impactful executive order titled, "Defending Women from Gender Ideology Extremism and Restoring Biological Truth to the Federal Government" (Exec. Order No. 14168, 2025) mandates that the federal government will now only recognize two sexes of male and female, which are "not changeable and grounded in fundamental and incontrovertible reality." This leaves TNB people in a perilous situation where they are not legally recognized, opening them up to further discrimination in the workplace, health care, housing, and education. This order also impacts TNB people's ability to access passports that reflect their gender identity, forces trans women to be housed in men's prisons, and could restrict access to public restrooms for TNB people in places such as federal offices, military bases, and national parks. Moreover, additional executive orders have been enacted that expand service bans for TNB military personnel, direct agencies to prevent gender-affirming medical care for youth under age 19, prohibit trans girls from participating on school sports teams, and eliminate "federal funding or support for illegal and discriminatory treatment and indoctrination in K-12 schools, including based on gender ideology" (The White House, 2025). In addition, there has been a tremendous loss for TNB rights at the Supreme Court level in the *United States v. Skrmetti* issued in June 2025 where they issued a decision effectively upholding state bans on gender-affirming care for TNB minors. As we go to press, there are additional cases that could be heard at the Supreme Court level that have the possibility of further restricting TNB rights.

We know attacks on TNB communities are not new, however, many of us are still unfamiliar with the roots of these attacks, which have been part of a coordinated effort to use TNB communities as a lightning rod to gain votes and swing elections. These legislative and executive attacks are incredibly disturbing on multiple levels, especially because TNB people comprise a small community who are often the target of other societal harm. For instance, TNB people often experience chronic stressors due to stigma, prejudice, harassment, discrimination, and victimization resulting from navigating oppressive, anti-TNB societal structures (Hendricks & Testa, 2012; Meyer, 2003). It is no surprise that, as a result, TNB people experience high rates of depression (Bockting et al., 2013; Fredriksen-Goldsen et al., 2014; Witcomb et al., 2018), anxiety (Bouman et al., 2017; Millet et al., 2017), suicidality (Dickey & Budge, 2020; James et al., 2016; Progovac et al., 2020), and substance use issues (Hughto et al., 2021; Mereish, 2019). For TNB people of color, when anti-TNB prejudice intersects with racism, the negative impacts can be magnified, resulting in increased victimization and violence (James et al., 2016). According to the initial report for the new 2022 *U.S Trans Survey* (James et al., 2024), 44% of respondents reported experiencing serious psychological distress in the past 30 days. Of the TNB respondents who saw a health care provider in the past 12 months, 48% reported negative experiences, such as being refused care, misgendering, providers using harsh or abusive language, or being physically rough with them.

In addition, mental health barriers for TNB people have been exacerbated due to a variety of issues, such as MHPs' lack of knowledge providing gender-affirming care to TNB people across the lifespan (Benson, 2013; Hall & DeLaney, 2019; McCullough et al., 2017; Sperber et al., 2005), and discrimination by MHPs (Bockting et al., 2013; Lyons et al., 2015; McCullough et al., 2017). TNB people have experienced MHPs pathologizing their gender identities (Bess & Stabb, 2009; Elder, 2016) and over- or underfocusing on their gender identities as a presenting issue (Hall & DeLaney, 2019; Sperber et al., 2005). Additionally, TNB people living in rural areas experience additional barriers, such as hostile climates, transportation issues, long wait times, and lack of available TNB-affirming MHPs and other health care providers (Loo et al., 2021). This book seeks to provide better frameworks to MHPs for understanding and providing higher quality care for TNB communities.

The Paradox of Trans Visibility

It is clear to many of us who work closely with and are in community with TNB clients, friends, coworkers, family, partners, and children that TNB folks thrive when their needs are met and they are granted inclusion in all facets of society, including education, health care, employment, legal rights, and human rights. Joy and flourishing are the result of working together to remove these barriers, allowing TNB people to be liberated from the confinement and constraints of oppression. It is important to keep in mind that as TNB visibility strengthens, community and connection spring forth. At the same time, increased TNB visibility activates danger and violence (both personal and legislative). Gossett and colleagues (2017), the editors of *Trap Door: Trans Cultural Production and the Politics of Visibility*, capture this paradox in the statement, "The representation of queer and trans bodies is at an all-time high, in both art and popular culture, manifesting what seems to be a great curiosity about gender-nonconforming subjects and an insatiable hunger for images of transgender bodies. Yet violence against trans people, particularly people of color, is also at an all-time high, showing how starkly such 'interest' plays out" (p. xiii). TNB representation is central to alleviating isolation and instilling feelings of hope, belonging, and affirmation. But we must remember to keep a close watch to hold violence at bay while supporting the cultivation of safety and community care.

Multifaceted Trans and Nonbinary Lives

As MHPs, it is important to keep the focus on TNB clients as individual people *and* as members of sociocultural groups (e.g., racial and ethnic groups, LGBTQ+, etc.). For instance, TNB people are experiencing the weight and impact of the tremendous movement to erase TNB identities in the United States. However, as MHPs we have the opportunity to deepen our understanding of TNB people as people who are not just experiencing sociopolitical headwinds. Rather,

TNB individuals and communities have agency and are living multifaceted and complex lives—certainly shaped by larger social and political structures—but also shaped by their own lived experiences of creativity, strength, relationships, unique and intentional cultural and community engagements, and their own likes and preferences. It is important that MHPs can move beyond the tropes of TNB people as tragic figures, victims, and hapless, unfortunate, and pitiable individuals, if we are to truly see TNB people clearly and be able to collaboratively support their whole personhood. As you engage with different aspects of this book, we ask you to expand your thoughts on what it means to be a TNB person living a meaningful and multilayered life at this time in history.

Addressing Continuing Trans and Binary Distrust of Mental Health Providers and Countering Gatekeeping Approaches

As we deepen our practice of TNB-affirming care, it is important for us as MHPs to understand that there is continued distrust of the mental health industry (and of health care in general) due to the harm of MHP gatekeeping that historically and currently exists for TNB people trying to access quality care. Gatekeeping is a paternalistic model of care that has persisted since the latter part of the 20th century. Since gender-affirming care was considered experimental when gender clinics began to emerge in the 1960s, few TNB people were permitted to access this care (Weigand, 2021). For instance, TNB people who did not conform to a cisgender-heteronormative gender binary (e.g., desire to have a career considered traditional for one's gender or to be in a heterosexual marriage and have children) were rejected from clinics. Out of nearly 1,200 applications at Johns Hopkins gender clinic in the 70s, only 23 were able to move forward (Siotos et al., 2019). In order to justify treatment for TNB people, medical providers and MHPs created a medicalized narrative. If TNB people needed medical treatment, they often needed to manipulate their own narratives or omit information so they could be approved for care (Weigand, 2021).

TNB people were required to express their gender in binary ways (e.g., living as a "woman" or as a "man"), leave their relationships, and take extensive personality and other psychological assessments to gain support for their desired social and medical transitions (Stryker, 2017). These gatekeeping practices were supported by formalized professional organizations (e.g., Harry Benjamin International Gender Dysphoria Association, now known as WPATH as of 2007) and MHP researchers that purported to support and serve TNB clients, but who also had inflicted immense harm on the lives of these same clients. The stories of this harm live on within TNB communities, and the aforementioned anti-TNB legislative and other societal attacks on TNB lives, alongside a larger health care system that has been slow to adopt TNB-affirming practices, have contributed to this distrust. Indeed, TNB clients still experience significant gatekeeping of their health care, as they often must access MHPs in order to get referrals to medical providers for hormone therapy and gender-affirming surgeries. Although it is beyond the scope of this chapter to discuss, it is important to note that the only two areas of medical care requiring such MHP letters of referral are for TNB health care and those seeking bariatric surgery, which reflects the distrust and restrictions health care has instituted on clients trying to access this type of care.

Because of the historical and continued harm of gatekeeping approaches, we strongly advocate for MHPs to challenge and resist gatekeeping efforts in health care wherever possible. You will see this echoed across the chapters within this book, as it is crucial that TNB communities have self-autonomy and MHP support and advocacy as they navigate societal systems (e.g., schools, health care; see Chapter 4 for interdisciplinary TNB-affirming care efforts MHPs can support and further with colleagues) that were not only not built with their needs in mind, but that also often actively work against their well-being. We also encourage MHPs to learn about existing mutual aid networks that TNB communities have created, as well as explore how MHPs can help expand access and material resources within these mutual aid networks (Singh & Awachie, 2025). In many ways, TNB-affirming care requires that we as MHPs consider a wide range of reparative acts (e.g., providing pro bono TNB client services, leading pro bono TNB-affirming practice professional development workshops, supporting local and community-based TNB organizations with financial or other material resources) we can engage in to address the long history of neglect, harm, and lack of access to care within our field.

HOW THIS BOOK IS ORGANIZED

We are deeply grateful for the extraordinary authors who wrote outstanding chapters for this second edition amidst unfolding and persistent anti-TNB attacks and erasure. As you read through this text, you will see that the chapters have been organized into three parts. In Part I: Foundations of Trans and Nonbinary-Affirming Care, you will find chapters on the diversity of gender identity within TNB communities (Chapter 1 by Rafe McCullough, Anneliese Singh, and Heidi Breaux), as well as chapters exploring ethical and legal foundations of TNB-affirming care (Chapter 2 by Cort M. Dorn-Medeiros, Sarah E. Burgamy, and Linda Campbell), the vital advocacy needed from MHPs in working with TNB communities (Chapter 3 by Robin M. Mathy), and a chapter exploring the collaboration networks MHPs develop in providing TNB-affirming care (Chapter 4 by Kelly Ducheny, Michael L. Hendricks, G. Nic Rider, and Colt M. St. Amand). This part on TNB-affirming care foundations ends with a chapter naming the harmful effects of bad science on TNB clients (Chapter 5 by Douglas Knutson, Bek Urban, and Aaron S. Breslow), reminding us of the vital importance of high-quality research and the role it plays in reinforcing TNB-affirming care by shifting societal culture to create a world that supports the joy and thriving of TNB communities.

In Part II: Working With Diverse Client Identities and Life Stages, there are chapters exploring specific TNB communities, such as chapters on TNB-affirming care with communities of color (Chapter 6 by Anneliese Singh, Sel J. Hwahng, Tochukwu Awachie, Aléx Bassi, Trae Brown, and Heidi Breaux), nonbinary communities (Chapter 7 by Em Matsuno, Jay Bettergarcia, and Nat L. Bricker), and TNB parents and caregivers (Chapter 8 by Daniel Walinsky, Julie M. Koch, and Anneliese Singh). In this part, you will also find chapters describing TNB-affirming care across life stages, such as the important role of MHPs in working with children (Chapter 9 by Aidan Key and Rafe McCullough), adolescents (Chapter 10 by Lisa Griffin), and TNB older adults (Chapter 11 by Kyle L. Bower and Mary Chase Mize).

Finally, in Part III: Clinical Skills and Interventions, we address areas of targeted focus for MHPs to deepen their TNB-affirming knowledge and skills. Chapter authors delve into the role of trauma (Chapter 12 by Theodore R. Burnes, Jan E. Estrellado, and Anneliese Singh) and how to address suicidality (Chapter 13 by Jayme Peta and Aspen Thomson) with TNB clients in supportive ways. We include chapters on how religion can often shape the life experiences of TNB clients (Chapter 14 by Ruben Hopwood and Jack Bruno) and how to support TNB clients participating in sports and recreation (Chapter 15 by John Gleaves, Matt Englar-Carlson, and Max Usman). We are grateful to all the chapter authors who remind us of the evidence base undergirding TNB-affirming care and how to translate this science into effective and supportive clinical work. Across each of the chapters, the authors have interspersed case examples to provide insights into the types of issues TNB clients encounter and offer MHPs ideas for how to work with them.

UPLIFTING TRANS AND NONBINARY JOY, LIBERATION, AND THRIVING

Ultimately, TNB-affirming practice should help us envision, build, sustain, and innovate MHP intervention and prevention efforts that center TNB joy, liberation, and thriving. We are excited to see new research examining these areas, but it is still nascent and thus critical to ensure we are following the lead of TNB community organizers and advocates who have long cultivated environments where TNB joy, liberation, and thriving are not just constructs to be defined, but rather are guideposts to be lived. As Raquel Willis (2023), a Black trans woman, author, and organizer, shares profoundly:

Trans liberation is . . .

beyond the field of expectations.

It's no more wondering who you could've been.

It's generations of elders, it's you and me

living longer than we thought.

It is our greatest hope that you not only find the information within this text helpful to furthering your own gender-affirming work with TNB communities, but that you also pass on this information to other MHPs in your sphere of influence. Indeed, the only way we have seen the field of TNB gender-affirming care shift towards more affirming (and in our view, ethical) approaches over the years has been because people like you have advocated for change in our field—change that responds to the calls to action made by many generations of TNB community organizers and clients who came before us. Therefore, an essential truth at this time is that the actions we take as MHPs—large and small—repeated over time to preserve, protect, expand, and innovate gender-affirming care will improve the care our next generations of TNB people and communities receive and know they deserve.

REFERENCES

Benson, K. E. (2013). Seeking support: Transgender client experiences with mental health services. *Journal of Feminist Family Therapy, 25*(1), 17–40. https://doi.org/10.1080/08952833.2013.755081

Bess, J. A., & Stabb, S. D. (2009). The experiences of transgendered persons in psychotherapy: Voices and recommendations. *Journal of Mental Health Counseling, 31*(3), 264–282. https://doi.org/10.17744/mehc.31.3.f6241546811133w50

Bockting, W. O., Minder, M. H., Swinburne Romine, R. E., Hamilton, A., & Coleman, E. (2013). Stigma, mental health, and resilience in an online sample of the U.S. transgender population. *American Journal of Public Health, 103*(5), 943–951. https://doi.org/10.2105/AJPH.2013.301241

Bouman, W. P., Claes, L., Brewin, N., Crawford, J. R., Millet, N., Fernandez-Aranda, F., & Arcelus, J. (2017). Transgender and anxiety: A comparative study between transgender people and the general population. *International Journal of Transgenderism, 18*(1), 16–26. https://doi.org/10.1080/15532739.2016.1258352

Crenshaw, K. (1991) Mapping the margins: Intersectionality, identity politics, and violence against women of color. *Stanford Law Review, 43*, 1241–1299. https://doi.org/10.2307/1229039

Delgado, R., & Stefancic, J. (2005). *The Derrick Bell reader.* New York University Press.

Dickey, L. M., & Budge, S. L. (2020). Suicide and the transgender experience: A public health crisis. *American Psychologist, 75*(3), 380–390. https://doi.org/10.1037/amp0000619

Exec. Order No. 14168, 90 FR 8615. (2025). https://www.whitehouse.gov/presidential-actions/2025/01/defending-women-from-gender-ideology-extremism-and-restoring-biological-truth-to-the-federal-government/

Fredriksen-Goldsen, K. I., Cook-Daniels, L., Kim, H.-J., Erosheva, E. A., Emlet, C. A., Hoy-Ellis, C. P., Goldsen, J., & Muraco, A. (2014). Physical and mental health of transgender older adults: An at-risk and underserved population. *The Gerontologist, 54*(3), 488–500. https://doi.org/10.1093/geront/gnt021

Ghorayshi, M. (2024, June 24). *Biden officials pushed to remove age limits for trans surgery, documents show.* Retrieved from https://www.nytimes.com/2024/06/25/health/transgender-minors-surgeries.html

Gossett, R., Stanley, E., & Burton, J. (Eds.). (2017). *Trap door: Trans cultural production and the politics of visibility.* Massachusetts Institute of Technology Press.

Hall, S. F., & DeLaney, M. J. (2019). A trauma-informed exploration of the mental health and community support experiences of transgender and gender-expansive adults. *Journal of Homosexuality, 68*(8), 1–20. https://doi.org/10.1080/00918369.2019.1696104

Hendricks, M. L., & Testa, R. J. (2012). A conceptual framework for clinical work with transgender and gender nonconforming clients: An adaptation of the minority stress model. *Professional Psychology: Research and Practice, 43*(5), 460–467. https://doi.org/10.1037/a0029597

Hughto, J. M., Quinn, E. K., Dunbar, M. S., Rose, A. J., Shireman, T. I., & Jasuja, G. K. (2021). Prevalence and co-occurrence of alcohol, nicotine, and other substance use disorder diagnoses among US transgender and cisgender adults. *JAMA Network Open, 4*(2), e2036512-e2036512. https://doi.org/10.1001/jamanetworkopen.2020.36512

James, S. E., Herman, J. L., Durso, L. E., & Heng-Lehtinen, R. (2024). *Early insights: A report of the 2022 US Transgender Survey.* https://transequality.org/sites/default/files/2024-02/2022%20USTS%20Early%20Insights%20Report_FINAL.pdf

James, S. E., Herman, J. L., Rankin, S., Keisling, M., Mottet, L., & Anafi, M. (2016). *The report of the 2015 U.S. Transgender Survey.* National Center for Transgender Equality. https://transequality.org/sites/default/files/docs/usts/USTS-Full-Report-Dec17.pdf

Loo, S., Almazan, A. N., Vedilago, V., Stott, B., Reisner, S. L., Keuroghlian, A. S. (2021). Understanding community member and health care professional perspectives on gender-affirming care: A qualitative study. *PLOS One, (16)*8, e0255568. https://doi.org/10.1371/journal.pone.0255568

Lyons, T., Shannon, K., Pierre, L., Small, W., Krusi, A., & Kerr, T. (2015). A qualitative study of transgender individuals' experiences in residential addiction treatment settings: Stigma and inclusivity. *Substance Abuse Treatment, Prevention, & Policy, 10*(17). https:// doi.org/10.1186/s13011-015-0015-4

Martín-Baró, I. (1994). *Writings for a liberation psychology* (A. Aron & S. Corne, Eds.). Harvard University Press.

Masten, A. (2001). Ordinary magic: Resilience processes in development. *American Psychologist, 56*(3), 227–238. https://doi.org/10.1037/0003-066X.56.3.227

Matsuno, E., & Budge, S. L. (2017). Non-binary/genderqueer identities: A critical review of the literature. *Current Sexual Health Reports, 9*(3), 116–120. https://doi.org/10.1007/s11930-017-0111-8

McCullough, R., Dispenza, F., Parker, L. K., Viehl, C. J., Chang, C. Y., & Murphy, T. M. (2017). The counseling experiences of transgender and gender nonconforming clients. *Journal of Counseling & Development, 95*(4), 423–434. https://doi.org/10.1002/jcad.12157

Mereish, E. H. (2019). Substance use and misuse among sexual and gender minority youth. *Current Opinion in Psychology, 30*, 123–127. https://doi.org/10.1016/j.copsyc.2019.05.002

Meyer, I. H. (2003). Prejudice, social stress, and mental health in lesbian, gay, and bisexual populations: Conceptual issues and research evidence. *Psychological Bulletin, 129*(5), 674–697.

Millet, N., Longworth, J., & Arcelus, J. (2017). Prevalence of anxiety symptoms and disorders in the transgender population: A systematic review of the literature. *International Journal of Transgenderism, 18*(1), 27–38. https://doi.org/10.1080/15532739.2016.1258353

Progovac, A. M., Mullin, B. O., Dunham, E., Reisner, S. L., McDowell, A., Sanchez Roman, M. J., Dunn, M., Telingator, C. J., Lu, F. Q., Breslow, A. S., Forstein, M., & Cook, B. L. (2020). Disparities in suicidality by gender identity among Medicare beneficiaries. *American Journal of Preventive Medicine, 58*(6), 789–798. https://doi.org/10.1016/j.amepre.2020.01.004

Ratts, M. J., Singh, A. A., Nassar-McMillan, S., Butler, S. K., & McCullough, J. R. (2016). Multicultural and social justice counseling competencies: Guidelines for the counseling profession. *Journal of Multicultural Counseling and Development, 44*(1), 28–48. https://doi.org/10.1002/jmcd.12035

Singh, A. A. (2016). Moving from affirmation to liberation in psychological practice with transgender and gender nonconforming clients. *American Psychologist, 71*(8), 755–762. https://doi.org/10.1037/amp0000106

Singh, A. A., & Awachie, T. (2025). Black, indigenous, and people of color trans and nonbinary liberation: A transcestral journey of critical consciousness, reckoning, and healing. *American Psychologist, 80*(4), 618–629. https://doi.org/10.1037/amp0001388

Singh, A. A., & dickey, l. m. (2017). Introduction. In A. A. Singh & l. m. dickey (Eds.), *Affirmative counseling and psychological practice with transgender and gender nonconforming clients* (pp. 3–18). American Psychological Association. https://doi.org/10.1037/14957-001

Singh, A. A., Hays, D. G., & Watson, L. S. (2011). Strength in the face of adversity: Resilience strategies of transgender individuals. *Journal of Counseling & Development, 89*(1), 20–27.

Singh, A. A., Parker, B., Aqil, A. R., & Thacker, F. (2020). Liberation psychology and LGBTQ+ communities: Naming colonization, uplifting resilience, and reclaiming ancient his-stories, her-stories, and t-stories. In L. Comas-Díaz & E. Torres Rivera (Eds.), *Liberation psychology: Theory, method, practice, and social justice* (pp. 207–224). American Psychological Association. https://doi.org/10.1037/0000198-012

Siotos, C., Neira, P. M., Lau, B. D., Stone, J. P., Page, J., Rosson, G. D., & Coon, D. (2019). Origins of gender affirmation surgery: The history of the first gender identity clinic in the United States at Johns Hopkins. *Annals of Plastic Surgery, 83*(2), 132–136. https://doi.org/10.1097/sap.0000000000001684

Sperber, J., Landers, S., & Lawrence, S. (2005). Access to health care for transgendered persons: Results of a needs assessment in Boston. *International Journal of Transgenderism, 8*(2–3), 75–91. https://doi.org/10.1300/J485v08n02_08

Stryker, S. D., Pallerla, H., Yockey, R. A., Bedard-Thomas, J., & Pickle, S. (2022). Training mental health professionals in gender-affirming care: A survey of experienced clinicians. *Transgender Health, 7*(1), 68–77. https://doi.org/10.1089/trgh.2020.0123

Trans Legislation Tracker. (2024). *2024 anti-trans bills tracker*. https://translegislation.com/

The White House. (2025, January 29). *Ending radical indoctrination in K–12 schooling* [Presidential action]. https://www.whitehouse.gov/presidential-actions/ending-radical-indoctrination-in-k-12-schooling/

Willis, R. (2023, June 29). What is trans liberation? *Them*. https://www.them.us/story/what-is-trans-liberation-raquel-willis-poem

Witcomb, G. L., Bouman, W. P., Claes, L., Brewin, N., Crawford, J. R., & Arcelus, J. (2018). Levels of depression in transgender people and its predictors: Results of a large matched control study with transgender people accessing clinical services. *Journal of Affective Disorders, 235*, 308–315. https://doi.org/10.1016/j.jad.2018.02.051

PART I: FOUNDATIONS OF TRANS AND NONBINARY-AFFIRMING CARE

1

GENDER DIVERSITY WITHIN TRANS AND NONBINARY COMMUNITIES

RAFE McCULLOUGH, ANNELIESE SINGH, AND HEIDI BREAUX

For mental health providers, the work lies in being the guiding mirror that leads trans and nonbinary people back home to themselves.

—Daniela Avila, trans woman

At this moment, one of the most exciting aspects of gender-affirming mental health care with trans and nonbinary (TNB) clients is that society, in general, is more familiar with the existence of TNB communities because of increased media representation. This does not mean that all of these representations are positive, accurate, kind, or respectful; nor does it mean that there is not significant anti-TNB prejudice amplifying societal anti-TNB bias and driving anti-TNB legislation (Feder, 2020). Despite these continuing challenges, mental health providers (MHPs) need to have a basic knowledge of TNB-affirming identity terms and also a firm understanding of the continued creativity and evolution of affirming language by TNB people across the lifespan and across cultural contexts. The way we use language has the power to demean, render invisible, and pathologize—or conversely—elevate, encourage, and liberate. MHPs need to not only have awareness and knowledge of TNB-affirming terms, but they must also have the desire to communicate with clients about which of those terms best defines them, affirms them, and lifts them up. Language is never

https://doi.org/10.1037/0000471-002
Affirmative Counseling and Psychological Practice With Trans and Nonbinary Clients, Second Edition, A. Singh and R. McCullough (Editors)
Copyright © 2026 by the American Psychological Association. All rights reserved.

fixed but rather always developing. As TNB communities continue to expand by creating new self-identification terms that honor and celebrate various queer identities, MHPs need to continuously evolve our language. This is more important than ever to transcend the backlash and setbacks that target TNB-affirming care. Language and terminology chosen for us, both by individuals and the TNB community, should always be prioritized over medicalized terms that were chosen for TNB by others, including in health and therapeutic settings.

In this chapter, we provide essential definitions of constructs, such as sex and gender, and highlight affirming glossaries from TNB community-based and mental health organizations that provide the foundations of TNB-affirming care. We also describe the use of affirming TNB terms originating within TNB communities (e.g., young people, people of color, older adults). In doing so, we look across the globe to history to note how TNB terminology has evolved pre- and postcolonization. We focus specifically on the terms *trans* and *nonbinary* because currently they are most commonly used in the United States, as terms like *gender nonconforming* and *gender diverse* have become socially antiquated. This also pays homage to the continued fight for our rights and recognition both inside and outside of the LGBTQIA+ community, where historically the "T" for transgender, as well as our community as a whole, has often been sidelined (Greer, 2018). We end the chapter with a discussion of the key aspects of ongoing learning about affirming TNB language, including the role of cultural humility and how competency and theoretical frameworks can help in the continuous process of mentoring and learning.

AFFIRMING LANGUAGE AND TERMINOLOGY WITH TRANS AND NONBINARY COMMUNITIES

As MHPs, we are working at a time when people in the world and within health care may be more familiar with the fact that TNB communities exist and have important needs; however, there is still a strong need to ensure our understanding of essential terms related to TNB communities. We will include some coverage of terminology, including culturally-specific TNB terms in the following section, but for resources on basic glossaries of terms used within TNB communities, we recommend the *Trans Lifeline Glossary* (https://translifeline.org/resource_category/glossary/), Trans Hub Language (https://www.transhub.org.au/language), *PFLAG National Glossary* (https://pflag.org/glossary/), *GLAAD LGBTQ+ Glossary of Terms* (https://glaad.org/reference/terms/), and the American Psychological Association's (2015) *Guidelines for Psychological Practice With Transgender and Gender Nonconforming People* for additional TNB terminology.

When providing TNB-affirming care, it is important to understand terms such as sex, gender, and sexual orientation. *Sex* is assigned at birth, usually based on the appearance of our external genitalia, and can be classified as female, male, or intersex. *Gender* or *gender identity* refers to a person's innate, felt sense of gender and can include being a women, man, or another gender that is not binary (e.g. nonbinary, agender, gender-nonconforming, gender-fluid, gender creative). Gender also refers to whether someone is trans (a person whose gender is not in alignment with the sex they were assigned at birth) or cisgender (a person whose gender is in alignment with the sex they were assigned at birth). *Sexual orientation* or *romantic orientation* relates to whom someone is sexually or intimately attracted to, if they are. It is essential for MHPs to understand the basic differences between gender identity and sexual orientation and realize that they are distinct constructs. When MHPs confuse these concepts, TNB clients can feel invalidated and misunderstood. Consider the following example of a participant in a qualitative study about TNB experiences with counselors. The trans male participant recounted his negative experience with an MHP who did not understand these differences:

> I'm on testosterone... I'm like kind of, early on in it. She [MHP] kept trying to get me to go to this women's [support] group, and I kept telling her, "No, I don't belong in a women's group." (McCullough et al., 2017, p. 429)

For some TNB people, gender identity and sexual orientation are interconnected and evolve together. Such is the case for TNB people who are romantically and sexually attracted to sameness. Their sexual orientation may not be static when they undergo a medical or social transition. For instance, a transfeminine person might have only dated men before medically transitioning and then exclusively dated women afterward. Similarly, a nonbinary person might be attracted solely to other nonbinary individuals after coming out as nonbinary, whereas previously they were attracted to cisgender people. Still, for some TNB people, their sexual orientations reflect even more fluidity over time. There are as many varied sexual romantic orientations for TNB people as there are for cisgender people. The use of correct terminology is important, but it may not be enough to fully understand what the correct identity term means to a TNB client.

Over a decade ago, a Wisconsin-based TNB education and advocacy organization created a document titled *The Terms Paradox* (FORGE, 2012). This document emphasized the importance of supporting TNB people in using their own identity terms to affirm their right to self-definition. However, it also acknowledged the fluidity throughout the evolution of TNB identities and the absence of standard definitions. Kate Bornstein (2016) published the book *Gender Outlaw: On Men, Women, and the Rest of Us*, which also examined intersections of femininity, sexuality, and the need to constantly critique societal paradigms. Thus, the terms discussed earlier are valuable only as far as they foster connection and deeper understanding of TNB people's lives, experiences, and needs. TNB communities have evolved significantly in their use of terminology over the years. An essential component of TNB-affirming care is MHPs' understanding that they may not be aware of rapidly evolving, affirming terms that TNB communities use. However, practicing cultural humility as a means to establish respect for clients' self-determination of terminology, and other aspects of the TNB experience, will help MHPs use terms that are most affirming for the TNB clients with whom they work. Further, MHPs should engage in dialogues with TNB clients about the personal meanings of their self-identification terms and mirror the terms the client uses for themselves. This should be done at all times, including in the presence of clients and in the presence of others when the client is not there. For some in the TNB community, the terminology traditionally used in TNB-affirming care can be too limiting. Some TNB activists are trying to address these limitations.

For instance, Florence Ashley (2022)—a transfeminine jurist, bioethicist, public speaker, and advocate—introduced the term *gender modality* to broaden the discussion of gender identity by considering the relationship between a person's gender identity and the gender assigned to them at birth. They advocate for the use of this term because it highlights the cultural context of gender and emphasizes that terms like transgender and cisgender do not fully capture the meaning of gender across different societies (Ashley, 2022). Additionally, the concept of a gender modality expands beyond just trans and cisgender categories, creating space for agender individuals (those who do not identify with any gender), intersex people, and those with culture-specific identities that may not align with Western gender notions (e.g., *Two-Spirit*, from Indigenous communities in North America, and *hijra*, recognized as a third gender on the Indian subcontinent). This approach is similar to how the understanding of sexual orientation has evolved to include options beyond gay and straight (Ashley et al., 2024).

It is important that MHPs avoid reducing TNB people to rigid or binary identity categories. Recently, there has been a trend to categorize TNB people into binary and nonbinary groups, often based on their medical transition decisions or how they appear. This can manifest in statements like, "They are nonbinary, but she is a binary trans person." However, TNB people who choose to medically transition and who may be perceived as cisgender in certain contexts can still identify as nonbinary or genderfluid. Nonbinary individuals may also use she/her or he/him pronouns and express their gender in more traditional masculine and feminine ways, therefore pronouns and gender expression should never be used as indicators of whether a TNB person identifies as binary or nonbinary. Unless a TNB client has self-identified with a particular label, such assigned descriptors are inherently limiting and detract from the diverse and expansive identities within TNB communities, which may include gender fluid, gender variant, genderqueer, gender expansive, agender, bigender, pangender, or combinations thereof. It is important for MHPs to embrace perspectives that broaden, rather than restrict, current understandings of gender.

Using Affirming Terminology Across the Trans and Nonbinary Lifespan and Across Cultural Contexts

For MHPs attempting to broaden their perspectives on gender, it is essential to understand lifespan and cultural contexts that shape how TNB people define and describe themselves. For example, younger TNB people may embrace the term *deadname* (the name given to a TNB person at birth but no longer used), whereas older TNB people may find this term disrespectful to their families who named them, including if they were named after someone in the family or someone important to the family. Similarly, the terms *assigned female at birth* (AFAB) and *assigned male at birth* (AMAB) may resonate positively with younger generations, but evoke negative feelings in older TNB people who recall times when doctors and MHPs urged them to forget their past, conceal their TNB histories, and move on with their lives. Even the ways in which TNB people define their histories can vary across generations. Younger TNB folks might assert that they were always male and that people are only now recognizing this fact, whereas older TNB people may initially conceptualize themselves as once female, but then see themselves as male or nonbinary after undergoing some type of transition (social or medical). *Nonbinary* is a newer term that older TNB folks may not use, and *queer* or *genderqueer* (meaning outside of the gender binary) may elicit past bullying experiences for older TNB people, but be embraced positively by younger TNB people (see Chapter 7 for a comprehensive discussion of affirming language within nonbinary communities).

MHPs should also be familiar with gender-affirming language that is generated from within communities of color. Some examples include the term *boi*, commonly used within Black and other communities of color (see *The Brown Boi Project* for more context at https://www.brownboiproject.org/). In addition, the term *stud* is often used in Black lesbian communities to describe a masculine AFAB person who may or may not transition medically or socially.

Additionally, *queen* and *reyna* are terms associated with Black and Latina trans women, particularly those who participate in pageants (Warri et al., 2021). There is not a direct Spanish to English translation for the word "transgender," however, *transgenero* is often socially used in the community.

In Native and Indigenous communities, settler colonialism introduced the concept of homophobia, patriarchy, and binary concepts of gender, which clashed with Indigenous acceptance of TNB and Two-Spirit people (Angelino et al., 2020). The influence of colonialism on Indigenous Polynesian people of the Hawaiian Islands, otherwise known as Native Hawaiians, or Kānaka Maoli, means that people have struggled not to conceptualize the gender term *māhū* (third gender) as negative (Minami, 2017). Hijras were considered dangerous to British colonial rule in India and were even criminalized (Hinchy, 2019). Due to their fighting back, hijras were able to preserve their cultural traditions, but they remain a minoritized group on the Indian subcontinent. Aléx Bassi, a nonbinary, transmasculine graduate student, who is a first-generation child of two immigrant parents (and a contributor to Chapter 6 of this volume on TNB people of color) offers their perspective:

> TNB clients are not a monolith. MHPs must lean into the intersectional lens and ensure the client is able to feel seen, heard, and supported in their identities. I feel this is especially important when working with TNB communities of color, where culture can have a deep influence on gender norms and roles.

By acknowledging and understanding these generational and cultural differences, MHPs can supply clients with more effective forms of support and demonstrate greater respect for the diverse identities within TNB communities.

MHPs should also be mindful that some terminology used to describe TNB people is considered problematic and is highly contextual, with certain terms being reserved exclusively for TNB community members. For instance, the term *tranny* may be used within the TNB community, but is off-limits for cisgender people. Further, terms like stealth and passing can be contentious, but many TNB people utilize such terms. *Stealth* refers to TNB people who do not disclose their TNB identities in specific contexts, often for safety reasons, but it can be misconstrued as implying deceit. This misinterpretation can expose TNB people to potential violence if someone reacts negatively upon discovering their TNB history. Similarly, *passing* refers to TNB individuals being perceived as the gender they identify with, but it can imply that they are not genuinely that gender, merely appearing as such. Despite their historical usage within TNB communities, these terms can be seen as problematic and may be rejected by some TNB people. Understanding these nuances allows MHPs to navigate the complexities of language and identity within the TNB community more thoughtfully and respectfully.

KEY ASPECTS OF ONGOING MENTAL HEALTH PROVIDER LEARNING

As we noted earlier, so much of being able to consistently evolve our affirming practice with TNB clients requires us to look to language generated from TNB communities themselves. This seems like a simple point, but it is actually one of the most complex aspects of providing TNB-affirming care. To do so, we must practice cultural humility and have deep commitments to growing our multicultural and social justice counseling competency in terms of the awareness, knowledge, skills, and actions we can take in evolving our foundations of affirming TNB terminology and language (Ratts et al., 2016). There is a distinction between cultural humility and cultural competency we can apply to TNB-affirming care (Ruud, 2018); whereas cultural competency implies that the MHP is the expert, the practice of cultural humility reminds MHPs to be aware of the limits of their knowledge and perspectives and to look to TNB clients and communities for some level of expertise. In essence, MHPs should follow the lead of the TNB clients with whom they work in terms of the language that feels affirming and true to their gender.

In regard to following the lead of TNB clients, there is finally a pathway for TNB people to pursue the mental health professions as practitioners themselves. Although it is important to acknowledge that TNB people have always influenced the mental health field through activism and community organizing, it is also crucial to understand that TNB people themselves are entering the mental health care field as providers, and their expectations should shape the next evolution of gender-affirming care. As Tochukwu Awachie, a Black, nonbinary doctoral student and a contributor to Chapter 6 of this volume shares,

> MHPs working with TNB communities of color must recognize that the therapeutic dynamic they create with clients has the potential to serve as an alternate reality. The counseling and psychological practice space can be a realm in which things that are inaccessible in larger society—such as gender and cultural affirmation, physical and emotional safety, or acknowledgement of an empathetic response to discriminatory experiences—become not simply more accessible but generously offered. To actualize this potential, MHPs must be deeply curious about the complexities of a client's concerns, as well as the larger world that informs them. We must strive to cultivate a unique healing sanctuary within the therapy space and to transform the world beyond it into a realm of greater safety, possibility, and liberation.

Tochukwu's urging reminds us that, in order to stay current with the diversity of sexual orientation and gender identity present within TNB communities, MHPs can be guided by both cultural humility and cultural competency in providing TNB-affirming care. MHPs can use the *Multicultural and Social Justice Counseling Competencies* (MSJCCs; Ratts et al., 2016) domains of awareness, knowledge, skills, and action to help deepen the cultural humility that Tochukwu says we need in order to provide TNB-affirming practice. As examples, we include questions under each of the following four domains of multicultural and social justice counseling competence:

Awareness

- How would I rate my awareness of TNB-affirming terminology on a scale of 1 to 10?
- How might TNB communities rate my awareness of TNB-affirming terminology on a scale of 1 to 10?

Knowledge

- What are opportunities to deepen my knowledge of TNB-affirming terminology within and outside of mental health continuing education, and are these professional development sessions led by TNB people?
- What are the sources of TNB-affirming terminology that I read or consume, and who are the people developing these sources (e.g., journals, social media)?

Skills

- How do I demonstrate cultural humility through learning TNB-affirming language across the TNB communities, including various TNB cultural contexts?
- Do I have the ability to apologize and repair relationships with TNB clients and communities when I make a mistake while using TNB-affirming language?

Action

- What are the actions needed to ensure the use of TNB-affirming language within the context in which MHPs work (e.g., practice, training, or research settings)?
- What are the long-term advocacy needs related to ensuring the use of TNB-affirming language in local, regional, national, or global contexts?

As MHPs, we can also use theoretical frameworks such as intersectionality, resilience, critical race theory, and liberation psychology to guide our practice of cultural humility with TNB clients. The tenets of these theories were shared in the introduction of this text. Below are questions MHPs can ask themselves in order to continuously explore and deepen both their cultural humility and competency in TNB-affirming care:

Intersectionality Theory

- What are the interlocking systems of power, privilege, and oppression that are influencing the context of a TNB client's presenting issues?
- How have these interlocking systems influenced a TNB client's experience of well-being?

Resilience Theory

- How has a client had to adapt and cope to adversity related to transprejudice and other intersectional oppressions as a TNB person?
- What individual and community resilience have they developed to navigate these oppressive systems?

Critical Race Theory

- What are the specific ways racism has impacted the mental health, resilience, coping, and overall well-being of a TNB client?
- How does systemic racism influence the access a TNB client has to needed resources, such as employment, money, housing, food, education, social support, and other critical needs?

Liberation Psychology

- Do the TNB clients we work with have knowledge of the rich lineage of TNB people in their local communities, as well as in other continents and cultures across the world? If not, how do we recover this memory and build this critical consciousness collaboratively to increase TNB well-being?
- How do we demystify MHP practice for TNB clients and ensure they have access to everyday psychological tools to amplify their well-being and thriving in the face of societal transprejudice and other interlocking oppressions?

CHAPTER SUMMARY

MHPs should be aware of the essential terms that comprise affirming TNB terminology. Gender-affirming mental health care will always evolve, and MHPs can actively practice cultural humility in a way that not only builds rapport and safety with TNB clients, but also transforms the contexts in which MHPs work that directly impact TNB well-being in the world. Cultural humility and cultural competency in gender-affirming care go hand-in-hand and shape foundational questions MHPs can ask themselves to ensure they are consistently growing and innovating their work with TNB clients. Theories of intersectionality, resilience, critical race theory, and liberation psychology are helpful guides in this growth and innovation of TNB-affirming care.

REFERENCES

American Psychological Association. (2015). Guidelines for psychological practice with transgender and gender nonconforming people. *American Psychologist, 70*(9), 832–864. https://doi.org/10.1037/a0039906

Angelino, A., Evans-Campbell, T., & Duran, B. (2020). Assessing health provider perspectives regarding barriers American Indian/Alaska Native transgender and Two-Spirit youth face accessing healthcare. *Journal of Racial and Ethnic Health Disparities, 7*, 630–642. https://doi.org/10.1007/s40615-019-00693-7

Ashley, F. (2022). 'Trans' is my gender modality: A modest terminological proposal. In L. Erickson-Schroth (Ed.), *Trans bodies, trans selves: A resource for transgender communities* (2nd ed., p. 22). Oxford University Press. https://www.florenceashley.com/uploads/1/2/4/4/124439164/florence_ashley_trans_is_my_gender_modality.pdf

Ashley, F., Brightly-Brown, S., & Rider, G. N. (2024). Beyond the trans/cis binary: Introducing new terms will enrich gender research. *Nature, 630*(8016), 293–295. https://doi.org/10.1038/d41586-024-01719-9

Bornstein, K. (2016). *Gender outlaw: On men, women, and the rest of us*. Vintage Books.

Feder, S. (Director). (2020). *Disclosure* [Film]. Netflix.

FORGE. (2012). *The terms paradox*. https://forge-forward.org/wp-content/uploads/2020/08/FAQ-06-2012-terms-paradox.pdf

Greer, E. (2018, October 29). Powerful gay rights groups excluded trans people for decades—leaving them vulnerable to Trump's attack. *The Washington Post*. https://www.washingtonpost.com/outlook/2018/10/29/trumps-attack-trans-people-should-be-wake-up-call-mainstream-gay-rights-movement/

Hinchy, J. (2019). *Governing gender and sexuality in colonial India: The Hijra, c. 1850–1900*. Cambridge University Press.

McCullough, R., Dispenza, F., Parker, L. K., Viehl, C. J., Chang, C. Y., & Murphy, T. M. (2017). The counseling experiences of transgender and gender nonconforming clients. *Journal of Counseling and Development, 95*(4), 423–434. https://doi.org/10.1002/jcad.12157

Minami, K. (2017). *Eh, you māhū? An analysis of American cultural imperialism in Hawai'i through the lens of gender and sexuality* [Unpublished undergraduate honors thesis]. Claremont McKenna College.

Ratts, M. J., Singh, A. A., Nassar-McMillan, S., Butler, S. K., & McCullough, J. R. (2016). Multicultural and social justice counseling competencies: Guidelines for the counseling profession. *Journal of Multicultural Counseling and Development, 44*(1), 28–48. https://doi.org/10.1002/jmcd.12035

Ruud, M. (2018). Cultural humility in the care of individuals who are lesbian, gay, bisexual, transgender, or queer. *Nursing for Women's Health, 22*(3), 255–263. http://doi.org/10.1016/j.nwh.2018.03.009

Warri, V., Bruno, J., Rapues, J. J., Keatley, J., & Sevelius, J. M. (2021). Transgender and gender diverse people who are Black, Indigenous, and people of color. In A. S. Keuroghlian, J. Potter, & S. L. Reisner (Eds.), *Transgender and gender diverse health care: The Fenway guide.* McGraw Hill.

2

ADDRESSING LEGAL AND ETHICAL ISSUES IN MENTAL HEALTH CARE FOR TRANS AND NONBINARY CLIENTS

CORT M. DORN-MEDEIROS, SARAH E. BURGAMY, AND LINDA F. CAMPBELL

Mental health providers (MHPs) frequently work with trans and nonbinary (TNB) clients navigating a landscape filled with critical ethical and legal considerations. TNB communities have persistently advocated for counseling practices that are both ethically sound and legally compliant. Their fervent advocacy, amplified across social media and news platforms, underscores their demand for a life in harmony with their public and private identities. This chapter explores the vital role of MHPs in supporting TNB clients through informed, affirming, and ethically grounded practices.

The demand for MHPs who work with TNB clients is increasing. Mental health professionals may develop a specialty practice with TNB clients; however, general practitioners with essential knowledge and skills can meet the standard of care for providing competent services. This chapter outlines the key elements of best practice from the perspective of generalist MHPs and addresses the application of ethical and legal standards of care. As authors, we have expertise in the ethical aspects of training students and working with TNB communities. Our own identities reflect both personal and professional relationships to TNB identities with both personal gender-diverse identities as well as over 20 years of clinical focus on TNB identities and human phenomenology.

https://doi.org/10.1037/0000471-003
Affirmative Counseling and Psychological Practice With Trans and Nonbinary Clients, Second Edition, A. Singh and R. McCullough (Editors)
Copyright © 2026 by the American Psychological Association. All rights reserved.

ETHICAL PRACTICE WITH TRANS AND NONBINARY CLIENTS

To provide ethical practice that affirms TNB communities, MHPs should be mindful that there are foundational ethical concepts that apply to counseling with TNB communities (e.g., respect for the rights of others, do no harm, social justice, beneficence, informed consent, confidentiality, and multiple relationships). In addition, there are ethical issues related to MHP competence, clinical practice, multiple relationships, informed consent, culture, race, minority stress, gender identity change efforts (GICE), and other diversity factors that are important to be addressed in the counseling relationship.

Competence

A crucial component of affirming care with TNB communities is respect and support of their autonomy to make decisions about their health care. It is crucial for MHPs to not make assumptions about TNB client counseling and life goals—making sure to avoid stereotyping and generalizations. Collaboratively exploring and identifying risk-benefit factors, and providing subsequent support for a TNB client's decision-making process, is critical. For instance, TNB clients may weigh decision factors about social or medical transition issues with varying priority and value; MHPs should follow the client's lead in determining the working issues and focus of counseling (Campbell & Arkles, 2017). The issues that TNB clients face when they seek counseling may or may not be directly related to their gender identities but rather to other financial, relational, academic, or work circumstances. A major ethical issue for MHPs working with TNB clients is to not necessarily attribute psychosocial concerns (such as depression or anxiety) to gender dysphoria—as these may be rooted in societal stressors, family discord, or other environmental conditions.

Another ethical challenge includes diagnosis. Gender dysphoria remains designated as a mental health disorder in the *Diagnostic and Statistical Manual of Mental Disorders (DSM-5-TR)* of the American Psychiatric Association (2022). Unlike the *DSM-5-TR*, the *International Statistical Classification of Diseases and Related Health Problems* (11th ed.; *ICD-11*; World Health Organization, 2019) classifies gender incongruence as a condition (not a mental disorder) that often results from historical and contemporary stigma, leading to minority stress which is societally based and not a function of TNB identity (Coleman et al., 2022). The *ICD-11* more accurately describes gender dysphoria as reinforced by external variables and environmental factors rather than a characteristic of the individual. Awareness of this contrast should result in the MHPs' use of the *ICD-11*, with the primary perspective of keeping with the principle of Respect for

Persons and Peoples and the standard of avoiding harm (American Counseling Association [ACA], 2014; American Psychological Association [APA], 2017).

Another ethical challenge includes the distinctiveness of gender identity and sexual orientation. For instance, MHPs can mistakenly conflate aspects of gender identity and sexual orientation in case conceptualizations. In providing competent care, MHPs should understand that (a) gender expression as well as gender identity are two separate aspects of a person's sense of self and may reside at any point on the gender identity spectrum, (b) gender identity is not necessarily the primary concern of the client, and (c) medical and social transitions can result in significant changes in privilege and social treatment based on relative stigmatized identities (Singh, 2013). Variables regarding specific identities, intersectionality, medical decisions, or historical trauma require an intentional perspective in providing affirmative care for TNB people. MHPs must approach all clients, regardless of gender presentation or sexual orientation, in a manner that recognizes and honors each client's personhood and unique qualities. No two TNB clients are alike, and TNB communities are not monolithic. Ethical practice requires MHPs to know and be aware of common risk factors, needs, potential clinical issues, and appropriate treatment interventions for TNB persons and understand that such issues will not apply to all TNB clients.

In addition, MHPs should ground their work in established scientific and professional knowledge in their respective disciplines (APA, 2017). As evidence-based practices developed explicitly for working with TNB communities are lacking, MHPs must adhere to the APA Presidential Task Force on Evidence-Based Practice (2006) definition of evidence-based practices as equal regard for research, clinical expertise, client characteristics, culture, and preferences. The elevation of the client's role in collaborating with the MHP, determining treatment, and decision-making underscores the importance of individualizing the therapeutic work to the uniqueness of the TNB clients. Understanding the historical and contemporary impact of stigma, discriminatory social attitudes, underlying laws and policies that reinforce bias, and other sociopolitical factors contributing to minority stress requires MHPs to expand their frame of reference and therapeutic stance to contribute to the health and well-being of TNB clients effectively.

Clinical Practice

Multiple factors are essential to understand when ethically working with TNB clients in clinical practice. Such factors can include working with interdisciplinary care teams, providing clinical assessments, and facilitating and supporting affirmative care across environments.

Interdisciplinary Practice

Interdisciplinary care is critically important for the competent care of TNB people in that multiple disciplines and areas of expertise are necessary for whole-person health care. Collaboration is incumbent upon MHPs' work with TNB people, given the necessity of access to specialty care such as primary care, endocrinology, physical therapy, pharmacy, gynecology, speech therapy, and others (APA, 2015, 2021). The role of MHPs in interdisciplinary care can include (a) necessary documentation to medical professionals in accessing TNB-affirming treatment, (b) educating specialty colleagues who are not fully knowledgeable, and (c) providing consultation on hormone treatment and other aspects of gender transition. In addition, MHPs may have more frequent contact with TNB clients than other health professionals, resulting in more timely and accurate client status information. If MHPs are not on the interdisciplinary team, the TNB person is disadvantaged in receiving integrated, affirming care. See Chapter 4 in this volume for more information on interdisciplinary collaborative care.

Assessment

MHPs should base their opinions, diagnoses, recommendations, and treatment plans on data and information that can substantiate their findings (ACA, 2014; APA, 2017). MHPs weigh many factors when rendering opinions and recommendations regarding aspects of the health and well-being of TNB clients. For example, psychosocial assessment can contribute to the understanding and differentiation of depression caused by external environments, gender dysphoria, incongruence, or other unrelated circumstances in the client's life, all of which can have overlapping symptoms. Only MHPs who have developed competency with TNB clients should assess TNB persons seeking treatment. Additionally, TNB-competent MHPs can (a) assess capacity to consent to treatment, (b) assess gender dysphoria and incongruence, (c) support and assist in social transition if applicable, and (d) adequately serve as a liaison on an interdisciplinary health team (Coleman et al., 2022). These additional competencies support the affirmative quality of care necessary to serve TNB communities.

Affirmative Care

MHPs can be instrumental in facilitating affirmative care for TNB clients through several means, including (a) conducting a psychosocial assessment that targets the client's needs with follow-up psychotherapy upon agreement by the client; (b) assisting clients in identifying social support among peers and building social support networks; (c) working with clients in determining when and how to disclose their gender identities to others and to be willing to negotiate family dynamics; (d) providing collateral services to family members in exploring family adjustment and promoting normalization of the family adjustment; and (e) working as a couple or individually with the significant other or others, making referrals, and providing resources to support the relationships (APA, 2015). Affirmative care upholds ethical practice in several ways, primarily by collaborating with clients to minimize their vulnerability to harm (APA, 2017).

Discrimination, Stigma, and Minority Stress

MHPs do not condone or engage in discrimination (ACA, 2014; APA, 2015, 2017) nor harass or demean someone based on gender identity (APA, 2015, 2017). MHPs treat and advocate for TNB persons who have experienced TNB prejudice and discrimination. MHPs recognize the impact of workplace discrimination, social stigma, and implicit bias on stress levels and develop treatment plans tailored to the client's specific therapeutic needs.

According to Hendricks and Testa's (2012) gender minority stress model, TNB persons often experience additional stressors from chronic encounters with societal stigma, discrimination, and prejudice that can lead to adverse physical and mental health outcomes. As such, TNB persons are vulnerable to both proximal and distal stressors. *Proximal stressors* typically involve thoughts, feelings, and emotional reactions following exposure to distal stressors. *Distal stressors* involve experiences of interpersonal and systemic rejection, discrimination, and violence. For example, a TNB person who is regularly harassed and bullied in the workplace due to gender identity experiences this distal stress. These stressors can result in shame, future risk avoidance, and internalized trans negativity (proximal stress). MHPs can intervene with proximal stressors through the therapeutic process. Distal stressors additionally call upon MHPs to support and advocate for institutional policy change, health and financial benefits, social services, and legal practices perpetuating discrimination.

The APA's (2015) *Guidelines for Psychological Practice With Transgender and Gender Nonconforming People* inform how MHPs may support their TNB clients. TNB clients may need support and assistance in many areas, given the complexity of navigating minority stress. Examples of support needs may include (a) direct therapeutic intervention targeting a trauma history of harassment or violence; (b) assistance in seeking social services that can identify TNB-affirming health professionals, housing, or religious communities; (c) addressing workplace discrimination and relational strain within the workplace; (d) coping techniques and methods for advocating to employers for a safe work environment; and (e) consulting with school administration, counselors, school nurses, and social workers to seek methods of increasing safety and improving the school environment for TNB students. Additionally, MHPs may assist students in identifying peer support from other TNB students (Bockting et al., 2013) by developing buddy systems and psycho-educational groups for allied cisgender students.

Culture, Race, and Other Identity Factors

Intersectionality theory (Crenshaw, 1989) is emerging as a core ethical factor in working with TNB persons; it is a theory that explores how interlocking oppressions such as racism and anti-TNB prejudice multiply one another. The shifting dynamic of the balance of power in varied contexts has gained recognition across minoritized communities. As historical power structures are increasingly critiqued, communities marginalized by intersecting systems of oppression are highlighting how institutional practices and societal norms have perpetuated inequity. This growing awareness has encouraged movements toward equity, advocacy, and inclusion that challenge dominant paradigms and uplift marginalized voices. MHPs understand the critical factors associated with age, gender, sexual orientation, gender identity and diversity, race, ethnicity, culture, national origin, religion, disability, language, and socioeconomic status, and they realize that competency in working with diverse clients is necessary (APA, 2017). Language is a vehicle to express acceptance and respect for diverse language clients. A culturally affirming language that reinforces principles of safety, dignity, and respect for others should be used when possible (APA, 2017). MHPs discuss the terminology they use or prefer with TNB and gender-diverse clients (Coleman et al., 2022).

Cultural competency conveys more than just knowledge; it provides a self-reflective stance in working with diverse clients. An essential aspect of cultural competence is *cultural humility*, defined as "the ability to maintain an interpersonal stance that is other-oriented (or open to the other) concerning aspects of cultural identity that are most important to the person" (Hook et al., 2013, p. 2). MHPs are alert to the impact of privilege and oppression represented in any given client's primary and salient identities.

Broaching refers to the MHP's ability to consider and bring into the counseling room how sociopolitical factors, including gender identity, race, and ethnicity impact clients' issues and concerns (Day-Vines et al., 2007). In such cases, it is critical to remain nuanced and refrain from speaking of universal terms such as male privilege and female privilege. Alternatively, the MHP can broach this topic using language related to *gender privilege* and attune to the client's use of gendered language about their past. For example, a Black trans woman has likely had to navigate anti-Black racism embedded in educational, health care, and other institutional systems throughout her entire life. However, experiences of sexism and transmisogyny (Serano, 2007) may be a newer experience for her. Depending on her previous gender presentation, she may have experienced a level of gender privilege during part of her life, particularly if she presented more masculine; however, this privilege is conferred by the perception of a culture and may not align with her lived experience.

A White trans man may appear to experience gender privilege because he is perceived as a White man. However, assuming his "male privilege" is equivalent to that of a White cisgender man overlooks essential nuances. This assumption disregards his past and present encounters with sexism and systemic gender inequities. As a trans man, he might still grapple with internalized sexism, anxiety about his body not being seen as male, and ongoing marginalization rooted in his potential socialization as a female.

White trans men, in particular, gain "male privilege" by conforming to socially accepted norms of White masculinity, which often includes adopting a traditionally masculine appearance (Anzani et al., 2022). The pressure to present in a traditionally masculine manner can create a struggle for such trans men to reconcile their upbringing and the "female" characteristics others may ascribe to them with their current male identity. It is also important to note that trans men of color frequently do not enjoy the same privileges as White trans men. Instead, trans men of color appearing traditionally masculine face a significantly higher risk of being perceived as criminals (Schilt, 2006). Ethical practice demands that MHPs take a person-centered, holistic approach to working with their TNB clients, which honors the complexity of their identities.

Consultation with a trusted colleague is also critical and vital to ethical work. For example, an MHP whose therapeutic focus with an Asian TNB client is on sexual identity could fail to see the cultural, religious, familial, and social impact imposed upon the client without consideration for the multiple identities of the person. MHPs and clients may also be unprepared for the impact on the person by unanticipated changes in acceptance or style of communication in long-standing social and friendship groups.

MHPs should recognize the importance of their clients' developmental history, identity of reference, and self-perception within their environments. MHPs must ensure they possess the knowledge and competence to grasp these complexities. By doing so, they can better support and treat the core identities of their clients, developing treatment plans that alleviate conflict and distress stemming from social, work, and school transitions. Additionally, MHPs can play a pivotal role in enhancing the competencies and resilience of TNB individuals as they navigate the intersection of stigmatized identities (Singh, 2013). Chapter 6 in this volume provides more detail on working with TNB people of color.

Multiple and Dual Relationships

TNB people frequently seek out communities in which they are safe, welcomed, and respected. Case examples regarding multiple or dual relationships often use scenarios about rural and small communities. However, clusters of culturally, ethnically, racially, and sexually diverse communities can remain small while flourishing in larger urban areas. MHPs who provide mental health services effectively to the TNB community are often in high demand. MHPs will realize that many of their clients frequently know each other. Further, it is not uncommon that MHPs who serve TNB communities may themselves be members of LGBTQ+ communities. Clients may be in other venues with the MHP outside the counseling setting, such as community events, advocacy projects, and social activities. It can be challenging for some MHPs to abide by multiple roles and ethical standards and have a social and community life beyond the therapy environment.

A key principle in mental health ethics codes (ACA, 2014; APA, 2017) is the need to be mindful of multiple relationships and their power dynamics. While some MHPs might interpret these guidelines as suggesting that all multiple relationships are unethical, the conversation has evolved. As we better understand the complexities of relationships, intersecting identities, and community affiliations—mainly as they apply to TNB communities—the focus has shifted to how MHPs can effectively navigate the challenges of holding multiple roles. For TNB people, these complexities involve navigating societal norms and biases, balancing multiple aspects of their identities, and maintaining connections within diverse communities. MHPs must consider the potential for exploitation and the loss of objectivity when determining whether a multiple-role relationship is acceptable, ensuring that they respect and support TNB clients.

TNB MHPs who provide behavioral health services to TNB clients may or may not choose to disclose their own gender identity in public venues such as websites or social media. If MHPs decide not to reveal their TNB identities, they should talk to their clients about the environmental and social factors that increase the likelihood of their encounter on the outside and discuss how to approach those occurrences. TNB MHPs may choose to disclose that they are TNB. Such disclosure and transparency may enhance the therapeutic alliance and comfort a TNB client. MHPs should be aware of the potential for countertransference. In the case of clients with meaningful, similar characteristics or life struggles to those of the MHP, a possible over-identification can obscure the client's individuality, resulting in an inaccurate treatment plan and poor decision-making.

Shared Community
For MHPs whose therapeutic work primarily focuses on TNB clients, the probability is high that clients will know each other and likely know that they have the same therapist. Confidentiality is a pillar of behavioral health services (APA, 2017), and MHPs cannot discuss their clinical work with clients or even acknowledge the identity of other clients. Even if a client says that the MHP is providing therapy for a friend and both friends have discussed and acknowledged the fact, the MHP must maintain strict confidentiality. Difficulties for the MHP can arise when a client's therapeutic work involves another client of the MHP.

When MHPs do not serve a specific community, retaining or transferring clients can solve the complexities of multiple roles. However, within a clustered community, client relationships may not be evident or existent for some time into the therapeutic process. In these situations, termination or referral is often not a viable solution given potentially limited resources in the area and likely the impact on the respective clients. MHPs are limited when a client belongs to a shared community, or the MHP is one of the few behavioral health specialists in the area. MHPs remain committed to confidentiality and compartmentalization of their work with clients.

A particular challenge may occur when an MHP has two clients in a personal or romantic relationship with each other. Should two clients bring up their shared activities, disagreements, and goals related to the relationship, the MHP may feel pulled between the two clients. For example, suppose one person, Jackson, and another, Brady, are in a romantic relationship, and both see the same MHP for regular, individual counseling.[1] Jackson discloses wanting to continue the relationship with Brady. Brady, however, reports wishing to end the relationship with Jackson. Jackson and Brady have only disclosed their feelings to their shared MHP and not each other. Jackson is a TNB person who sees this specific MHP due to her expertise working with the TNB community.

In this case example, the MHP has several options for proceeding. She could continue to see both clients while remaining vigilant to confidentiality issues. She could terminate and refer out either Jackson or Brady. She could terminate and refer out both Jackson and Brady. During individual sessions with Jackson and Brady, she could also discuss the option of either or both people signing a release of information (ROI) for the other to discuss the relevant clinical matters. Should Jackson and Brady decide to sign an ROI and both continue to see

---
[1] The case examples in this chapter have been modified to disguise clients' identities and protect their confidentiality.

the MHP, the MHP mustn't disclose the identity of the other partner until an ROI is obtained. The ROI should be presented as a standard protocol for the client's desire to share information with a spouse or partner.

In another scenario, an MHP may learn information about a client that the client did not disclose. For example, one client, Sam, discloses in therapy that they and another client, Liam, went out last month to a bar, and each drank several beers. Liam has a history of an alcohol use disorder and had just last week reported in a session that he had maintained 6 months of sobriety. The MHP and Liam celebrated his sobriety in session. The MHP now has contradictory information based on Sam's report of the night out drinking. They struggle with what to do with this new information. The MHP is now uncomfortable discussing Liam's reported sobriety and may even develop feelings of mistrust and resentment towards Liam. In this case, the MHP should seek out professional consultation or supervision. Consultation or supervision will give a platform for the MHP to process feelings towards both Sam and Liam ethically, discuss options according to a chosen ethical decision-making model (Juntunen et al., 2023), and strategize the best way to move forward focusing on client health and wellbeing.

Informed Consent
A foundational ethical principle in behavioral health is respect for people's rights and dignity (ACA, 2014; APA, 2017; National Association of Social Workers, 2021). Embedded in this principle is the concept of informed consent.

> Informed consent speaks to the value of respect for others in ensuring that recipients of our services understand fully the purpose and course of treatment, involvement of third parties, limits of confidentiality, potential outcomes and expectations the client may reasonably have of the MHP. (Campbell & Arkles, 2017, p. 102)

To ensure comprehension, MHPs must use clear and understandable language when discussing informed consent with clients.

MHPs should invite TNB clients to collaborate on the informed consent process, including confidentiality and the exceptions to confidentiality. Examples of exceptions to confidentiality that must be included in an informed consent are a court order for the release of client records, reported or suspected child or elder abuse, and imminent threat of harm to self or others. During the informed consent process, MHPs should clearly and transparently discuss the limits of confidentiality and invite the client to ask questions. The age of consent to engage in therapy will vary depending on the state where the MHP practices. In working with clients under the age of consent, respective to the state of practice, MHPs will make every effort to gain a minor client's assent and ensure the minor client is aware of parent consultation and decision-making. It is essential to be transparent with clients under 18 that unless they have been emancipated, their parents or legal caregivers can request clinical or medical records until the client turns 18.

Additionally, the MHP should discuss releases of information during the informed consent process. Releases of information allow the client to consent to share information with others. For example, a release of information allows the MHP to share relevant information for outside referrals to specialists or medical providers or to include family or friends in the therapeutic process if so desired by the client. For TNB clients, for example, documented therapy or other mental health evaluation may be required for the client to pursue TNB-affirming medical procedures, including hormone therapy or other surgical interventions. The MHP providing this documentation or evaluation must receive client consent and a signed release of information before sending out any requested documentation, even if the client has given verbal consent.

MHPs may encounter situations where advocating for TNB clients becomes necessary. The parameters, boundaries, and scope of such advocacy should be thoroughly discussed and agreed upon during the informed consent process. For instance, a TNB individual might encounter obstacles in obtaining insurance coverage for medical interventions. In such cases, they may seek assistance from their MHP to advocate for appropriate coverage. Before embarking on advocacy efforts, the MHP should establish clear expectations with the client, refraining from guaranteeing specific outcomes. It is crucial to involve the client in the advocacy process to the greatest extent possible. This may involve the MHP negotiating with the insurance company to secure coverage for necessary TNB-affirming care. Suppose the MHP decides to proceed with advocacy. In that case, they should first obtain the client's consent by having them sign an ROI to authorize communication with the insurance company. Alternatively, if the client receives a denial letter with an option to appeal, the MHP could offer support in drafting the appeal and providing a separate letter of support.

There may be circumstances where written consent or an ROI is unnecessary. For example, a client may be engaged in a large, multidisciplinary agency where they work with an MHP, a case worker, and a life skills trainer. In this setting, the client usually only signs one informed consent for the agency. Typically, the client does not need to sign a separate consent or ROI for each of these parties as they are all a part of the same agency. However, in such a context, the MHP must always confirm the consent protocols with their supervisor or agency of practice, as many still opt to exceed the basic requirements of consent and release of information. MHPs understand that informed consent is an ongoing process, and routinely revisiting informed consent with clients is a part of best practice.

LEGAL CONCERNS WHEN WORKING WITH TRANS AND NONBINARY CLIENTS

MHPs must often navigate complex legal landscapes to provide competent and effective TNB-affirming care. Such navigation can lead to a crossroads of clinical practice and legal implications in professional work, particularly with TNB clients. This section identifies common legal concerns and implications that may arise while working with TNB clients. Common legal concerns for MHPs on gender-related care may include various presenting concerns. Some of these include but are not limited to (a) concerns about legal client identification documents (e.g., birth certificates, social security cards, passports, state identification cards, and driver's licenses); (b) navigating access to public accommodations such as restrooms, locker rooms, prisons, and jails; (c) supporting incarcerated TNB persons; and (d) helping those TNB persons who may be seeking asylum, at least in part, due to gender identity status.

MHPs must understand and consider how TNB clients' social identities and related experiences of interlocking oppressions will influence their exposure to, and consequences from, the legal system (Galupo & Orphanidys, 2022). Most TNB clients may experience a minoritized status due to their gender identity. Still, other aspects of their identity such as race, sexual orientation, ability status, socioeconomic status, and age can significantly affect access to resources, the likelihood of involvement in the legal system, and physical safety in public and private spheres. For example, over half of all violence targeting LGBTQ+ communities is perpetrated against trans women. Further, trans women of color are statistically more likely to be the victims of violence perpetrated towards TNB people (National Center for Transgender Equality, 2015). The additional interlocking oppression of systemic racism with anti-TNB bias, misogyny, and sexism places trans women of color facing notably higher rates of homicide, homelessness, and incarceration among LGBTQ+ persons. Black trans women, in particular, are significantly overrepresented in the homicide rates of trans people (Momen & Dilks, 2021). MHPs must consider the whole person of their client and all intersecting identities when providing therapeutic services, support, and advocacy. See Chapter 6 for further discussion of the experiences of TNB communities of color.

A significant area of advocacy for MHPs may be around access to health care. TNB people often struggle to access adequate, competent, TNB-affirming health care. The lack of access to health care is simultaneously both an issue of health care disparity based on too few TNB competent health care providers (Kachen & Pharr, 2020), as well as a proliferating legal issue as the current sociopolitical context in the United States and globally (Ghorayshi,

2022) has become increasing contentious around TNB-affirming health care access.

At the time of writing, legislation to ban access to TNB-affirming care, especially for TNB youth under 18 years old, has been passed, is pending, or is being introduced in state legislatures (American College of Physicians, 2022). MHPs are often instrumental in facilitating access to TNB-affirming health care for TNB people. Applicable clinical care guidelines such as the World Professional Association for Transgender Health (WPATH) Standards of Care, Version 8 (SOC8; Coleman et al., 2022) also delineate specific roles for MHPs in the process of client acquisition of gender-affirming medical and surgical treatment (GAMST). MHPs routinely provide documentation, often in the form of a letter, to medical and surgical providers. This documentation is essential in providing TNB clients access to crucial medical interventions and, if applicable, insurance coverage.

Identity Documents

Many TNB people seek to change their gender marker or designation on legal documents, such as a state-issued driver's license or social security card. The process by which a TNB client can change their gender designation on legal documents varies from state to state. In many states, a licensed MHP may be asked to provide an attestation of a TNB client's gender identity. This attestation is often limited to a medical provider, with a few exceptions. While MHP services are not usually required to make legal document changes, clients may request support navigating these processes as they can be cumbersome and overwhelming, especially for young TNB clients.

In some states, such as Alabama, Arkansas, and Michigan, the ability to change the gender marker on a birth certificate is limited to those who have acquired TNB-affirming surgery, often still delineated in state laws as *sex reassignment surgery*. For example, Alabama requires a certified copy of a court order stating the applicant's "sex . . . has been changed by surgical procedure" and will then only amend the birth certificate but will not replace the original (National Center for Transgender Equality, n.d.). This requirement may limit the ability to acquire an accurate and authentic primary legal document for those for whom surgery is not indicated, not accessible due to financial constraints or lack of access to medical resources, or not desired (Movement et al., n.d.-b; National Center for Transgender Equality, n.d.). While the number of youth and adolescents identified under the TNB umbrella has increased recently, surgical intervention with this population is still considered rare (Vandermorris & Metzger, 2023). As such, surgical requirements for changes to legal documents may particularly impact TNB youth and adolescents. See Chapters 9 and 10 for further discussion of TNB children and adolescents.

From 2020 to 2025, over two dozen states have attempted to pass, or have passed, legislation that bans some form of gender-affirming care for persons under 18 years old. Several states, such as Georgia, Kentucky, and Texas, are currently undergoing litigation and challenges to these proposed bans. However, a couple of states have been successful in enacting some form of a ban, including Arizona, which prohibits doctors from performing gender-affirming surgery on minors, and Wyoming, which bans any form of gender-affirming health care for minors (Human Rights Campaign, n.d.). MHPs must learn about the requirements for changing legal documents in the state they practice to know how to support their TNB clients in navigating these processes.

Over time, 21 states and Washington, DC, have begun to offer the gender designation "X" as a nonbinary gender identification option rather than solely an "M" or (male) and "F" designation (female; Migdon, 2022). Due to standardization, the process of changing federal documents such as social security cards and passports no longer requires evidence of surgical intervention. The individual may attest to the identified gender without a physician or health care provider documentation (Zapote, 2022; see also Bureau of Consular Affairs, n.d.). Processes to change one's legal name vary on a state-by-state and even county-by-county basis.

In many locations, TNB persons must publish their intention to change their legal name, along with their current legal name and requested legal name, in a local, public announcement publication (e.g., newspaper), effectively requiring TNB people to disclose their identities publicly. An MHP may provide attestation documentation to the court, noting an individual's status as a TNB person as the reason for the name change request (National Center for Transgender Equality, n.d.). Navigating legal requirements and bureaucratic systems to align one's legal identity with one's authentic gender identity can be complicated and daunting. As such, MHPs should be aware of applicable state and federal laws on legal identity factors.

Documentation or Letters in Health Care Access

Prevailing clinical care guidelines, such as the WPATH SOC8 (Coleman et al., 2022), describe an instrumental role for many MHPs in providing culturally competent care for TNB people. According to the WPATH SOC8, the MHP remains a supportive health care service provider (psychotherapy, consultation, psychoeducation) and a facilitator of health care advocacy. Examples of facilitating health care advocacy can include fostering a TNB-inclusive environment using TNB-affirming language, particularly in client-facing interactions and materials; systemic use of correct client names and pronouns; and proactively assisting TNB clients in navigating complex medical and health care systems (Hostetter et al., 2022).

MHPs must understand their profession's historical role and respective ethical responsibilities in a TNB person's ability to access gender-affirming medical care. By understanding how ethical obligations have changed, MHPs can provide more informed care for their TNB clients. In previous iterations of clinical care guidelines (e.g., WPATH SOC6), MHPs were positioned as gatekeepers of clients' access to TNB-affirming medical care, especially in earlier versions of the WPATH *SOC* (e.g., version 6 and earlier; Budge, 2015). Historically, TNB persons had to undergo extensive psychotherapy to access TNB-affirming medical care. In TNB communities, it was thus understood that MHPs were often barriers to accessing care. Only with a MHP's approval could a TNB person receive desired medical interventions, such as hormone therapy and gender-affirming surgery. Some medical providers and insurance companies have moved to a patient consent model for adult TNB clients. Others still require MHP support to approve coverage for medical interventions.

Medical professionals and MHPs were historically under rigid guidelines from WPATH and other governing bodies in treating TNB patients and clients. TNB persons, for example, were required to "prove" their gender identity to medical and mental health professionals as a necessary pathway to receive hormone therapy or surgery. TNB people had to live socially as the "opposite sex" for up to 2 years while in therapy to prove they were serious about transitioning and could handle the personal and social consequences. This process required the person to live in a stereotypically binary presentation where trans women had to present as feminine, trans men as masculine, and heterosexuality was required. In other words, trans women should be attracted to men and trans men to women. Otherwise, it was assumed the TNB person was confusing their sexuality as gay or lesbian with their gender identity. TNB people were also encouraged to select "gender-appropriate" names (Meyer et al., 2002).

Historically, gender identity was viewed as a basis for pathology, with a focus on the identity aspect of gender (e.g., gender identity disorder in the *DSM-IV-TR* [text rev.]). Diagnoses such as gender identity disorder in children and transsexualism in adolescents and adults with a specified sexual orientation outcome both preceded in *DSM-III* (American Psychiatric Association, 1980). This perspective often led MHPs to see TNB clients through a lens of affliction and despair. However, advancements in psychological science now highlight positive outcomes for TNB individuals who receive affirming care (Olson-Kennedy et al., 2018; Wiepjes et al., 2018). This evolving understanding of gender identity, which transcends a binary sociocultural construct, has transformed the role of MHPs from gatekeepers to facilitators in TNB health care. Despite this progress, the continued inclusion of gender dysphoria in the *DSM-5-TR* still frames a normative aspect of human diversity (gender identity) as a potential psychological pathology. Nonetheless, a unilateral perspective regarding these diagnostic categories does not exist. Some TNB clients may express a feeling of validation of their experience, especially regarding gender dysphoria, and regard the diagnosis as a means to access medically necessary health care. Additionally, diagnoses frequently serve as a means to access insurance reimbursement for gender-affirming health care. At times, some TNB clients may express frustration or feelings of invalidation at an MHP's failure to utilize a diagnosis for fear of being unable to acquire health care (Mizock & Lundquist, 2016).

Although the shift from focusing on identity to dysphoria has encouraged MHPs to prioritize alleviating distress over pathologizing identity itself, the presence of this diagnosis perpetuates the association of TNB identity with pathology. MHPs have an ethical and professional duty to distinguish diagnostic misclassification from the external and environmental origins of dysphoria and to communicate these distinctions clearly in their professional practice.

Letters and documentation will serve as both a form of provider-to-provider communication (e.g., MHP to physician) and, likely, as documentation of the client's necessity for GAMST for insurance purposes. These letters and documentation are vehicles for advocacy for TNB clients in the health care and health insurance systems. Competency requires MHPs to learn the specifics of legal, state, and medical guidelines to ethically provide thorough and accurate documentation that meets the criteria to support the TNB client's medical needs. During this process, the MHP may need to work across disciplines and advocate for the client to medical and insurance providers.

Competent and informed letters and documentation are critical tools for MHPs working for TNB clients. A sufficient form of documentation works as an ethical and legal balancing act of providing adequate information regarding the TNB client's gender identity, psychosocial history, and current mental and emotional health considerations. Also essential is information on client and MHP processes regarding informed consent, or assent of the client and consent of legal decision maker(s), in the case of minors.

Documentation must clearly outline that the client had the opportunity for a meaningful exploration of their gender, indicated an interest in GAMST, and has realistic expectations of the probable outcomes of psychological and medical interventions. MHPs may be pivotal advocates of TNB access to gender-affirming health care. Such advocacy can come in the form of aiding clients in identifying TNB-affirming and competent medical providers, thus creating an ad hoc multidisciplinary care team around TNB clients and ensuring financial access to care through insurance coverage. Some MHPs may find themselves engaging with a client's insurance provider in such a way as to protect client privacy and confidentiality while helping acknowledge the necessity of GAMST for TNB persons.

Historically, MHPs have expressed confusion or uncertainty about their role regarding documentation in facilitating TNB-affirming health care for clients (APA, 2015). Frequently, MHP insecurity regarding documentation for clients seeking GAMST is related to a need for formal clinical competency education in working with TNB people during graduate training programs (APA, 2015). A lack of culturally competent education results in disenfranchisement for the MHP and their role as facilitative health care providers working for their TNB clients. This lack of training and competency is an ethical, legal (i.e., nondiscrimination), and advocacy issue. Thus, MHPs must seek education, both initial competency and continuing, to align with ethical and legal tenants of psychological care (APA, 2017).

In addition to the documentation required to access GAMST, MHPs may be called upon to provide assessment documentation regarding a TNB client's fitness to perform a professional vocation. Such vocations can include medicine, law enforcement, aviation, and firefighting. It is important to note that these vocations often require psychological assessment of all job applicants, not only those with a reported history of gender identity disorder, gender transition, or TNB identity. In cases of psychological assessment for a specific vocation, the MHP should be very attentive to the informed consent process. In this context, informed consent includes discussing all possible outcomes of a psychological assessment and the ethical responsibility of the MHP to be thorough and accurate in their reporting. The MHP should be careful not to guarantee any particular outcome of the psychological assessment or that the client's assessment will pass the employer's criteria to enter the desired vocation.

Access to Public Accommodations

Given that gender identity does not always conform to the traditional male and female binary, MHPs need to be equipped to support TNB people as they navigate a cisgender-centric world entrenched in the gender binary as it relates to accessing public accommodations such as restrooms and locker rooms. Processing and validating safety concerns, both physical and emotional, with TNB clients may be frequent therapeutic foci. For example, TNB people often face minority stress due to inadequate access to essential public and private facilities, such as being able to use gender-inclusive restrooms and locker or changing rooms.

Additionally, TNB people may be disproportionately vulnerable in corrections settings, encountering assignments in correctional environments based on their sex assigned at birth rather than on their gender identity (National Commission on Correctional Health Care [NCCHC], 2020). According to the NCCHC (2020), TNB persons in correctional facilities are disproportionately more likely to be discriminated against—as well as to experience emotional and physical abuse. MHPs can play crucial roles in writing TNB-affirming attestations or identifying specific gender-related health care needs, such as psychological and behavioral health needs or GAMST.

Between 2020 and 2025, so-called "bathroom bills" have been introduced in many states (ACLU, n.d.). These bills have sought to limit access to binary gendered restrooms for TNB people, according to assumptions of sex assigned at birth. An early example of a "bathroom bill" is North Carolina's Public Facilities Privacy & Security Act (HB2) in 2016, which garnered national attention and began an onslaught of other such bills proposed across the United States (e.g., Arkansas House Bill 1156, Iowa Senate File 482, Idaho Senate Bills 1100 and 1016; Atwood et al., 2024). Such efforts within the legal and governmental systems continue as a form of identity-based discrimination often propagated by the falsehood that permitting TNB-affirming restroom and locker room access would compromise the safety of those using the facility. In reality, reports of privacy and safety concerns within the context of public toilets, locker rooms, and changing rooms are scarce (Hasenbush et al., 2019). Despite these claims, which lack any evidence or scientific basis, such prejudice persists. Consequently, MHPs may engage in supportive therapeutic care with TNB people, managing anxiety and stress related to primary access to public accommodations.

Asylum and Refugee Status

As the number of people forcibly displaced across the globe continues to grow, including refugees and asylum seekers, MHPs should be aware of how to support TNB clients who are applying for asylum and refugee status (United Nations High Commissioner for Refugees [UNHCR], 2022). TNB asylum seekers may face many forms of persecution in their countries of origin, including but not limited to (a) physical, sexual, or psychological violence; (b) forced change of a sexual orientation or gender identity; (c) laws that criminalize LGBTQ+ relationships; (d) harmful practices that reflect the traditions, social norms, or values of the culture or country of origin; and (e) "severe or cumulative instances of discrimination or restrictions on exercising human rights" (UNHCR, 2022, p. 5).

Notably, in seeking asylum based on persecution due to gender identity, TNB persons must disclose their gender identity status, which may present a dilemma. On the one hand, the person needs to disclose their gender identity in pursuit of protection. On the other hand, the person fears further persecution based on their disclosed identity. Even once engaged in the asylum process, the American Civil Liberties Union (ACLU) estimates that upwards of 20% of sexual abuse cases in the custody of U.S. Immigration and Customs Enforcement involve a TNB person (APA, Committee on Sexual Orientation and Gender Diversity, 2019, p. 2). MHPs who may encounter or routinely work with TNB asylum seekers should be aware of the many facets of minority stress and the possibility of mistreatment of the asylum seeker because of the individual's gender identity. In detention centers, for example, TNB detainees who do not receive gender-affirming treatment or appropriate medical care are likely to experience severe physiological and psychological harm (APA, Committee on Sexual Orientation and Gender Diversity, 2019).

MHPs must actively support TNB refugees by addressing their unique challenges through an ethical, gender-affirming approach. TNB refugees often experience compounded trauma stemming from both their displacement and their gender identity, making it crucial for MHPs to provide care that is not only trauma-informed but also affirming of their gender identity (D'souza et al., 2022). This means acknowledging and validating their experiences, advocating for their access to gender-affirming health care, and ensuring their identities are respected in all aspects of their resettlement process. Ethically, MHPs must navigate these complexities sensitively, advocating for policies and practices that protect TNB refugees from further harm. By fostering an inclusive and supportive environment, MHPs can help TNB refugees rebuild their lives with dignity, resilience, and a sense of belonging, while holistically promoting their mental and emotional well-being.

This chapter should not be considered by MPHs as clinical guidance. Instead, this should remind MHPs of the unique challenges of TNB asylum seekers. MHPs should seek out additional resources, including *LGBTQ Asylum Seekers: How Clinicians Can Help* (APA, Committee on Sexual Orientation and Gender Diversity, 2019), which provides further guidance and education regarding many facets of gender diverse asylum seekers and is inclusive of the various roles a MHP may assume, including assessor, supportive therapist, and advocate.

Gender Identity Change Efforts

MHPs should be aware that TNB clients have been subjected to gender identity change efforts (GICE), often called *conversion therapy*. GICE continues to be practiced by some MHPs, religious clergy, and churches who inaccurately espouse a pathology-based model regarding diverse gender identities. These efforts refer to a "range of techniques used by MHPs and nonprofessionals to change gender identity, gender expression, or associated components of these to be in alignment with gender role behaviors that are stereotypically associated with the sex assigned at birth" (APA, 2021, p. 1; see also Hill et al., 2010; Substance Abuse and Mental Health Services Administration, 2015).

GICE is a misguided, unethical, and harmful practice that causes significant mental and emotional harm (Rivera & Pardo, 2022). For example, TNB adults previously exposed to GICE demonstrate a significantly higher rate of severe psychological distress, including past suicide attempts, compared to TNB adults who did not experience GICE (Turban et al., 2020). The 2021 APA Resolution on Gender Identity Change Efforts summarizes applicable evidence and research supporting the APA policy to "oppose discrimination based on gender identity, gender expression, and trans and gender nonbinary identities, and actively opposes the adoption of discriminatory legislation" (APA, 2021, p. 3). The APA Resolution also opposes GICE because "such efforts put persons at significant risk of harm" (p. 3). Additionally, the policy resolution "promotes professional training in TNB-affirming practices and opposes professional training in GICE in any stage of the education of psychologists, including graduate training, continuing education, and professional development" (p. 3).

Despite this policy statement and that of other prevailing professional mental health and health care organizations delineating strong opposition for GICE practices (American Counseling Association, 2014; Substance Abuse and Mental Health Services Administration, 2015; and World Health Organization, n.d.), legislatures continue to debate whether GICE and sexual orientation change efforts (SOCE) are a form of free speech or parental rights issues. Fortunately, many states have sought, outright, to ban these harmful and ineffective practices with minors aged under 18 in most states (Movement Advancement Project, n.d.-a). MHPs should be aware of their local state laws and the prevailing evidence debunking the efficacy of GICE and further acknowledging the significant risk of harm.

Current Sociopolitical Context

It is critical that MHPs are aware of the current sociopolitical context around TNB-affirming health care. MHPs must be knowledgeable about laws on TNB clients to provide ethical, competent, and informed care in a challenging legal environment. TNB-affirming health care is under increased scrutiny across the United States. As societal knowledge around TNB communities and related issues has increased, so has anti-TNB social and political sentiment.

Federal, state, and local-level bills and laws restricting TNB persons' access to TNB-affirming health care facilitate anti-TNB attitudes. Specifically, TNB-affirming health care, including mental and behavioral health care, has been targeted where it concerns treatment for children and minor adolescents. In some states, TNB-affirming health care has been declared "child abuse" (e.g., *Doe v. Abbott*, 2022; see also ACLU, 2023b).

Legislators have introduced bills and laws in other states that criminalize health care providers offering TNB-affirming services. Still, others have aimed to both eliminate youth access to TNB-affirming health care, prohibit the use of state funds (e.g., Medicaid), and ban health insurance companies from covering such care (ACLU, 2023a; *Brandt v. Rutledge*, 2022). The ethical landscape for culturally competent care for TNB people has become increasingly fraught with legal considerations.

Abreu et al. (2022) cited specific negative impacts of anti-TNB laws and bills on TNB youth, including depression, suicidal ideation or risk of suicide, anxiety, increased gender dysphoria, decreased safety and increased stigma, and lack of access to medical care. Despite ample evidence of the positive psychosocial outcomes of TNB-affirming care for TNB youth (Wiepjes et al., 2018) and adults (APA, 2015; Hughto et al., 2020), MHPs will need to continue to be aware of the ever-shifting landscape of gender-based health care as well as be engaged in advocacy for best practices and evidence-based TNB-affirming health care. MHPs may also derive evidenced-based support for and recommendations concerning gender-affirming care from such policy statements as the *APA Policy Statement on Affirming Evidence-Based Inclusive Care for Transgender, Gender Diverse, and Nonbinary Individuals, Addressing Misinformation, and the Role of Psychological Practice and Science* (APA, 2024). MHPs working in states where such care has been restricted or banned may benefit from cultivating wide referral networks of affirming providers in states where such care is unrestricted and, where appropriate and necessary, refer TNB individuals to seek care in other states or via telehealth when legally possible. Ongoing efforts to expand interjurisdictional practice (e.g., PSYPACT) are vital to ensure adequate, gender-competent care for all TNB individuals regardless of location.

Recommendations for Diagnosing Gender Incongruence

As guidelines, best practices, diagnostic categories, and classification of diverse genders and distress arising from gender incongruence continue to evolve, mental health practice is at the center of these shifts. In the coming years, the *ICD-11* will reach full adoption by the United States. With the advent of full adoption, coding regarding gender dysphoria will have moved out of the "Mental, behavioral and neurodevelopmental disorders" section (under gender identity disorder in *ICD-10-CM*) into a new chapter on "Conditions related to sexual health" (Chapter 17) as "Gender Incongruence of adolescence and adulthood," "gender incongruence of childhood," and "gender incongruence not specified" (World Health Organization, 2019). It is unknown what impact this change may have on accessibility to TNB-affirming health care. As of this writing, MHPs often diagnose gender dysphoria, still coded as "gender identity disorder of childhood" and "transsexualism" in adults as part of a model of health care access. It may be that MHPs will turn attention to diagnosing symptoms arising from distress related to gender incongruences, such as depression and anxiety, versus the need to diagnose gender incongruence or dysphoria as a primary classification or disorder.

SUMMARY

MHPs should know that TNB health care is rapidly evolving in terms of opportunities and challenges to ensure ethical and legal TNB-affirming care. As society's awareness of TNB communities, the nonbinary nature of gender, and the visibility of TNB people continue to increase, MHPs can continuously pursue TNB cultural competency and understanding of legal and ethical considerations that guide TNB-affirming care. Once relegated to the idea of a specialized area of competency, MHPs can no longer ethically bypass care for TNB people—especially since all of the clients with whom MHPs work have a gender identity and often experience mental health distress due to gender binary assumptions and remaining cissexist societal attitudes. Gender identity diversity is a normative and varied aspect of human diversity and it is imperative that all MHPs possess competency across gender identifications.

REFERENCES

Abreu, R. L., Sostre, J. P., Gonzalez, K. A., Lockett, G. M., Matsuno, E., & Mosley, D. V. (2022). Impact of gender-affirming care bans on transgender and gender diverse youth: Parental figures' perspective. *Journal of Family Psychology, 36*(5), 643–652. https://doi.org/10.1037/fam0000987

American Civil Liberties Union. (n.d.). *Mapping attacks on LGBTQ rights in U.S. state legislature.* https://www.aclu.org/legislative-attacks-on-lgbtq-rights?impact=public

American Civil Liberties Union. (2023a, February 9). *Court cases: Brandt et al v. Rutledge et al.* https://www.aclu.org/cases/brandt-et-al-v-rutledge-et-al

American Civil Liberties Union. (2023b, February 10). *Court cases: Doe v. Abbott.* https://www.aclu.org/cases/doe-v-abbott

American College of Physicians. (2022, November 11). *Attacks on gender-affirming and transgender health care.* https://www.acponline.org/advocacy/state-health-policy/attacks-on-gender-affirming-and-transgender-health-care

American Counseling Association. (2014). *ACA code of ethics.* https://www.counseling.org/docs/default-source/default-document-library/ethics/2014-aca-code-of-ethics.pdf

American Psychiatric Association. (1980). *Diagnostic and statistical manual of mental disorders* (3rd ed.).

American Psychiatric Association. (2022). *Diagnostic and statistical manual of mental disorders* (5th ed., text rev.). https://doi.org/10.1176/appi.books.9780890425787

American Psychological Association. (2015). Guidelines for psychological practice with transgender and gender nonconforming people. *American Psychologist, 70*(9), 832–864. https://doi.org/10.1037/a0039906

American Psychological Association. (2017). *Ethical principles of psychologists and code of conduct.* https://www.apa.org/ethics/code/principles.pdf

American Psychological Association. (2021). *APA resolution on gender identity change efforts.* https://www.apa.org/about/policy/resolution-gender-identity-change-efforts.pdf

American Psychological Association. (2024). *APA policy statement on affirming evidence-based inclusive care for transgender, gender diverse, and nonbinary individuals, addressing misinformation, and the role of psychological practice and science.* https://www.apa.org/about/policy/transgender-nonbinary-inclusive-care.pdf

American Psychological Association, Committee on Sexual Orientation and Gender Diversity. (2019, June). *LGBT asylum seekers: How clinicians can help.* https://www.apa.org/pi/lgbt/resources/lgbtq-asylum-seekers.pdf

American Psychological Association, Presidential Task Force on Evidence-Based Practice. (2006). Evidence-based practice in psychology. *American Psychologist, 61*(4), 271–285. https://doi.org/10.1037/0003-066X.61.4.271

Anzani, A., Decaro, S. P., & Prunas, A. (2022). Trans masculinity: Comparing trans masculine individuals' and cisgender men's conformity to hegemonic masculinity. *Sexuality Research & Social Policy, 20*(2), 539–547. https://doi.org/10.1007/s13178-021-00677-5

Atwood, S., Morgenroth, T., & Olson, K. R. (2024). Gender essentialism and benevolent sexism in anti-trans rhetoric. *Social Issues and Policy Review, 18*(1), 171–193. https://doi.org/10.1111/sipr.12099

Bockting, W. O., Miner, M. H., Swinburne Romine, R. E., Hamilton, A., & Coleman, E. (2013). Stigma, mental health, and resilience in an online sample of the US transgender population. *American Journal of Public Health, 103*(5), 943–951. https://doi.org/10.2105/AJPH.2013.301241

Brandt v. Rutledge, 47 F.4th 661 (8th Cir. 2022).

Budge, S. L. (2015). Psychotherapists as gatekeepers: An evidence-based case study highlighting the role and process of letter writing for transgender clients. *Psychotherapy, 52*(3), 287–297. https://doi.org/10.1037/pst0000034

Bureau of Consular Affairs. (n.d.). *Selecting your gender marker.* U.S. Department of State. https://travel.state.gov/content/travel/en/passports/need-passport/selecting-your-gender-marker.html

Campbell, L. F., & Arkles, G. (2017). Ethical and legal concerns for mental health professionals. In A. A. Singh & l. m. dickey (Eds.), *Affirmative counseling and psychological practice with transgender and gender nonconforming clients* (pp. 95–118). American Psychological Association. https://doi.org/10.1037/14957-005

Coleman, E., Radix, A. E., Bouman, W. P., Brown, G. R., de Vries, A. L. C., Deutsch, M. B., Ettner, R., Fraser, L., Goodman, M., Green, J., Hancock, A. B., Johnson, T. W., Karasic, D. H., Knudson, G. A., Leibowitz, S. F., Meyer-Bahlburg, H. F. L., Monstrey, S. J., Motmans, J., Nahata, L., . . . Arcelus, J. (2022). Standards of care for the health of transgender and gender diverse people, version 8. *International Journal of Transgender Health, 23*(Suppl. 1), S1–S259. https://doi.org/10.1080/26895269.2022.2100644

Crenshaw, K. (1989). Demarginalizing the intersection of race and sex: A Black feminist critique of antidiscrimination doctrine, feminist theory, and antiracist politics. *University of Chicago Legal Forum, 1*(8), 138–167.

Day-Vines, N. L., Wood, S. M., Grothaus, T., Craigen, L., Holman, A., Dotson-Blake, K., & Douglass, M. J. (2007). Broaching the subjects of race, ethnicity, and culture during the counseling process. *Journal of Counseling and Development, 85*(4), 401–409. https://doi.org/10.1002/j.1556-6678.2007.tb00608.x

D'souza, F., Blatman, Z., Wier, S., & Patel, M. (2022). The mental health needs of lesbian, gay, bisexual, and transgender (LGBT) refugees: A scoping review. *Journal of Gay & Lesbian Mental Health, 26*(4), 341–366. https://doi.org/10.1080/19359705.2022.2109333

Galupo, M. P., & Orphanidys, J. C. (2022). Transgender black, indigenous, and people of color: Intersections of oppression. *International Journal of Transgender Health, 23*(1-2), 1–4. https://pmc.ncbi.nlm.nih.gov/articles/PMC8986269/

Ghorayshi, A. (2022, July 28). *England overhauls medical care for transgender youth: The National Health Service is closing England's sole youth gender clinic, which had been criticized for long wait times and inadequate services.* The New York Times. https://www.nytimes.com/2022/07/28/health/transgender-youth-uk-tavistock.html

Hasenbush, A., Flores, A. R., & Herman, J. L. (2019). Gender identity nondiscrimination laws in public accommodations: A review of evidence regarding safety and privacy in public restrooms, locker rooms, and changing rooms. *Sexuality Research & Social Policy, 16*(1), 70–83. https://doi.org/10.1007/s13178-018-0335-z

Hendricks, M. L., & Testa, R. J. (2012). A conceptual framework for clinical work with transgender and gender nonconforming clients: An adaptation of the Minority Stress Model. *Professional Psychology: Research and Practice, 43*(5), 460–467. https://doi.org/10.1037/a0029597

Hill, D. B., Menvielle, E., Sica, K. M., & Johnson, A. (2010). An affirmative intervention for families with gender variant children: Parental ratings of child mental health and gender. *Journal of Sex & Marital Therapy, 36*(1), 6–23. https://doi.org/10.1080/00926230903375560

Hook, J. N., Davis, D. E., Owen, J., Worthington, E. L., Jr., & Utsey, S. O. (2013). Cultural humility: Measuring openness to culturally diverse clients. *Journal of Counseling Psychology, 60*(3), 353–366. https://doi.org/10.1037/a0032595

Hostetter, C. R., Call, J., Gerke, D. R., Holloway, B. T., Walls, N. E., & Greenfield, J. C. (2022). "We are doing the absolute most that we can, and no one is listening": Barriers and facilitators to health literacy within transgender and nonbinary communities. *International Journal of Environmental Research and Public Health, 19*(3), 1229. https://doi.org/10.3390/ijerph19031229

Hughto, J. M. W., Gunn, H. A., Rood, B. A., & Pantalone, D. W. (2020). Social and medical gender affirmation experiences are inversely associated with mental health problems in a U.S. non-probability sample of transgender adults. *Archives of Sexual Behavior, 49*(7), 2635–2647. https://doi.org/10.1007/s10508-020-01655-5

Human Rights Campaign. (n.d.). *Map: Attacks on gender-affirming healthcare by state.* https://www.hrc.org/resources/attacks-on-gender-affirming-care-by-state-map

Jane Doe v. Greg Abbott, No. 03-22-00126-CV, 2022 WL 837956 (Tex. App. 3d Dist. Aug. 29, 2022).

Juntunen, C. L., Crepeau-Hobson, F., Riva, M. T., Baker, J., Wan, S., Davis, C., III, & Caballero, A. M. (2023). Centering equity, diversity, and inclusion in ethical decision-making. *Professional Psychology: Research and Practice, 54*(1), 17–27. https://doi.org/10.1037/pro0000488

Kachen, A., & Pharr, J. R. (2020). Health care access and utilization by transgender populations: A United States transgender survey study. *Transgender Health, 5*(3), 141–148. https://doi.org/10.1089/trgh.2020.0017

Meyer, W., III, Bockting, W. O., Cohen-Kettenis, P., Coleman, E., DiCeglie, D., Devor, H., Gooren, L., Hage, J. J., Kirk, S., Kuiper, B., Laub, D., Lawrence, A., Menard, Y., Patton, J., Schaefer, L., Webb, A., & Wheeler, C. C. (2002). The Harry Benjamin International Gender Dysphoria Association's standards of care for gender identity disorders, sixth version. *Journal of Psychology & Human Sexuality, 13*(1), 1–30. https://doi.org/10.1300/J056v13n01_01

Migdon, B. (2022, May 31). *Here are the states where you can (and cannot) change your gender designation on official documents.* The Hill. https://thehill.com/changing-america/respect/diversity-inclusion/3507206-here-are-the-states-where-you-can-and-cannot-change-your-gender-designation-on-official-documents/

Mizock, L., & Lundquist, C. (2016). Missteps in psychotherapy with transgender clients: Promoting gender sensitivity in counseling and psychological practice. *Psychology of Sexual Orientation and Gender Diversity, 3*(2), 148–155. https://doi.org/10.1037/sgd0000177

Momen, R. E., & Dilks, L. M. (2021). Examining case outcomes in US transgender homicides: An exploratory investigation of the intersectionality of victim characteristics. *Sociological Spectrum, 41*(1), 53–79. https://doi.org/10.1080/02732173.2020.1850379

Movement Advancement Project. (n.d.-a). *Equality maps: Conversion "therapy" laws.* https://www.lgbtmap.org/equality-maps/conversion_therapy

Movement Advancement Project. (n.d.-b). *Equality maps: Identity document laws and policies.* https://www.lgbtmap.org/equality-maps/identity_documents

National Association of Social Workers. (2021). *Code of ethics.* http://www.socialworkers.org/About/Ethics/Code-of-Ethics/Doce-of-Ethics-English

National Center for Transgender Equality. (n.d.). *ID documents center.* https://transequality.org/documents

National Center for Transgender Equality. (2015). *The report from the 2015 U.S. transgender survey.* http://www.ustranssurvey.org/reports

National Commission on Correctional Health Care. (2020, November). *Transgender and gender diverse health care in correctional settings* [Position statement]. https://www.ncchc.org/wp-content/uploads/Transgender-and-Gender-Diverse-Health-Care-in-Correctional-Settings-2020.pdf

Olson-Kennedy, J., Warus, J., Okonta, V., Belzer, M., & Clark, L. F. (2018). Chest reconstruction and chest dysphoria in transmasculine minors and young adults: Comparisons of nonsurgical and postsurgical cohorts. *JAMA Pediatrics, 172*(5), 431–436. https://doi.org/10.1001/jamapediatrics.2017.5440

Rivera, D. P., & Pardo, S. T. (2022). Gender identity change efforts: A summary. In D. C. Haldeman (Ed.), *The case against conversion "therapy": Evidence, ethics, and alternatives* (pp. 51–68). American Psychological Association. https://doi.org/10.1037/0000266-003

Schilt, K. (2006). Just one of the guys? How transmen make gender visible at work. *Gender & Society, 20*(4), 465–490. https://doi.org/10.1177/0891243206288077

Serano, J. (2007). *Whipping girl: A transsexual woman on sexism and the scapegoating of femininity*. Emeryville.

Singh, A. A. (2013). Transgender youth of color and resilience: Negotiating oppression, finding support. *Sex Roles, 68*(11-12), 690–702. https://doi.org/10.1007/s11199-012-0149-z

Substance Abuse and Mental Health Services Administration. (2015, October). *Ending conversion therapy: Supporting and affirming LGBTQ youth* (HHS Pub. No. SMA 15-4928). https://store.samhsa.gov/sites/default/files/sma15-4928.pdf

Turban, J. L., Beckwith, N., Reisner, S. L., & Keuroghlian, A. S. (2020). Association between recalled exposure to gender identity conversion efforts and psychological distress and suicide attempts among transgender adults. *JAMA Psychiatry, 77*(1), 68–76. https://doi.org/10.1001/jamapsychiatry.2019.2285

United Nations High Commissioner for Refugees. (2022, September). *UNHCR's views on asylum claims based on sexual orientation and gender identity: Using international law to support claims from LGBTQ+ people seeking protection in the U.S.* https://www.unhcr.org/en-us/631f45ad9.pdf

Vandermorris, A., & Metzger, D. L. (2023). An affirming approach to caring for transgender and gender-diverse youth. *Paediatrics & Child Health, 28*(7), 437–448. https://doi.org/10.1093/pch/pxad045

Wiepjes, C. M., Nota, N. M., de Blok, C. J. M., Klaver, M., de Vries, A. L. C., Wensing-Kruger, S. A., de Jongh, R. T., Bouman, M. B., Steensma, T. D., Cohen-Kettenis, P., Gooren, L. J. G., Kreukels, B. P. C., & den Heijer, M. (2018). The Amsterdam cohort of gender dysphoria study (1972–2015): Trends in prevalence, treatment, and regrets. *The Journal of Sexual Medicine, 15*(4), 582–590. https://doi.org/10.1016/j.jsxm.2018.01.016

World Health Organization. (n.d.). *Gender incongruence and transgender health in the ICD*. https://www.who.int/standards/classifications/frequently-asked-questions/gender-incongruence-and-transgender-health-in-the-icd

World Health Organization. (2019). *International statistical classification of diseases and related health problems* (11th ed.). https://icd.who.int/

Zapote, A. (2022, October 20). *Social Security implements self-attestation of sex marker in Social Security number records*. Social Security Administration. https://blog.ssa.gov/social-security-implements-self-attestation-of-sex-marker-in-social-security-number-records

3

INTEGRATING ADVOCACY INTO GENDER-AFFIRMING CARE WITH TRANS AND NONBINARY CLIENTS

ROBIN M. MATHY

Advocacy is an important aspect of mental health providers' (MHPs') roles when working with trans and nonbinary (TNB) clients—members of a vulnerable and marginalized community facing escalating and pervasive anti-TNB stigma, bias, discrimination, and harassment across health care and other societal institutions. Therefore, MHPs need to be able to contextualize how advocacy may play an integral role in helping reduce the harm of these sociopolitical contexts that influence many of the mental health issues for which TNB clients present for counseling (Compton & Morgan, 2022; Pepping et al., 2025). For clarity, this chapter defines *advocacy* as "the pursuit of influencing outcomes—including public policy and resource allocation decisions within political, economic, and social systems and institutions—that directly affect people's current lives" (Snyder & Iton, 2020, p. 4). Numerous mental health organizations have asserted the importance of MHP advocacy in the provision of gender-affirming care (e.g., American Counseling Association [ACA], 2010; American Psychological Association [APA], 2015; World Professional Association for Transgender Health, 2018). In this chapter, the need for TNB advocacy is reviewed and different types and models of advocacy are described. Finally, the ACA Advocacy Competencies (ACA, 2018) are applied to TNB advocacy with and on behalf of TNB clients.

---

https://doi.org/10.1037/0000471-004
Affirmative Counseling and Psychological Practice With Trans and Nonbinary Clients, Second Edition, A. Singh and R. McCullough (Editors)
Copyright © 2026 by the American Psychological Association. All rights reserved.

THE CRITICAL NEED FOR MENTAL HEALTH PROVIDERS TO DEVELOP TRANS AND NONBINARY ADVOCACY SKILLS

The field of TNB health care has changed over time because of the advocacy efforts of TNB people and their allies within and outside of health care. MHPs have an ethical responsibility to be active agents of efforts to achieve social equity (C. C. Lee, 2018). MHPs can make strong contributions to TNB advocacy by actively staying up to date on the most current information about TNB-affirming practices and research that identifies positive counseling outcomes with TNB clients. TNB advocacy for MHPs, like clinical practice, will be contingent upon person, place, time, circumstances, goals, and objectives.

MHPs can play a crucial role in advocating for TNB clients and communities by staying informed about policies that restrict access to gender-affirming care or limit TNB participation in public life. For example, research indicates that hostile legislative environments are associated with increased anxiety, depression, and suicidality among TNB people (Hughto et al., 2022; W. Y. Lee et al., 2024; Restar et al., 2024). By leveraging their expertise, MHPs can effectively communicate these adverse mental health outcomes to policymakers and community leaders. MHPs "can speak out for transgender community members' safety and actively engage in fighting anti-transgender legislation at the local level" (Witt & Medina-Martinez, 2022, p. 31). For example, consider a scenario where a school board proposes a policy mandating that TNB students use bathrooms corresponding to their sex assigned at birth. An MHP, recognizing the potential psychological harm of such a policy, could present empirical evidence to the board demonstrating the adverse consequences of exclusionary bathroom policies. Legislative advocacy is not limited to the local level. At the state level, psychiatrist and researcher Dr. Jack Turban has provided critical expert testimony about risks of suicidality and legislative restrictions such as *Doe v. Ladap* (2023) and *L. W. v. Skrmetti* (2023)—a case seeking to challenge the Tennessee ban on gender-affirming care for minors.

PRINCIPLES OF EFFECTIVE ADVOCACY

A systematic review (Guerrero et al., 2024) identified several principles of effective advocacy campaigns that MHPs can use in strategies supporting TNB people and communities. First, effective advocacy involves both structural and individual levels, which are examined in greater detail later. Second, for effective advocacy to occur, MHPs can draw on their professional role as health care providers. For example, MHPs can integrate advocacy into their clinical practice by helping clients navigate systemic barriers, such as assisting with medical documentation for gender marker changes or providing referrals for other forms of gender-affirming care such as speech therapy, electrolysis (or laser hair removal), reliable sources of chest binders, endocrinologists, or surgeons. This advocacy can be accomplished by integrating the multilevel and multidisciplinary gender-affirming services discussed later. Perhaps the most critical advocacy competency for MHPs to develop is the ability to effectively engage in multilevel, multisystem, collaborative activities that extend care beyond the immediate clinical context and into the communities and environments in which TNB people experience their lived realities.

Guerrero et al. (2024) also highlighted several notable risks associated with collaborative advocacy for vulnerable clients, which are also relevant to TNB people and communities. They emphasized the need for clear guidelines in education and practice to help mitigate these possibilities. First, an MHP engaging in advocacy can be prepared to address concerns from TNB clients and communities that they are advocating based on their own perceptions of social pressures rather than the actual needs of the community. This may be problematic because TNB clients and communities may seek or prefer advocacy that supports long-term, systemic change rather than responses shaped by shifting political and social trends. For example, TNB people may want MHPs to advocate for passing legislation that protects their right to serve openly in the United States Armed Forces rather than focusing more narrowly on advocacy related to issuing or rescinding relevant executive orders (Mathy & Mirreghabie, 2025).

Conversely, MHPs who do not align the intensity of their advocacy to those of the clients and communities with whom they work face the risk of being perceived as overly protective in their attempts to shield clients from the stigma that limits TNB socioeconomic opportunities. TNB people may perceive this as paternalistic and threatening to clients' rights to self-determination. For example, an MHP may well intend to protect a client from potential harm by assuming a gatekeeper role rather than supporting the client's self-determination and right to exercise their informed consent for care. Notably, many TNB clients and their MHP allies are increasingly advocating against the assessment and referral process endemic in the gatekeeping model, arguing that it is dehumanizing, unethical, and reflects mistrust and suppression of TNB people's diverse experiences (Ashley, 2019).

Finally, the adverse sequelae of stigma often become apparent in research regarding the social determinants of health rather than the immediate symptoms with which TNB clients present (Guerrero et al., 2024). Therefore, MHPs can learn to apply advocacy skills to mitigating underlying causes of stressors such as the disproportionately high and interlocking issues of poverty, unemployment, homelessness, and food insecurity in TNB communities (Russomanno & Tree, 2020). There are many avenues MHPs can take to actively engage in advocacy. For example, MHPs can strive to change government policies, practices, regulations, and statutes; develop and deploy ballot initiatives; engage in collective action; or support litigation (Snyder & Iton, 2020). Carr et al. (2023) note that although MHPs are not specifically prepared or trained to engage in advocacy, their overall training uniquely positions them to do so.

AMERICAN COUNSELING ASSOCIATION ADVOCACY COMPETENCIES

Once familiar with the principles of effective advocacy discussed in the previous section, MHPs can use the *ACA Advocacy Competencies* (ACA, 2018) to tailor their advocacy strategies to TNB communities. Importantly, the ACA Advocacy Competencies are especially distinct from other professional organization standards, as they provide a clear framework that can be applied to a wide variety of communities and advocacy issues (see Figure 3.1). In these competencies, there are two primary ways that MHPs can engage in advocacy, both of which can be applied to TNB clients: (a) advocating with TNB clients (micro individual client level of empowerment advocacy, mezzo community collaboration advocacy, and macro public collective action level of advocacy) and (b) advocating on behalf of TNB clients (micro individual client advocacy level, mezzo systems of advocacy level, and macro public social or political advocacy levels).

By applying the ACA Advocacy Competencies when working with TNB clients and communities, MHPs can advocate effectively at individual, community, and systemic levels, ensuring that mental health services and policies are equitable and affirming for TNB people across the following 10 areas:

1. Client empowerment and self-advocacy skills
   - educating TNB individuals on their legal rights and health care protections
   - enhancing TNB self-advocacy skills for navigating discriminatory health care, education, and workplace environments
   - providing trauma-informed and culturally competent psychological support to help TNB clients manage distress caused by discrimination
   - utilizing the ACA Advocacy Competencies to support TNB individual and systemic client advocacy

FIGURE 3.1. ACA Advocacy Competency Domains

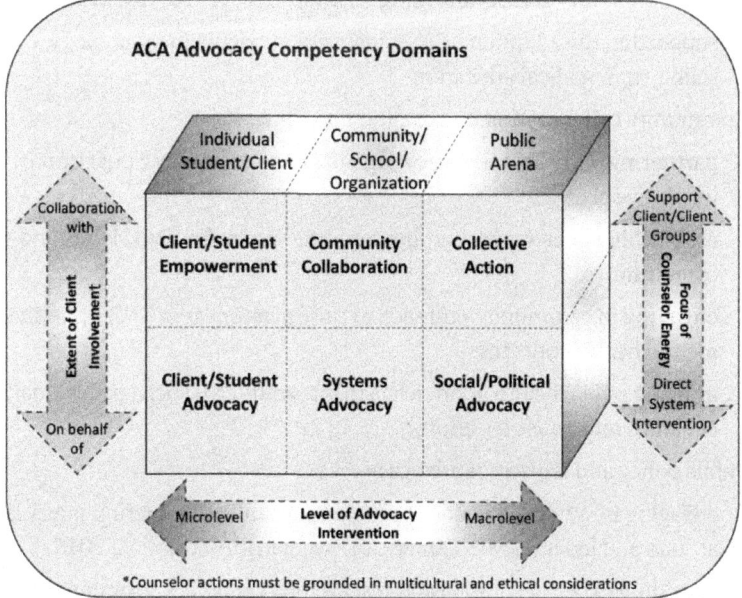

Note. ACA = American Counseling Association. See American Counseling Association (2018). Adapted from *ACA Advocacy Competencies: A Social Justice Framework for Counselors* (p. 3), by M. J. Ratts, R. L. Toporek, and J. A. Lewis, 2010, American Counseling Association. Copyright 2010 by the American Counseling Association. Adapted with permission.

2. Clinical and ethical advocacy in mental health settings
   - practicing affirming, evidence-based psychological care for TNB clients (APA, 2024)
   - implementing gender-affirming treatment protocols in clinical practice (American Psychiatric Association, 2020)
   - addressing TNB implicit bias in mental health assessments and interventions
   - applying multicultural and social justice counseling competencies to ensure inclusive therapy (Ratts et al., 2015)
   - challenging discriminatory diagnostic or treatment policies within mental health organizations (American Psychiatric Association, 2022)
3. Systems and institutional advocacy
   - advocating for policy changes in health care systems to eliminate barriers to TNB-inclusive care
   - ensuring TNB competency training for medical and mental health professionals

- pushing for TNB-inclusive workplace policies, such as nondiscrimination protections and gender-affirming health care coverage (ACA, 2024)
- supporting the adoption of TNB-inclusive curricula in psychology, counseling, and medical education

4. Community collaboration and coalition building
   - partnering with TNB advocacy organizations to promote policy and legislative changes
   - establishing peer support groups and safe spaces for TNB clients and communities
   - engaging in community outreach to raise awareness of TNB rights and mental health concerns
   - utilizing public health approaches to integrate TNB social determinants of health into advocacy efforts

5. Public policy and legislative advocacy
   - engaging in systems advocacy by addressing anti-TNB discriminatory laws at state and federal levels (American Psychiatric Association, 2018a)
   - providing expert testimony and research-based policy recommendations to policymakers about gender-affirming care
   - advocating for legal protections against TNB discrimination in housing, employment, health care, and education (American Psychiatric Association, 2018b)
   - supporting legislation that promotes gender-affirming medical and psychological care (American Psychiatric Association, 2012)

6. Public awareness and media advocacy
   - addressing misinformation about TNB identities and health care through public education campaigns (APA, 2024)
   - engaging in TNB media advocacy by writing op-eds, participating in interviews, and sharing accurate information
   - using narrative advocacy to humanize TNB experiences and influence public opinion

7. Organizational leadership and professional advocacy
   - encouraging professional organizations to adopt TNB-affirming policies
   - advocating for diverse representation of TNB voices in leadership and decision-making positions
   - developing best practice guidelines for TNB-inclusive mental health care (APA, 2015)

8. Research and data-driven advocacy
   - conducting empirical research on TNB mental health disparities to inform policy
   - utilizing evidence-based practice to counter anti-TNB pseudoscience and politically motivated restrictions on TNB care
   - promoting data transparency in research on TNB health outcomes
9. Social and political advocacy
   - engaging in policy reform efforts to expand TNB protections in mental health and social services
   - advocating against TNB grassroots organizing and direct action campaigns
   - lobbying legislators and engaging in direct political advocacy to advance TNB rights
10. Evaluation and sustainability in advocacy
    - continuously assessing the effectiveness of TNB advocacy strategies and making necessary adjustments
    - engaging in long-term relationship building with TNB advocacy efforts to remain adaptive to changing political and social landscapes so they support TNB safety, wellness, and thriving

The following case study provides an example of how to apply the ACA Advocacy Competencies to an individual client.

Case Study: Advocacy for Alex, a Nonbinary College Student

Alex, a 19-year-old nonbinary college student, sought counseling after experiencing significant mental health distress due to gender-related discrimination on their campus.[1] Despite the institution's public commitment to inclusivity, Alex frequently encountered misgendering by faculty, lack of access to gender-neutral restrooms, and resistance from the administration when requesting a name change on school records. In therapy, Alex expressed feelings of isolation, anxiety, and depression, compounded by the fear of academic repercussions if they pursued formal complaints. Their MHP recognized the urgency of Alex's situation and began integrating advocacy competencies at multiple levels.

---

[1] The case of Alex has been modified to disguise the client's identity and protect their confidentiality.

At the individual level, the MHP empowered Alex by helping them build self-advocacy skills, such as scripting conversations with professors about pronouns and understanding their legal rights under Title IX and local nondiscrimination policies. Recognizing that systemic barriers were limiting Alex's access to resources, the MHP engaged in systems advocacy, reaching out to campus administrators to advocate for a formalized gender-affirming policy. The therapist also used community collaboration, connecting Alex with an on-campus LGBTQ+ student organization to amplify their concerns collectively. As the advocacy expanded, the therapist leveraged political and social advocacy strategies, including assisting student groups in drafting a policy proposal for gender-inclusive housing and restroom accessibility. Applying these evidence-based advocacy skills helped the MHP transform Alex's individual struggle into a broader institutional movement, demonstrating how multilevel advocacy can create lasting systemic change.

ADDITIONAL CONSIDERATIONS IN TRANS AND NONBINARY ADVOCACY

In addition to having proficiency in using the ACA Advocacy Competencies, MHPs can play a pivotal role in mental health advocacy across local, state, and national levels. MHP advocacy efforts often involve collaborating with mental health professional organizations to influence policy, enhance services, and raise public awareness.

Levels of Advocacy

When working at the local level of TNB advocacy, MHPs can take referrals from trans advocacy and service organizations. For example, New York–based Gays and Lesbians Living in a Transgender Society (https://www.glitsinc.org) is a "Black trans-led advocacy and direct services organization that is dedicated to fighting systematic discrimination against marginalized communities, in New York City and beyond." Among other services, they provide crisis management, health care advocacy, and referrals to MHPs and health care providers for hormone replacement therapy and other medical issues. They value knowing MHPs who can provide gender-affirming care for their intersectional clientele (anonymous mental health advocate, personal communication) or volunteer to provide crisis management and community outreach services. In sum, to make valuable contributions at the local level, MHPs can network with local advocacy organizations to provide gender-affirming care, volunteer crisis services, and community outreach.

At the state level, MHPs can actively engage in TNB health coalitions or initiate one if one does not exist. The Massachusetts Transgender Health Coalition, part of the Massachusetts Transgender Political Coalition (2025), provides an exemplar of how this can be accomplished:

> The Massachusetts Transgender Health Coalition (MTHC) includes active memberships from LGBTQ+ and health advocacy organizations that serve transgender and gender diverse people throughout the state. The coalition works to increase access to quality, equitable health care for trans and gender diverse people. Members meet monthly to discuss bills, laws, policies, and other issues related to trans-inclusive health care and services, coordinate responses, troubleshoot barriers in patient navigation, and share resources and information. (para. 1)

Developing Skills in Legislative and Policy Advocacy

MHPs can increase the effectiveness of their advocacy by developing skills in policy analysis, legislative engagement, and strategic activism. These skills can be acquired through additional postgraduate education, continuing education, noncredit certificate courses, participation in advocacy groups, and mentorships with recommended readings. For example, professional bodies such as the APA and the ACA regularly offer advocacy toolkits and position statements that MHPs can leverage to support TNB-inclusive policies (Singh & dickey, 2017). Furthermore, MHPs should be prepared to articulate the mental health consequences of discriminatory policies in legislative and community forums.

Using Intersectionality Theory

Intersectionality theory (Crenshaw, 1991) can provide a helpful, overarching perspective that MHPs can use to apply to their advocacy efforts with and on behalf of TNB communities. MHPs can take a more holistic approach to TNB advocacy by acknowledging how transprejudice intersects with other interlocking oppressions (e.g., racism, ableism, classism, xenophobia). For instance, intersectionality theory helps MHPs remember that advocacy confronts hierarchies of power and privilege that are interconnected, as opposed to mutually exclusive aspects of TNB people's lives. Instead, they are part of a complex system of interlocking power dynamics and oppressions that influence TNB mental health, physical health, and overall well-being. For instance, to be able to advocate with and on behalf of TNB communities of color, MHPs must be able to acknowledge that racism is not only real but that racism also multiplies the barriers TNB people of color face when accessing counseling and other health care services and providers (see Chapter 6 for further discussion of MHP practice and advocacy with TNB communities of color). Intersectionality theory additionally guides MHPs to understand and reflect on their own experiences of privilege and oppression related to multiple social identities, influencing how MHPs engage in or avoid advocacy for TNB people (Chang et al., 2018).

Strengthening Interdisciplinary Collaboration

Advocating effectively with and on behalf of TNB clients and communities often necessitates interdisciplinary collaboration, as noted earlier. Oransky et al. (2019) point out that mental health disparities are multidetermined. Because of this, meeting the needs of TNB youth necessitates multilevel interventions in their lives. Their multidisciplinary model includes macrolevel advocacy "including efforts to implement social change" (p. 603), mezzo-level interventions that ensure the health care milieu is gender affirming, as well as microlevel interventions that include gender-affirming cognitive behavioral therapy, such as dialectic behavior therapy, family therapy, and support groups. Oransky et al.'s article includes more specific details about ways to implement this model.

In addition, Rafferty et al. (2023) and Coyne et al. (2023) emphasize that comprehensive multidisciplinary care involves both medical providers and MHPs working collaboratively with TNB youth and their caregivers. The authors argue that such collaborative efforts are essential for assessing gender-related support needs and facilitating access to developmentally appropriate medical and mental health interventions. Additionally, Coyne et al. (2023) discuss the role of multidisciplinary teams in community training, education, outreach, and advocacy for TNB youth, aligning with the argument that partnerships with organizations like the National Center for Transgender Equality and the World Professional Association for Transgender Health can enhance advocacy efforts by connecting mental health professionals with legal experts, policymakers, and grassroots activists.

Relevant to advocacy with and on behalf of TNB youth and their families, Coyne et al. (2023) underscore the importance of integrating advocacy with multidisciplinary care in which MHPs work collaboratively with medical providers, TNB youth, and their families in ways that extend beyond direct services and into "community training, education, community outreach, [and] nonmedical programming" (p. 479). In essence, it can be helpful for MHPs to think of advocacy as a process, one which is an integral part of their professional role. By combining process with role, they can be ideally situated in a collaborative network with other health care providers and professionals with expertise in areas such as law, education, community organizing, etc., all working with and on behalf of TNB people and communities. See also Chapter 4 in this volume for more information on interdisciplinary collaborative care.

EVIDENCE-BASED PUBLIC POLICY ADVOCACY MODELS AND SKILLS

MHPs engaging in TNB advocacy can also benefit from knowing about advocacy models and skills that use strategic approaches, integrate research, engage in coalition building, and seek to influence policymaking to drive systemic change. Multiple evidence-based models guide advocacy efforts, each providing frameworks that MHP advocates can employ. Five of the most prominent evidence-based public policy advocacy models are presented next.

Kingdon's Multiple Streams Framework

The multiple streams framework (MSF; Kingdon, 1984, 1995) provides a foundational model for understanding how policy change occurs by aligning three critical streams: (a) the *problem stream* (public recognition of an issue), (b) the *policy stream* (viable policy solutions), and (c) the *political stream* (governmental and public willingness to act). According to this framework, policy change happens when these three streams converge, creating a *policy window* where advocates can push for reforms. MSF is particularly useful for MHPs seeking to influence legislative processes by strategically timing advocacy efforts.

To effectively engage in advocacy within the MSF, three essential skills are required. First, *problem identification and framing* are crucial, as they involve defining social issues in ways that attract policymakers' and the public's attention. Second, *strategic timing and political analysis* are necessary to assess when political coalitions are most receptive to policy change. Third, *agenda-setting* is integral to advocacy, as it combines empirical research with public discourse to elevate the importance of an issue and situate it within ongoing policy debates. These skills allow MHPs to effectively advocate for policies that advance TNB rights, particularly in areas such as health care, education, and sports inclusion.

Harris et al. (2023) provide an example of how MHPs can use the MSF to advocate for TNB policy issues, specifically analyzing legislative efforts targeting transgender athletes. Their study examines state-level legislation restricting

TNB participation in interscholastic sports using qualitative data from public records to document how these policies were justified. The research highlights how national interest groups played a critical role in the diffusion of policies across states, leveraging the problem window by exploiting high-profile sports events, judicial rulings, and political debates to frame TNB participation as a policy issue. This dynamic created "solutions searching for problems" (Harris et al., 2023, p. 575), demonstrating how symbolic politics, rather than empirical evidence, shaped legislative responses. The study underscores the importance of agenda setting and coalition building, as advocates must be prepared to counter misinformation and strategically engage with policymakers to ensure that policies are grounded in research and equity rather than reactionary political maneuvering.

Narrative Policy Framework

The narrative policy framework (NPF) recognizes the power of storytelling in shaping policy discourse (Shanahan et al., 2018). Unlike purely data-driven advocacy models, the NPF emphasizes how narratives influence policymaker decision-making and public opinion. It argues that effective advocacy involves crafting compelling stories that humanize policy issues, making them emotionally and politically resonant. Flores et al. (2022) note that policy narratives operate at micro-, mezzo-, and macrolevels simultaneously, considering individuals, actions of groups and coalitions, and culture and institutions, respectively.

The NPF has three essential advocacy skills: (a) *framing and messaging* focuses on constructing persuasive narratives that convey policy goals effectively, (b) *public engagement and communication* underscores the use of storytelling to mobilize support from diverse audiences, and (c) *evidence-based persuasion* combines qualitative narratives with empirical data to strengthen advocacy efforts. An MHP might apply the NPF to advocacy through framing and messaging by crafting a narrative that positions inclusive mental health policies as a critical component of the well-being and dignity of TNB individuals. For instance, they might use a tagline like "Healthy Minds, Inclusive Lives" to encapsulate the idea that gender-affirming care is not only a matter of clinical best practices but also a fundamental human right. For public engagement and communication, an MHP advocate could strive to build widespread support by engaging both the TNB community and the broader public through multiple channels, such as organizing community forums, webinars, or panel discussions where TNB people share their lived experiences in a safe, respectful setting. In addition, the MHP might write op-eds and use social media campaigns to disseminate clear, empathetic messages about needed policy changes. To use evidence-based persuasion, an MHP advocate can complement narratives with public outreach, compiling robust research that supports their advocacy efforts. By linking qualitative personal narratives with quantitative research data, the MHP can build a compelling case for policy reform that appeals to both the heart and mind.

Advocacy Coalition Framework

The advocacy coalition framework (ACF), developed by Sabatier and Jenkins-Smith (1993), describes how long-term policy change occurs through coalitions of actors with shared beliefs and policy goals. The framework posits that policy learning (i.e., the process of adapting to new evidence and political realities) plays a crucial role in sustaining advocacy over time. The ACF is particularly relevant in highly polarized policy environments where competing coalitions influence decision making.

Essential advocacy skills for the ACF include the following: (a) *coalition building and networking,* which entails developing alliances among advocacy groups, legislators, and community organizations; (b) *policy learning and adaptability,* which focuses on adjusting advocacy strategies based on evolving research and political shifts; and (c) *skills for political negotiation and stakeholder engagement,* which concentrates on finding common ground with policymakers and opposition groups. MHPs who join policy advocacy coalitions have substantial power to influence legislation and other policies (Campau, 2024). The author discusses efforts MHPs have made to influence social acceptance of sexual and gender minorities using the ACF and theories of policy analysis. The ACF offers MHPs a valuable lens for promoting social justice for TNB individuals by identifying and mobilizing diverse stakeholders—ranging from community advocates to policymakers—in a shared pursuit of equitable social change. By mapping the belief systems and policy subsystems that influence economic disparities, MHPs who use the ACF can effectively collaborate with others for strategic policy learning and challenge discriminatory practices and structural barriers. This coordinated approach not only empowers TNB communities to articulate their needs but also drives systemic policy reforms aimed at creating inclusive economic opportunities and reducing social inequities.

Unified Model of Advocacy

The Unified Model of Advocacy (Hoefer, 2019) provides a structured framework for engaging in evidence-based advocacy at multiple levels, from individual interventions to broad policy initiatives. The model consists of five interconnected phases: (a) getting involved, (b) understanding the issue, (c) planning, (d) advocating, and (e) evaluating. These phases ensure that advocacy efforts are strategic, data-driven, and sustainable. The *getting involved* phase requires a psychological commitment to advocacy, including a willingness to invest time and resources in promoting TNB rights. The *understanding-the-issue* phase entails conducting in-depth research to critically analyze policies, assess their impact, and challenge personal and societal biases regarding gender roles, identities, and expressions. The *planning* phase involves identifying key decision-makers, formulating targeted advocacy strategies, and determining the optimal time for action. The *advocating* phase focuses on executing the advocacy plan, leveraging persuasion, negotiation, and strategic communication to influence policymakers. Finally, the *evaluation* phase is essential for assessing advocacy outcomes, refining strategies, and preparing for future initiatives.

The Unified Model of Advocacy requires several key advocacy skills. Policy analysis and research interpretation are fundamental, as effective advocacy relies on a thorough understanding of how policies impact marginalized populations, particularly TNB individuals. Stakeholder engagement and coalition building are also essential, as advocacy efforts are most successful when multiple stakeholders—including MHPs, legal experts, and advocacy organizations—work collaboratively. In the advocating phase, skills such as public speaking, lobbying, and media engagement are critical for influencing policy discussions and public narratives. Strategic messaging and storytelling enhance advocacy effectiveness, as decision-makers often respond to compelling personal narratives combined with empirical data. Finally, sustainability and long-term planning ensure that advocacy efforts remain adaptable and responsive to shifting political climates, maximizing the long-term impact.

MHPs can apply the Unified Model of Advocacy to support TNB people at both micro- and macrolevels. At the microlevel, MHPs can advocate within clinical settings by facilitating support groups for TNB clients experiencing stress due to anti-TNB policies and discrimination. The understanding-the-issue phase involves engaging in self-reflection on personal biases and acknowledging how cisnormativity may shape therapeutic approaches. In the planning phase, MHPs can identify advocacy targets such as school boards, hospital administrators, and local policymakers to promote inclusive policies (e.g., gender-affirming health care access, TNB student protections). During the advocating phase, MHPs can testify at public hearings, publish op-eds, or collaborate with legal and policy experts to challenge discriminatory legislation. The evaluation phase ensures that advocacy efforts remain effective and responsive, allowing MHPs to refine their approaches based on policy changes and community feedback. By adopting this structured approach, MHPs can actively contribute to systemic change and the advancement of TNB rights within mental health and public policy domains.

Social Determinants of Health Policy Model

The social determinants of health (SDOH) policy model contends that health outcomes are largely shaped by social, economic, and environmental factors rather than individual behaviors alone (Braveman & Gottlieb, 2014). This framework promotes advocacy that addresses root causes of health disparities through policy reform. Key skills of the SDOH policy model include: (a) *systems thinking*, which can be considered the identification of connections between social policies and health outcomes; (b) *multisector engagement*, which necessitates collaboration across different policy arenas, such as housing, employment, and health care; and (c) *structural advocacy*, which promotes legislative changes that address inequities at the systemic level.

Goldsen et al. (2022) conducted a population-based study to analyze between and within group disparities by cisgender, transgender binary, and transgender nonbinary adults. They found considerable heterogeneity in inequities across the subgroups. This suggests that MHPs who engage in advocacy using the SDOH policy model can provide stakeholders with a more nuanced picture of the health disparities that people with various gender identities experience. Ultimately, the epidemiology of health problems varies as the identified group membership under study changes. What may be true for an aggregate group may not be accurate for the heterogenous subgroups. This is particularly important when considering intersectionality when advocating.

Each of the five evidence-based advocacy models discussed here provide a structured approach to influencing public policy and systemic change. Although the models differ in focus—some emphasizing coalition building, others leveraging storytelling or public health data—they all underscore the importance of strategic advocacy skills such as policy analysis, framing and messaging, coalition building, and stakeholder engagement. MHPs, advocates, and policymakers can apply these models to advance social justice, health equity, and systemic reform to diverse policy areas affecting TNB people and communities.

CHAPTER SUMMARY

Advocacy is a central role of TNB-affirming care noted across TNB professional competencies, guidelines, and standards. MHPs providing TNB-affirming care

are in powerful positions to advocate for TNB clients and communities. In this regard, MHPs can engage in advocacy in multiple ways—from teaching clients self-advocacy skills to navigating family, school, and health care settings, to networking with medical and mental health providers to create coordinated care networks and challenge anti-TNB policies and legislation. Regardless of how long MHPs have been striving to develop the awareness, knowledge, and skills to advocate effectively with and on behalf of clients, the ultimate focus should be on cultivating TNB-affirming contexts that support TNB mental health and overall well-being.

REFERENCES

American Counseling Association. (2018). *ACA advocacy competencies*. https://www.counseling.org/docs/default-source/competencies/aca-advocacy-competencies-updated-may-2020.pdf

American Counseling Association. (2024). *Approved advocacy for transgender and nonbinary issues and concerns*. https://www.counseling.org/about/values-statements/advocacy-for-transgender-and-nonbinary-issues-and-concerns#

American Psychiatric Association. (2012, July). *Position statement on access to care for transgender and gender variant individuals*. https://media.kjzz.org/s3fs-public/Position-2012-Transgender-Gender-Variant-Access-Care-1.pdf

American Psychiatric Association. (2018a, July). *Position statement on access to care for transgender and gender diverse individuals*. https://www.psychiatry.org/getattachment/d3ef4763-8a0e-4da3-ab01-efe932ca9478/Position-2018-Access-to-Care-for-Transgender-and-Gender-Diverse-Individuals.pdf

American Psychiatric Association. (2018b, July). *Position statement on discrimination against transgender and gender diverse individuals.* https://www.psychiatry.org/File%20Library/About-APA/Organization-Documents-Policies/Policies/Position-2018-Discrimination-Against-Transgender-and-Gender-Diverse-Individuals.pdf

American Psychiatric Association. (2020, July). *Position statement on treatment of transgender (trans) and gender diverse youth*. https://www.psychiatry.org/getattachment/8665a2f2-0b73-4477-8f60-79015ba9f815/Position-Treatment-of-Transgender-Gender-Diverse-Youth.pdf

American Psychiatric Association. (2022). *Diagnostic and statistical manual of mental disorders* (5th ed., text rev.). https://doi.org/10.1176/appi.books.9780890425787

American Psychological Association. (2015). Guidelines for psychological practice with transgender and gender nonconforming people. *American Psychologist, 70*(9), 832–864. https://doi.org/10.1037/a0039906

American Psychological Association. (2024, February). *APA policy statement on affirming evidence-based inclusive care for transgender, gender diverse, and nonbinary individuals, addressing misinformation, and the role of psychological practice and science.* https://www.apa.org/about/policy/transgender-nonbinary-inclusive-care

Ashley, F. (2019). Gatekeeping hormone replacement therapy for transgender patients is dehumanising. *Journal of Medical Ethics, 45*(7), 480–482. https://doi.org/10.1136/medethics-2018-105293

Braveman, P., & Gottlieb, L. (2014). The social determinants of health: It's time to consider the causes of the causes. *Public Health Reports, 129*(Suppl. 2), 19–31. https://doi.org/10.1177/00333549141291S206

Campau, S. (2024). Policy perspectives on efforts to end conversation practices. *Cognitive and Behavioral Practice, 31*(1), 31–34. https://doi.org/10.1016/j.cbpra.2023.09.001

Carr, E. R., Davenport, K. M., Murakami-Brundage, J. L., Robertson, S., Miller, R., & Snyder, J. (2023). From the medical model to the recovery model: Psychologists engaging in advocacy and social justice action agendas in public mental health. *American Journal of Orthopsychiatry, 93*(2), 120–130. https://doi.org/10.1037/ort0000656

Chang, S. C., Singh, A. A., & dickey, l. m. (2018). *A clinician's guide to gender-affirming care: Working with transgender & gender nonconforming clients*. Context Press. https://bit.ly/3QJcgoP

Compton, E., & Morgan, G. (2022). The experiences of psychological therapy amongst people who identify as transgender or gender non-conforming: A systematic review of qualitative research. *Journal of Feminist Family Therapy, 34*(3–4), 225–248. https://doi.org/10.1080/08952833.2022.2068843

Coyne, C. A., Yuodsnukis, B. T., & Chen, D. (2023). Gender dysphoria: Optimizing healthcare for transgender and gender diverse youth with a multidisciplinary approach. *Neuropsychiatric Disease and Treatment, 19*, 479–493. https://doi.org/10.2147/NDT.S359979

Crenshaw, K. (1991). Mapping the margins: Intersectionality, identity politics, and violence against women of color. *Stanford Law Review, 43*(6), 1241–1299. https://doi.org/10.2307/1229039

Doe v. Ladapo, No. 4:23-cv-00114-RH-MAF (N.D. Fla. 2023). Retrieved from https://storage.courtlistener.com/recap/gov.uscourts.flnd.460963/gov.uscourts.flnd.460963.113.0.pdf

Flores, A., Boden, D., Haider-Markel, D., Lewis, D., Miller, P., & Taylor, J. (2022). Taking perspective of the stories we tell about transgender rights: The narrative policy framework. *Policy Studies Journal, 51*(1), 123–143. https://doi.org/10.1111/psj.12475

Goldsen, K. I. F., Romanelli, M., Hoy-Ellis, C. P., & Jung, H. (2022). Health, economic and social disparities among transgender women, transgender men and transgender nonbinary adults: Results form a population-based study. *Preventive Medicine, 156*, 106988. https://doi.org/10.1016/j.ypmed.2022.106988

Guerrero, Z., Iruretagoyena, B., Parry, S., & Henderson, C. (2024). Anti-stigma advocacy for health professionals: A systematic review. *Journal of Mental Health, 33*(3), 394–414. https://doi.org/10.1080/09638237.2023.2182421

Harris, S., Jedlicka, S., Pielke, R., & Ryan, H. (2023). The politics of exclusion: Analyzing U.S. state responses to interscholastic transgender athletes. *International Journal of Sport Policy and Politics, 15*(4), 757–778. https://doi.org/10.1080/19406940.2023.2242878

Hoefer, R. (2019). *Advocacy practice for social justice* (4th ed.). Oxford University Press.

Hughto, J. M., Meyers, D. J., Mimiaga, M. J., Reisner, S. L., & Cahill, S. (2022). Uncertainty and confusion regarding transgender non-discrimination policies: Implications for the mental health of transgender Americans. *Sexuality Research and Social Policy, 19*, 1069–1079. https://doi.org/10.1007/s13178-021-00602-w

Jacobs, S., Thomas, W., & Lang, S. (Eds.). (1997). *Two-spirit people: Native American gender identity, sexuality, and spirituality*. University of Illinois Press.

Kingdon, J. W. (1984). *Agendas, alternatives, and public policies*. Little, Brown and Co.

Kingdon, J. W. (1995). *Agendas, alternatives, and public policies* (2nd ed.). HarperCollins.

Lee, C. C. (2018). *Counseling for social justice* (3rd ed.). American Counseling Association Foundation.

Lee, W. Y., Hobbs, J. N., Hobaica, S. DeChants, J. P., Price, M. N., & Nath, R. (2024). State-level anti-transgender laws increase past-year suicide attempts among transgender and nonbinary young people in the USA. *Nature Human Behaviour, 8*, 2096–2016. https://doi.org/10.1038/s41562-024-01979-5

L. W. v. Skrmetti, 679 F. Supp. 3d 668 (M.D. Tenn. 2023). Retrieved from https://casetext.com/case/l-w-v-skrmetti-1

Massachusetts Transgender Political Coalition. (2025). *MA Trans Health Coalition*. https://www.masstpc.org/what-we-do/ma-trans-health-coalition/

Mathy, R. M., & Mirreghabie, N. (2025). A precarious policy: Executive Order 14,004 involving U.S. trans military service. *Journal of Social Work and Social Welfare Policy, 3*(1), Article 130. https://doi.org/10.33790/jswwp1100130

Oransky, M., Burke, E. Z., & Steever, J. (2019). An interdisciplinary model for meeting the mental health needs of transgender adolescents and young adults: The Mount Sinai Adolescent Health Center approach. *Cognitive and Behavioral Practice, 26*(4), 603–616. https://doi.org/10.1016/j.cbpra.2018.03.002

Pepping, C. A., Cronin, T. J., & Davis, A. W. (2025). Mental health care for transgender and non-binary adults: An investigation of affirmative practice, therapy experiences and outcomes, and reasons for treatment termination. *Sexuality Research and Social Policy*, Advance online publication. https://doi.org/10.1007/s13178-024-01065-5

Rafferty, J., Adelson, S. L., & Makadon, H. (2023). Optimizing healthcare for transgender and gender diverse youth: A position paper. *Journal of Adolescent Health, 72*(4), 411–420. https://doi.org/10.1016/j.jadohealth.2022.12.002

Ratts, M. J., Singh, A. A., Nassar-McMillan, S., Butler, S. K., & Rafferty, J. (2015). *Multicultural and social justice counseling competencies*. American Counseling Association. https://www.counseling.org/docs/default-source/competencies/multicultural-and-social-justice-counseling-competencies.pdf?sfvrsn=20

Ratts, M. J., Toporek, R. L. & Lewis, J. A. (2010). *ACA advocacy competencies: A social justice framework for counselors*. American Counseling Association.

Restar, A., Layland, E. K., Hughes, L., Dusic, E., Lucas, R., Bambilla, A. J. K., Martin, A., Shook, A., Karrington, B., Schwarz, D., Shimkin, G., Grandberry, V., Xanadu, X., Street, C. G., Operario, D., Gamarel, K., & Kershaw, T. (2024). *JAMA Network Open*, Article e2431306. https://doi.org/10.1001/jamanetworkopen2024.31306

Russomanno, J., & Jabson Tree, J. M. (2020). Food insecurity and food pantry use among transgender and gender non-conforming people in the Southeast United States. *BMC Public Health, 20*(1), 590. https://doi.org/10.1186/s12889-020-08684-8

Sabatier, P. A., & Jenkins-Smith, H. C. (1993). *Policy change and learning: An advocacy coalition approach*. Westview Press.

Schena, D., II, Rosales, R., & Rowe, E. (2022). Teaching self-advocacy skills: A review and call for research. *Journal of Behavioral Education, 32*, 641–689. https://doi.org/10.1007/s10864-022-09472-7

Shanahan, E. A., Jones, M. D., Mcbeth, M. K., & Radalli, C. M. (2018). The narrative policy framework. In C. M. Weible & P. A. Sabatier (Eds.), *Theories of policy process* (4th ed., pp. 173–200). Routledge.

Singh, A. A., & dickey, l. m. (Eds.). (2017). *Affirmative counseling and psychological practice with transgender and gender nonconforming clients.* American Psychological Association. https://doi.org/10.1037/14957-000

Smith, A. (2005). *Conquest: Sexual violence and American Indian genocide.* South End Press.

Snyder, H. M., & Iton, A. B. (2020). *Advocacy for public health policy change: An urgent imperative.* American Public Health Association Press.

Witt, H., & Medina-Martinez, K. (2022). Transgender rights & the urgent need for social work advocacy. *Social Work in Public Health, 37*(1), 28–32. https://doi.org/10.1080/19371918.2021.1970685

4

AFFIRMATIVE INTERDISCIPLINARY COLLABORATIVE CARE WITH TRANS AND NONBINARY CLIENTS

KELLY DUCHENY, MICHAEL L. HENDRICKS, G. NIC RIDER, AND COLT M. ST. AMAND

In this chapter, we discuss the important role mental health providers (MHPs) have in ensuring holistic affirmative interdisciplinary collaborative care (ICC) with trans and nonbinary (TNB) communities. For instance, MHPs working with TNB communities are regularly called upon to help their clients navigate uninformed, oppressive, demeaning, and damaging systems (Keo-Meier et al., 2018). To be effective, MHPs must be aware of systemic discrimination and invalidation of TNB identities and will need to determine when and how they address this in ways that best benefit their TNB clients.

In addition, MHPs must become proficient at helping clients navigate and access necessary services outside of their areas of expertise (e.g., medical treatments, insurance appeals, identity documentation, etc.). Through advocacy and collaborative care, MHPs become a strong voice for TNB affirmative care and help lay a foundation for the safest passage through the range of obstacles and barriers TNB clients regularly encounter (Keo-Meier et al., 2018). This is especially critical given the deluge of legislative attacks and insurance coverage restrictions that have occurred since 2020 that were designed to pathologize and interrupt medically necessary health care for TNB youth and adults (Kuper et al., 2022). Interdisciplinary collaborative advocacy can be a powerful tool to demonstrate the positive impact of gender-affirming care and the research base

---

https://doi.org/10.1037/0000471-005
Affirmative Counseling and Psychological Practice With Trans and Nonbinary Clients, Second Edition, A. Singh and R. McCullough (Editors)
Copyright © 2026 by the American Psychological Association. All rights reserved.

it is built upon. In this chapter, we describe models of ICC and discuss the critical importance of ICC in TNB affirmative care. In addition, we discuss MHPs' roles in TNB-affirming ICC throughout a range of settings and systems including school, childcare, religious and spiritual settings, legal and correctional facilities, work, travel, primary care, and overall access to gender-affirming medical interventions.

OVERVIEW OF INTERDISCIPLINARY COLLABORATIVE CARE

MHPs are well positioned to serve an essential role in ICC and to facilitate effective and respectful communication across disciplines that results in improved treatment for TNB people (Coyne et al., 2023; McIntosh, 2016). MHPs have a fluid understanding of the interplay of biological, psychological, and social factors that affect clients' lives and others' understanding of gender identity and gender expression (Hendricks & Testa, 2012). In addition to sharp assessment and diagnostic skills, MHPs possess several abilities which aid in the development and cohesion of interdisciplinary teams and make MHPs extremely effective collaborators, which include (a) identifying contextual factors and barriers impacting treatment effectiveness; (b) understanding language, values, and perspectives of different disciplines; (c) effectively communicating client treatment goals across disciplines; (d) understanding and integrating client cultural and gender identity into treatment planning; and (e) educating others to improve multicultural competence and integrate intersectionality into care planning.

Interdisciplinary communication in ICC can be oral or written, bidirectional (exchange), multidirectional (collaboration of multiple disciplines), or unidirectional (release of information from one provider to another). Best practice offers TNB clients fully informed consent about the information to be shared and actively engages clients as members of the interdisciplinary care team. The simplest and most common form of ICC occurs when an MHP and a medical provider or psychiatrist discuss issues related to a client's medication regimen, or when two MHPs doing individual and family counseling with the same client collaborate. Most MHPs have engaged in some kind of ICC even if it is not focused on TNB affirmative care (Torrence et al., 2014). When working with the TNB community, ICC is a more involved and more consistent part of working with clients (Coyne et al., 2023; Lee et al., 2022). Because many TNB clients require services from a broad range of professionals—including primary care providers, endocrinologists, obstetrics and gynecology providers, surgeons, school personnel, employers, religious leaders, and attorneys—it is important that MHPs are in communication with others involved in their clients' care. Additionally, the MHP will likely interact with systems that clients need to access to obtain necessary documentation to maneuver through daily activities (American Psychological Association [APA], 2015). These may include local, state, and federal offices that issue identification documents (i.e., driver's license, ID, birth certificate, passport, U.S. permanent resident card, social security card), school record offices, and the Transportation Security Administration (World Professional Association for Transgender Health [WPATH], 2015).

There are two main settings within which TNB-affirming ICC occurs. A centralized setting includes clinics, hospitals, or health centers that employ an interdisciplinary team of health care professionals to work as a treatment team providing care to TNB clients (Koehler et al., 2021; Reisner et al., 2015). Many large U.S. cities have one or more of such clinics or hospital-based programs. Many TNB clients receive their care from these centralized systems, with some Two-Spirit, lesbian, gay, bisexual, trans, and queer or questioning (2SLGBTQ+) health centers providing medical and behavioral health care for thousands of TNB clients each year. While many services can be coordinated under one roof at such health centers, these organizations still coordinate care with outside providers when clients work with providers across multiple systems or require care or resources that are not provided by the health care center (e.g., surgery, oncology, electrolysis, legal assistance).

A decentralized system exists when providers who are in separate locations (e.g., private practice or hospital-based establishments) build working relationships and collaborative networks to facilitate efficient cross-referral and communication to ensure the best coordinated care for TNB clients (Koehler et al., 2021). In some major cities, providers across a range of disciplines have developed formal or informal networks. Networks expand and contract as new TNB-affirming providers are identified and other providers leave the area or change their practice availability. Such networks facilitate cross-referral and prompt care as clients navigate the complex and often daunting health care system to obtain needed services (Stroumsa, 2014). Decentralized systems are more common in rural areas and in cities that do not have health care systems that specifically serve 2SLGBTQ+ or TNB communities (Denaro et al., 2023) but can also exist side-by-side with centralized systems in many cities. Within the range of centralized and decentralized systems, ICC may take many forms for MHPs. Among the various health care professionals working with TNB clients, MHPs often have the most contact with clients and are in the best position to understand how care across multiple domains and across a TNB client's lifespan should be linked. MHPs may also have more contact with family members, be more aware of the lived experiences of clients, and have a deeper awareness of important cultural issues and individualized client needs that must be incorporated into care.

Recent increases in telehealth spurred by COVID-19 have improved access to TNB affirmative care, especially for people in rural areas or small towns (Renner et al., 2021). Telehealth has also improved access to care for people living in poverty, people of color seeking care with culturally aligned providers, and people benefiting from care in alternate languages. For psychologists, in particular, the introduction of PSYPACT—the interstate compact for licensed psychologists—has allowed qualified psychologists in these states to provide telehealth services in other participating states (Association of State and Provincial Psychology Boards, n.d.), as of this writing, over 42 states, DC, and Guam are part of the PSYPACT compact. Other behavioral health professions have an established interstate compact (i.e., psychiatry, psychiatric nursing, counseling) or are seeking to create one (i.e., social work; Adashi et al., 2021; Counseling Compact, 2023; National Association of Social Workers, 2023). In addition, video consultation has become much more common and has expanded access to TNB care and consultation (Nieder et al., 2022). Several electronic consultation (e-consultation) systems have been developed. Some systems support providers from multiple locations in one organization like the Veterans Administration e-consultation service (Shipherd, Kauth, & Matza, 2016) and ICC education (Shipherd, Kauth, Firek, et al., 2016); some systems provide voluntary consultation to any interested provider via email request like TransLine (see http://project-health.org/transline/).

Within centralized care systems, a separate release of information may not be required for communication between providers. However, different disciplines work under different requirements for release of information outside of their respective care system. For example, it is standard practice for medical providers to exchange information with an external referral source without a signed release, while MHPs are required to obtain a written release before communicating with an outside entity. MHPs involved in an ICC team should ensure that they have met their legal requirements for release from clients or their guardians, in addition to meeting requirements within their care systems (Chang et al., 2018).

WHY INTERDISCIPLINARY COLLABORATIVE CARE IS CRITICAL FOR TRANS- AND NONBINARY-AFFIRMING CARE

ICC improves client health outcomes and the quality of care that clients receive (Mabel et al., 2019). A range of professional organizations have strongly endorsed the need for interdisciplinary care and comprehensive integrated services for TNB clients (APA, 2015; Byne et al., 2012; Coleman et al., 2022). In addition, multiple studies have demonstrated that ICC enhances the effectiveness of treatment for TNB clients (Hembree et al., 2009). Client health outcomes and service quality are enhanced by the improved continuity of care that ICC offers and better communication between shared providers. Transparent, effective, and supportive ICC can also help minimize the retraumatization of TNB clients in health care settings given the protective historical mistrust and suspicion TNB communities may experience when engaging with health care systems that have done significant historical harm (APA, 2015). Without ICC, clients are sometimes expected to carry messages and questions between providers and care systems, often leading to confusion and frustration on the part of the client and providers, and sometimes resulting in delayed care (McIntosh, 2016). When health care professionals work collaboratively, colleagues can communicate directly with each other to develop a comprehensive treatment plan that coordinates the client's biopsychosocial care and more efficiently addresses client needs (Mabel et al., 2019)—while client engagement and retention are also improved. Many, if not most, TNB clients have at some point had to obtain services from providers who were ill-informed regarding gender and their needs as TNB people (Panchal et al., 2022). As a result, TNB people have often felt dissatisfied with or even harmed by the health care they received (James et al., 2024; Panchal et al., 2022). When clients feel that their providers are attentive, competent, and respectful, clients may more actively engage in their treatment and remain in care, which in turn helps ICC teams amplify TNB clients' voices and needs.

When care involves contact with TNB clients' families, significant others, or chosen intimate circles, ICC can facilitate the management of complex systems issues. Close collaboration is also especially important in complex cases that require careful consideration—and clear and consistent communication—to provide clients with affirmative and empowering care that effectively addresses the causes of distress or dysfunction clients may be experiencing. In such cases, a TNB client's history or diagnoses may be complicated and problems that clients face might not be resolved without the close collaboration that comes with ICC. In addition, cultural backgrounds (e.g., religion and spirituality—see Chapter 14, this volume) and interlocking oppressions (e.g., racism and transprejudice—see Chapter 6, this volume) can have a profound effect on clients, their families, and communities, significantly impacting how care can be most responsive and best aligned with clients' goals and needs (Wesp et al., 2019). Social and structural factors based on a person's identities and social positions, especially if multiple identities are marginalized, can deeply impact a client's lived experiences, experienced discrimination, and access to and engagement in care (Bowleg, 2012; Collins, 1991; Crenshaw, 1991; Wesp et al., 2019). The following case example illustrates some of these complexities.

Case Example: Working With a Youth and Family

Michael, a 16-year-old TNB young man who was assigned female at birth, has begun counseling at his parents' insistence.[1] Michael's parents immigrated from Pakistan, with Michael born and educated in the United States. Michael began assertively requesting hormone therapy (HT) after being attacked by a peer and severely hurt at a school social event. Michael's parents are hesitant to proceed with medical transition; they believe that "their daughter" hasn't carefully explored gender identity issues and don't want Michael to discuss gender identity issues with anyone outside the immediate family. A high school administrator has contacted Michael's parents to identify concerns about Michael's bathroom choice, his request that others call him Michael instead of his legal name, his increasing anger and frustration in the classroom, and the bullying and fights that are occurring as other youth become aware of Michael's requests. Michael's primary care provider is concerned about the discord in the family, will not prescribe HT without parental consent, and is growing progressively more worried about Michael's use of nonprescribed hormone medications and supplements to effect physical changes he desperately wants.

In this case, ICC is a critical aspect of care with the MHP in an ideal position to communicate with other systems and coordinate a shared treatment plan. This treatment plan will be influenced by the family's cultural values, Michael's intersectional experiences related to his social identities and social positions, his parents' intersectional identities, and the systems that Michael's parents rely on for support and guidance (i.e., extended family, spiritual leaders, and communities). An understanding of the interlocking systems of oppression Michael's parents are experiencing as Pakistani immigrants in the United States will offer profoundly important context for communication and treatment planning with them for their child. It will be critical to explore the parents' cultural understanding of gender and hijra identities, cultural binary gender norms, and fears of continued harm and discrimination Michael (and his family) may experience (Majid et al., 2023). Michael's intersectional experiences and needs based on his identities as a Pakistani American, gender expansive young person are also critical to understand. A collaborative treatment plan will need to navigate generational and acculturation differences between Michael and his

---

[1] The case examples in this chapter are composites of multiple clients which have been modified to disguise all client identities and protect their confidentiality.

parents, acknowledging how cultural and religious values may be influencing family functioning and health care choices. The MHP could support discussion between Michael's parents and school administrators to address the bullying and harm Michael is experiencing and to create a plan for name, pronoun, and bathroom use at school and at home. In addition, the MHP (in partnership with the primary care provider), could support the family to explore and understand Michael's lived experience when considering the next steps in care.

As in all instances of ICC, it is important to clarify and secure any release of information needed for collaborative communication between providers, Michael, Michael's parents, and the school system. Aspects of the treatment plan or ICC approach will vary depending on a family's religious or spiritual background, race and ethnicity, country of origin, level of acculturation, socioeconomic status, primary language, and beliefs about the cause and impact of a TNB identity (Golden & Oransky, 2019). See Chapter 10 for in-depth information on working with TNB adolescents.

DEVELOPING PROFESSIONAL AND ORGANIZATIONAL GROWTH IN INTERDISCIPLINARY COLLABORATIVE CARE

ICC enhances professional and organizational growth and development in ways that ultimately benefit TNB clients, as well as the providers and organizations that serve them. In addition, ICC allows professional colleagues to teach and learn from each other, rather than relying on clients to teach their providers how to offer TNB affirmative care (Soled et al., 2022). Through this interdisciplinary exposure, providers become progressively more informed and better prepared to facilitate communication and transitions between disciplines—which offers providers the ability to better prepare their clients for interaction with different disciplines and to identify circumstances that may warrant a specific interdisciplinary referral or course of action. Through ICC, MHPs are also able to reinforce care instructions offered by other providers. For example, an MHP who regularly collaborates with surgeons might speak with a client who has chosen to disregard the vaginal dilation directions received from their surgeon following a vaginoplasty. As a result of ICC, the MHP understands the significant impact of such a decision (permanent closure of the newly formed vaginal canal) and can facilitate communication between client and surgeon to discuss long-term physical, psychological, and sexual impacts.

By working in close collaboration with an interdisciplinary team, providers constantly hone and update their knowledge and clinical skills. This is especially critical in TNB health in which the knowledge and evidence base is growing rapidly (APA, 2015). This continually improves providers' ability to guide and inform clients. In this way, ICC minimizes barriers to care for current and future TNB clients and makes care more TNB affirmative. Because the learning that is gained from working with an ICC team impacts all team members, the systems in which the team members work are also impacted (Coyne et al., 2023). The learning that is gained through ICC can also positively impact colleagues in other organizations and other providers, and this learning can inform current practice models and the fields as a whole and inform policy and advocacy efforts.

Finally, it is important to note that despite an increasing amount of information available about TNB people and the care that they require, only a small percentage of health care providers across disciplines have developed the expertise needed to provide TNB affirmative care and few graduate or postgraduate programs offer specialized training in TNB affirmative care (Coyne et al., 2023; Rodriguez-Wallberg et al., 2022; Soled et al., 2022). At this point in time, clinicians with solid expertise in working with TNB clients are uncommon and are unique in their respective fields. At the same time, the lack of training opportunities for health care professionals in TNB health has resulted in some providers across disciplines offering services to TNB clients or claiming expertise without adequate training or exposure. With ICC, it becomes possible to include practitioners who are at different levels of development and knowledge, allowing them to learn from ICC team members that are more experienced in offering TNB affirmative care. This provides a training and supervision mechanism ensuring more health care providers receive affirming TNB training (Coyne et al., 2023).

COMMON ROLES OF MENTAL HEALTH PROVIDERS IN INTERDISCIPLINARY COLLABORATIVE CARE

ICC teams can be made up of a variety of professionals, both within and outside of health care professions, and the TNB client (Chang et al., 2018). Depending on the setting and the situation, ICC teams may include MHPs (e.g., psychologists, psychiatrists, mental health counselors, social workers, family therapists, case managers, school counselors, university counseling staff), medical professionals (e.g., primary care providers, internists, obstetrics and gynecology providers, endocrinologists, surgeons, nurses, nutritionists, pharmacists, physical therapists, speech therapists), and allied professionals (e.g., electrologists, laser hair removal technicians, acupuncturists, speech and language pathologists, case managers or patient navigators, school personnel, religious or spiritual leaders, lawyers, ethicists; Lee et al., 2022; Mabel et al., 2019; Soled et al., 2022). Because MHPs often spend the greatest amount of time with clients and have the skills to develop a deep understanding of clients' needs, wishes, and barriers to care, they serve a critical role in ensuring that all members of the team have a fuller picture of the client and understand that the client is a critical member of the ICC team. This, in turn, helps to ensure that decisions made and actions taken are fully aligned with both the client's desires and their best interests. The role of the MHP is influenced by the client's willingness to consent to release information outside of the MHP's health care system and the client's comfort working with an ICC team. Many TNB clients enthusiastically support ICC models if they trust that their providers are honest, transparent, and genuinely invested in supporting their access to necessary care. In this way, TNB clients often view MHPs as advocates for their overall health care. It is important for the client and MHP to specifically discuss and agree to any limitations on the information that will be shared with the ICC team, as well as possible outcomes.

Schools and Childcare Settings

Special expertise in child and adolescent mental health, in addition to expertise in providing TNB affirmative care, is required when working with TNB and gender questioning youth (Coleman et al., 2022). TNB and gender questioning youth can present with a complicated clinical picture and with complex system issues (Keo-Meier & Ehrensaft, 2018; Magalhães et al., 2022). MHPs may be called upon to assist young clients and their families to coordinate a care and education plan with a youth's school system or, for younger children, a youth's childcare setting. The collaboration may include participation in a meeting with the youth, the youth's parents or guardians, school administrators, and school counselors to create a plan for respectful, supportive treatment of the youth in the educational or childcare setting (APA & National Association of School Psychologists, 2014; Coyne et al., 2023; Gay, Lesbian and Straight Education, n.d.; Warwick & Shumer, 2023). The requested plan may be developed with school staff or may be created with the family and communicated to the school through a letter. The development and implementation of a plan can help the school better understand the youth's needs, educate school staff about gender identity and gender expression, and solicit support for the youth. A letter to the school might describe the youth's experience of gender, specify names and pronouns to be used when addressing the youth, clarify bathroom and locker room use, and describe conditions (e.g., uniform) that would facilitate a more affirmative learning environment for the youth in the school or childcare setting. MHPs may also be asked to provide education about gender identity to staff, teachers, parents, and students (Coyne et al., 2023).

Religious and Spiritual Systems

Many TNB people were raised in a faith tradition that they may wish to maintain throughout their lives (Erickson-Schroth, 2022). Although quite a few faith traditions openly discourage, ignore, or pathologize TNB identities, MHPs may be able to assist their clients in the process of reconciling their faith with their gender identity and finding new outlets for spiritual growth. MHPs can use faith-based family guidance to help families learn to support their child's TNB identity in the context of their religious and cultural values (Glassgold & Ryan, 2022). This can be especially critical support for families of color given a frequent deep integration of family, community, faith, and the importance of spiritual connection, guidance, and acceptance in families' lives (Glassgold & Ryan, 2022). MHPs can create a network of gender-affirming religious and spiritual guides, including pastoral counselors, chaplains, priests, rabbis, nuns, pastors, imams, and shamans. MHPs can gather information about how sacred texts of various faith traditions discuss gender and TNB people and different faiths groups' comfort in welcoming TNB people into their community, discuss issues of gender identity with religious and spiritual leaders, or facilitate a meeting with the client and their religious leader to improve communication and mutual understanding. Common intrapersonal challenges include internalized transprejudice related to a belief that being TNB is inherently sinful or disordered and resulting trauma from excommunication or religious ritual, exorcism, or prayer to change one's TNB identity. Additional challenges include families feeling that they must choose between supporting their TNB family member or maintaining their faith. See Chapter 14 for more information on TNB clients and faith traditions.

Legal and Correctional Systems

MHPs may be called upon to interact with various personnel in correctional or legal systems to ensure the well-being of their clients. If a client has been incarcerated or jailed, an MHP can provide a letter to the jail or correctional setting staff with client consent. The letter can describe the client's gender identity, specify names and pronouns to be used when addressing the client, clarify bathroom and shower use, and describe conditions that would facilitate a safe and respectful environment for the client (e.g., ability to wear a bra, permission to have facial hair). The letter may also offer housing recommendations (i.e., general population housing, women's section, men's section). It can be important to specifically address the possibility that the correctional system will choose to place a TNB client in isolation, instead of general population housing, as a protective measure. If the client is incarcerated, it may also be necessary to inform medical personnel at the facility of the client's need for continuation of HT and facilitate proof of prescription through the client's medical provider to support the client's access to necessary medication. In some cases, clients who are facing sentencing on criminal charges may require a letter to the judge that describes the client's gender identity and the treatment needs of the client. The following case example illustrates some issues an MHP might encounter when a client is in a correctional or legal setting.

Case Example: Working With an Incarcerated Trans Woman
Vanessa, a 29-year-old African American trans woman, was incarcerated at a local jail for engaging in sex work. On her third day, after being cleared for housing in the general population and placed on a male unit, she sought an emergency mental health appointment. Vanessa reported that she had been taking "off market" hormones for 15 years. For the last five years, she had engaged in sex work to support herself; in that time, more than a dozen of her friends (also transgender women of color) had been brutally assaulted, two had been stabbed, and one had been murdered. Vanessa had not taken her hormones for several days and was reporting symptoms consistent with early menopause. More urgently, she had received three serious threats from male inmates in her new housing unit, causing her to reexperience trauma-related symptoms and to fear for her safety. When she reported her concerns to the correctional officers on her unit, she was told that she belonged on a male unit because she had "male" genitalia and that she would have to solve her own problems with the placement.

In this case, an ICC approach would be critical to address the client's previously undocumented medical and mental health needs, and immediate safety issues in her assigned jail unit. An MHP could work with jail officials to advocate for the client's placement on a female unit to improve the client's safety and to align her placement with her identity. In addition, collaboration with the jail's medical director to offer a hormone prescription and ensure the client's receipt of those medications could dramatically improve the client's access to medically necessary care. An MHP could also collaborate with the client's lawyer to advocate for ongoing mental health support and to highlight the traumatic effect of continued incarceration on a male unit and the misgendering the client is experiencing by jail staff and other inmates. If the client has not committed a violent offense, an MHP could collaborate with a client's attorney to submit a request with justification to a judge to advocate for house arrest as opposed to incarceration.

Child Custody Evaluation

When a TNB or gender questioning youth or TNB parent or caregiver is the subject of a child custody evaluation, an MHP may be called upon to offer documentation to inform the evaluation. The child custody evaluator is often not trained in TNB affirmative care and may not understand that gender identity and gender expression are significant issues to be addressed in the evaluation (Kuvalanka et al., 2019). Whenever a TNB or gender questioning youth is the subject of such an evaluation, the role of the MHP can involve educating the evaluator about gender identity issues, describing the youth's gender identity and expression, identifying the level of support received from different caregivers, and describing work with the youth or caregivers. A similar communication can occur with the guardian ad litem who has been assigned to represent the child or adolescent's best interests. In this case, it is important that the guardian ad litem understand the youth's best interests from the perspective of the youth (Kuvalanka et al., 2019). A letter can also be provided to the evaluator when a TNB parent or caregiver is involved in a child custody evaluation. A helpful addition to the letter can include noting there is no indication that children of TNB parents experience short- or long-term negative impact because of their parent's gender identity and that research shows good quality child–parent relationships and few behavioral or emotional concerns in children with TNB parents (Imrie et al., 2020).

Updating Important Documents

In other cases, an MHP may be called upon to write a letter or complete a form to assist a client to change their gender marker on vital documents, such as a driver's license, social security card, passport, or birth certificate. Information regarding the specific requirements for various identity documents in different states can be found on websites such as the National Center for Transgender Equality. It is important to determine whether there is a prescribed format that must be followed and whether information must be submitted on a specific form. There may also be verbatim language that must be included in a letter for it to be considered valid; this may differ by federal, state, county, and city regulations. For example, some Department of Motor Vehicle offices require a letter designating the client's current gender, that this gender is stable, and that it is not likely to change in the foreseeable future. While in the past, the U.S. Department of State would only accept a verbatim letter from a physician to change the gender marker on a U.S. passport, people may now self-select a gender marker and can select male (M), female (F), or unspecified (X) for another gender identity.

Work and Travel Settings

At times, clients may be interested in changing their expression of their gender identity at work. In these situations, a letter from the MHP to human resources personnel or the client's supervisor may be both instructive and helpful in gaining understanding and support in the work environment (Chang et al., 2018). For clients who decide to transition while remaining at their current place of employment, a letter can help prepare the employer for upcoming changes (APA, 2015). A letter to an employer might explain gender identity, describe the client's experience of gender, specify correct client names and pronouns, clarify bathroom and locker room use, and describe conditions facilitating an affirmative work environment. In certain high-security jobs (e.g., law enforcement, security, airline pilots), additional information may be required to ensure that the client is allowed to continue working in their position during and after transition.

MHPs can also write a letter to assist clients in their safe passage, particularly when traveling on commercial airlines or crossing borders. Because current screening procedures can reveal anatomical features that may not conform to the client's gender presentation, a safe passage letter can help to explain the discrepancy that may be observed to security staff. Clients can carry such a letter and produce it if necessary. The same letter can be used if a client is detained by police or pulled over for a traffic violation, or if a client is approached in a gender-specific public space or bathroom and asked about the appropriateness of their presence.

Medical Systems and Access to Medical Procedures

Collaboration with medical professionals is perhaps the most common instance of ICC (Coyne et al., 2023). TNB people have the same basic health care needs as cisgender people in terms of screening, prevention, and treatment, while also having health care needs that are associated with their gender identity. ICC can actively contribute to TNB people's engagement and retention in primary care, linking trusted providers and services to the TNB client (Denaro et al., 2023; Lee et al., 2022). While many TNB people tend to focus on their gender-related health care needs, it is important that MHPs support them in accessing affirmative general health care as well, including primary, dental, and behavioral health care.

For gender-affirming care, the MHP's role involves the following: to ensure readiness and understanding of the medical procedures or treatments; evaluate a client's ability to grant informed consent; advocate for informed and TNB-affirming medical care; assist the client to integrate the medical procedures and body changes into their identity; help prepare a TNB client for mental, physical, and social changes that may occur; maximize the success of medical interventions and the client's satisfaction with those interventions; assist the TNB client to access necessary care; and help the ICC team interpret and apply the client's unique needs and desires for their health care and life (APA, 2015).

Historically, MHPs have been placed in the role of gatekeepers rather than ICC team members (Soled et al., 2022), as many medical providers would not prescribe HT or perform surgery without "approval" letters from MHPs that indicated that clients were ready for these procedures and had demonstrated their readiness by meeting restrictive prescribed criteria, including "lived experience" as the "opposite" gender (Weigand, 2021). There were numerous problems with this practice, not the least of which was that it dictated the conditions under which clients were allowed to obtain needed services. Thus, clients often reported a rigid and stereotypical gender binary narrative allowing them to access the letter they needed, disregarding their own gender identity and expression (Meyerowitz, 2004).

Since the early 2000's, models of TNB affirmative care have improved and clinical practice has evolved to include a deeper understanding of nonbinary gender identities (see Chapter 7, this volume, on working with nonbinary clients) and approaches to care that personalize treatment to meet each TNB client's unique gender and embodiment goals (Coyne et al., 2023). Revised systems of care actively include clients as ICC team members, avoid strict gatekeeping roles for any ICC team member, apply a broader understanding of gender identity and expression, recognize that there is no correct process of transition, and position clients to play a much larger role in deciding the procedures that they will undergo (Coleman et al., 2022). The development of the ICC model has not only reduced the gatekeeping role, thereby removing a substantial barrier in the ability of clients to obtain needed services, but has also resulted in a model in which collaborative team members trust each other enough to identify challenges and barriers, working together to improve and innovate the way they offer TNB affirmative care (Denaro et al., 2023; Soled et al., 2022). Some providers and systems, however, still utilize a gatekeeper process (Soled et al., 2022) and reify the gender binary.

Within medical systems, the most common collaboration involves working with primary care providers, endocrinologists, and surgeons to facilitate clients' access to HT and surgical procedures. The focus of the ICC interaction is the same whether providers work as a centralized, preexisting interdisciplinary team or constitute a decentralized network of independent professionals, although formality of the documentation may differ (i.e., a short, internal electronic health record note vs. a letter from an independent colleague to include in the health record). The content of HT and surgery letters is influenced by the medical provider's requirements, with some having strict qualification requirements (i.e., only a doctoral level MHP or only a psychiatrist) and some guided by the client's insurance company requirements.

When writing letters for HT or surgery, MHPs follow a fairly standard format, with surgical letters offering greater detail and depth (Coleman et al., 2022; Keo-Meier et al., 2018). In these letters, MHPs should briefly describe the training and experience that they have working with TNB clients. The letters should also indicate the amount of time that the MHP has known or worked with the client, the frequency or number of times the client has been seen, and the nature of the relationship with the client. A description of the client's gender identity and gender expression, some gender history, and a comment about how the requested treatment will help the client to achieve congruence and authenticity are commonly included (Keo-Meier et al., 2018). MHPs should describe any psychological or psychiatric conditions and note whether these present a contraindication for HT or surgery.

Hormone Therapy for Adults
There are two basic models of HT: a more traditional Standard of Care (SOC) model and an informed consent model (Coleman et al., 2022; Deutsch, 2012). The two models are not in conflict but are instead at different places on a continuum of assessment for HT (Coleman et al., 2022). A traditional SOC model requires a qualified health care professional to conduct an assessment that evaluates whether a client meets specific criteria that would warrant a referral for HT, one element of which is the client's ability to grant informed consent (Coleman et al., 2022). An informed consent model reduces barriers for an adult client to access HT while still requiring them to demonstrate a knowledge of the effects and risks of HT, the ability to apply that knowledge to medical decision making, and the ability to grant informed consent. A growing number of health centers and interdisciplinary teams are utilizing an informed consent model for HT prescription for adults 18 and over (Coleman et al., 2022). An informed consent model requires that clients requesting HT receive comprehensive, accessible information about the effects and risks of HT, and are screened to ensure their ability to understand the information and to apply that information in their decision-making process. Providers or MHPs screen for conditions that may interrupt informed consent and work with clients to expeditiously

establish informed consent when possible (Coleman et al., 2022). An MHP's role in this process may include screening to ensure clients can grant informed consent, offering information about HT effects and risks, and identifying any suggestions to maximize a positive HT experience.

Many providers prescribing HT are not located in an informed consent clinic and may be more likely to require a letter from an MHP that follows a traditional SOC model. Many endocrinologists or primary care providers request letters from MHPs because they lack adequate training in mental health to diagnose gender dysphoria or incongruence and differentially distinguish symptoms and conditions that may mimic gender dysphoria or incongruence (Coleman et al., 2022; McIntosh, 2016). In such cases, interdisciplinary colleagues are working to ensure that the care they are providing will have the intended beneficial effect. The length and level of detail in these letters will depend on the requirements of each HT provider. MHPs may need to offer HT providers information about a client's unique experience and transition plan, helping providers to understand clients' need and readiness for HT when they do not offer stereotypical narratives or goals. MHPs can also support HT providers in understanding clients' unique transition plans that may include a request for low levels of HT to achieve a more androgynous appearance or certain psychological benefits, or a plan to discontinue HT after specific permanent physical changes have occurred.

When working with clients who are seeking HT, MHPs can be especially helpful in preparing clients for the effects of treatment (e.g., helping clients to understand the effects of HT, what it will not do, which effects are permanent or temporary, and possible influence on mood, identity, and expression). MHPs can collaborate with medical professionals who are prescribing HT by educating clients and ensuring clients are able to make fully informed decisions prior to starting HT (Coleman et al., 2022; Deutsch, 2012). MHPs can help clients understand that HT may cause infertility and facilitate a discussion about whether clients want to cryogenically store eggs or sperm (dickey et al., 2016). Once clients have begun HT, MHPs can assist them in understanding the effects, as well as the changes they can expect across time, including HT's impact on emotional functioning (Keo-Meier et al., 2015). By monitoring these effects, MHPs can also help clients understand when it may be appropriate to contact their medical provider if they experience an unusual response pattern. If clients are considering the possibility of discontinuing HT, MHPs can help them prepare for the loss of the temporary HT changes.

Puberty Suppression and Hormone Therapy for Youth
In the past, HT and puberty suppression have followed a very formal SOC process in clinical settings that serve TNB and gender questioning youth.

However, as some of these clinical settings mature, providers have adapted the decision-making process to the needs and situation of each youth or family (McIntosh, 2016). The interplay of psychological, physical, and social development makes it critical to have interdisciplinary care teams when working with TNB and gender questioning youth (Chen et al., 2016; Warwick & Shumer, 2023). MHPs play an important role on these teams due to cognitive and social development considerations, as well as family dynamics, including the degree of support within the family for the youth's gender identity and expression (Glassgold & Ryan, 2022). This is crucial when conducting a mental health evaluation to determine the appropriateness and timeliness of a medical intervention (APA, 2015). MHPs can also help when adolescents present with a late-onset (i.e., postpubertal) nonbinary or gender diverse identification with no childhood history of gender role nonconformity or gender questioning (Ehrensaft, 2020). Parents, school staff, and medical providers are often not well-informed, and a thorough assessment can establish the appropriateness of HT or puberty suppression. MHPs can also assist the ICC team when complex family dynamics exist, such as parent and youth disagreement about the speed or type of medical care a youth has requested. MHPs can assist the ICC team in exploring the fear and burden of responsibility that parents and caregivers may feel as they make health decisions (Coyne et al., 2023; Wagner & Armstrong, 2020).

Surgeries
Surgeons typically require at least one letter or opinion from an MHP prior to initiating gender-affirming surgery (Coleman et al., 2022). In some surgeries, or as a preference by some surgeons, two letters from independent MHPs may be required. Surgeons may request letters from MHPs when they lack adequate training in mental health to make a diagnosis of gender dysphoria or incongruence and differentially distinguish symptoms and conditions that may mimic gender dysphoria (Coleman et al., 2022). Many surgeons require a detailed letter that follows SOC protocol and may only accept letters from specific types of MHPs. This type of letter may be nuanced to write for a nonbinary client who does not endorse a binary gender identity because some surgeons may require assurance that the client has an established identity that stereotypically aligns with the surgery being considered (i.e., a client requesting vaginoplasty is a TNB woman, has consistently identified as a woman and "dresses" as a woman). In other cases, the client may desire a modified surgical procedure, such as a "zero depth" vaginoplasty.

Nonetheless, if the client wishes to utilize this surgeon, the letter must conform to the surgeon's expectations. MHPs can offer surgeons information about a client's unique experience and transition plan, helping surgeons to understand clients' readiness for and the appropriateness of gender-affirming surgery when clients do not offer stereotypical narratives or goals. Surgery letters for nonbinary clients should carefully balance a client's unique identity and needs with the information surgeons need to feel confident that surgery is psychologically appropriate, and that the client will not retroactively regret their decision to undergo the procedure (Schechter & Schechter, 2018). Involving the client as an active ICC team member and discussing letter requirements can empower clients to participate in the creation of the letter and the personal gender narrative it presents. When working with those interested in surgical procedures, MHPs ensure they have realistic expectations of costs, logistics, risks, and potential surgery results (e.g., appearance, use, sensate response). Discussion should also include what clients can expect to experience in the recovery period after surgery, including the length of expected recovery time. Clients should also be aware that there are different surgical techniques in common practice (i.e., nipples, clitoris), and only some may retain nerve connection.

Primary Care and Other Specialty Care
When communicating with a medical provider offering HT, puberty suppression or gender-affirming surgery, an MHP is frequently speaking to an informed colleague. MHPs who work within an ICC model interact regularly with clients' primary care providers, gynecologists, internists, pharmacists, endocrinologists, and other medical or allied professionals such as fertility specialists, nurses, speech therapists, occupational therapists, and health educators. Collaboration in an ICC model can be bidirectional. Just as medical providers may rely on MHPs to provide documentation that TNB clients will use to initiate a medical transition and to address the psychological and social aspects of transition with the client before, during, and after HT or surgery, MHPs also often refer clients to medical providers for assessment and treatment (Coleman et al., 2022; Coyne et al., 2023).

Given the lack of informed TNB-affirming medical and allied health providers, clients will frequently receive care from providers who have not worked with TNB people. Communicating and collaborating with colleagues who are unfamiliar with or intimidated by TNB health care requires a supplemental set of skills. MHPs may need to offer support, information, and education to interdisciplinary colleagues who are unfamiliar with issues of gender identity and gender expression to assist their clients in obtaining TNB affirmative care (APA, 2015; Coyne et al., 2023). For example, an MHP assisting a TNB person obtain a vaginoplasty could contact the client's new gynecologist in preparation for the client's first office visit. This could include providing the gynecologist with general information about the client's gender history, coaching on respectful ways to communicate with and about the client, and discussing how both providers could most affirmatively raise the continued need for appropriate health checks to ensure the client's best physical health (APA, 2015; Unger, 2014).

MHPs can also play an important role in helping interdisciplinary colleagues who are less familiar with TNB affirmative care understand TNB clients' presentations and reframe their behavior, if necessary, to assist the colleague in providing the best care possible. Many TNB clients have fought extremely hard to access care with uninformed providers in a system that fails to appreciate the medical necessity of their requests (James et al., 2024). As a result, TNB clients may be perceived as aggressive, insistent, angry, and unwilling to compromise (Soled et al., 2022). In these instances, it can be helpful to reframe their presentation as stemming from fear, a fight for body integrity, and self-advocacy in a predominantly oppressive and discriminatory health care system (Ducheny et al., 2019).

When communicating with providers who may not regularly engage in ICC, MHPs should be intentional about the mode of communication they choose and the method in which information is given, received, and shared. It may help to clarify how the information exchange could improve the care provided to the client by all treating professionals, clearly define roles, and discuss the various levels of expertise in TNB care that each provider brings to the exchange. It can also be of assistance to offer the interdisciplinary colleague the opportunity to communicate with an ICC team member with strong TNB affirmative care experience in the same profession if available, especially if the colleague is in need of specific treatment guidance that an MHP may not have or if the colleague fails to value the expertise and support an MHP can offer. MHPs are encouraged to remember that learning and expanding one's understanding of the gender spectrum can be uncomfortable and anxiety-provoking (Ducheny et al., 2019), and that some providers may find it difficult to manage issues of gender identity while also recognizing and respecting other cultural identities of the client. Providing TNB affirmative care may require difficult or uncomfortable personal and professional change by the colleague. In providing care to TNB clients, colleagues will need to confront previously unexamined stereotypes, implicit bias, fears, and anti-TNB prejudice (Ducheny et al., 2019; Soled et al., 2022) and it may take years for a colleague to become competent in TNB affirmative care.

For the MHPs, it may be particularly difficult to work with colleagues who say or do things that are not TNB-affirming, that diminish TNB clients' lives and choices, or disregard how difficult it can be for TNB clients to remain in care. MHPs are encouraged to lead by example, remaining alert for any receptive teaching moments with their colleagues, using affirmative language, and gently suggesting ways for colleagues to improve care of TNB clients. Using a colleague's professional language and couching elements of TNB affirmative care in language that aligns with their values (i.e., health outcomes, client's ability to consent to pelvic exam, improve patient retention in care, treatment adherence, reduced no-show rate) can also improve the care they offer to TNB clients. When things get difficult, it can often be helpful to seek consultation from a trusted colleague who can offer support and a reminder of why the effort will ultimately improve the care TNB clients receive.

Special Considerations in Interdisciplinary Collaborative Care

Between 2010 and 2024, an increasing number of health insurance plans began explicitly covering gender-affirmative care and various procedures (e.g., Stroumsa, 2014), including Medicaid, Medi-Cal, and Medicare plans. However, because insurance plans were unfamiliar with TNB affirmative care and were slow to revise previous exclusions and restrictions, clients sometimes encountered difficulty obtaining reimbursement for health care costs, including prescribed medications, procedures, and surgery. In these cases, a letter to the insurance company from an ICC team member could sometimes facilitate the reimbursement process or support an appeal when coverage had been denied. Before communicating with an insurance company, it is important to know exactly what the client's insurance policy says about coverage for the specific procedures, and to then pair that language with treatment protocols received by the client. It is unclear how insurance coverage for TNB care will evolve going forward and how this will affect access to care. As care constrict, ICC will be even more crucial in supporting TNB communities, clients, and colleagues.

While ICC may require more administrative time from providers on the front end of treatment, it can provide care that is ultimately more efficient, effectively utilizing funding and other scarce resources. As insurance carriers increasingly cover TNB affirmative care (Stroumsa, 2014), the costs of the various treatments and procedures will come under closer scrutiny. Because most TNB health care involves providers across a range of health care disciplines, ICC will be a necessary component in ensuring coverage for this medically necessary care and providing such care in the most cost-efficient way possible. For example, many insurance policies require one or two letters from MHPs that establish a diagnosis of gender dysphoria to justify the medical treatment or surgical intervention, even though the WPATH *Standards of Care Version 8* only recommends a single qualified health care professional's opinion to access such treatment (Coleman et al., 2022). MHPs who engage in ICC have the distinct advantage of knowing when a letter is needed and what must be included for the client to obtain medical or surgical services through collaborative discussion with the care team.

The experience of practicing as an ICC team within the same organization and across a range of organizations or practices can differ. Preexisting relationships can enhance the MHP's ability to discuss TNB affirmative care issues but can also create pressure and discomfort when those discussions impact all professional activities that the colleagues share. MHPs may have less ability to impact a system from the outside, but they can partner with key colleagues with whom they work well and who enhance their ability to provide quality TNB client care. When MHPs are not part of an existing interdisciplinary setting or team, and especially when they practice in isolated or rural communities, it is still possible to identify interdisciplinary colleagues with whom they may collaborate or refer, if only by phone or video conference (Nieder et al., 2022). For example, a rural MHP could identify a TNB-affirming pediatrician in a surrounding area and collaborate with the pediatrician to work with parents raising concerns about their gender questioning or TNB youth. MHPs can help create a network of resources that can be used for referral to assist clients (i.e., support groups, community centers, hair stylists, makeup artists, tailors, electrologists, lawyers, intimate apparel fitters, physical therapists, massage therapists; Simmons et al., 2025). MHPs may also be able to collaborate with social service colleagues to provide their clients with TNB-affirming referrals for housing, financial support, vocational or educational counseling and training, TNB-affirming faith communities, peer support, and other community resources (Chang et al., 2018; Warwick & Shumer, 2023).

ICC work with and for TNB clients is challenging on many levels, but it can also be profoundly rewarding (Ducheny et al., 2019; McIntosh, 2016). MHPs who are fortunate enough to work on a preexisting ICC team are encouraged to make use of the available resources. Those who do not have this benefit will need to intentionally create a network of interdisciplinary colleagues to consult on issues of treatment, exchange resources, and utilize e-consultation services when helpful (Coyne et al., 2023; Simmons et al., 2025; Soled et al., 2022). This will improve MHP care and help reduce and soothe secondary traumatization, as well as the discouragement MHPs can encounter as they champion TNB affirmative care. Few sanctioned TNB credentialing or certification programs exist, although a widely recognized one is the WPATH Global Education Initiative (https://www.wpath.org/gei/GEI-Certification). Training opportunities from professional organizations (APA, 2015) are available and online opportunities exist for individual and systems learning (e.g., TNB care ECHO program offering health care teams interactive, case-based learning with an expert ICC team;

National LGBTQIA+ Health Education Center, n.d.; Shipherd, Kauth, Firek, et al., 2016). Completion of such in-depth learning is becoming more common, and MHPs should critically assess the expertise of their colleagues with whom they collaborate.

CHAPTER SUMMARY

As we have discussed, ICC is an integral aspect of care when working with TNB clients and communities as it significantly improves health outcomes and TNB people's quality of life. The specifics of surgery and HT change quickly and will require MHPs to frequently refresh their knowledge. While those specifics may shift, the need for this work is deep and abiding, and will only grow in the future as more TNB people seek care and as more systems learn to offer this care in a TNB-affirming way.

REFERENCES

Adashi, E. Y., Cohen, I. G., & McCormick, W. L. (2021). The interstate medical licensure compact: Attending to the underserved. *JAMA, 325*(16), 1607–1608. https://doi.org/10.1001/jama.2021.1085

American Psychological Association. (2015). Guidelines for psychological practice with transgender and gender nonconforming people. *American Psychologist, 70*(9), 832–864. https://doi.org/10.1037/a0039906

American Psychological Association, & National Association of School Psychologists. (2014). *Resolution on gender and sexual orientation diversity in children and adolescents in schools.* http://www.apa.org/about/policy/orientation-diversity.aspx

Association of State and Provincial Psychology Boards. (n.d.). *PSYPACT participating states map.* Retrieved April 6, 2024, from https://psypact.org/mpage/psypactmap

Bowleg, L. (2012). The problem with the phrase women and minorities: Intersectionality-an important theoretical framework for public health. *American Journal of Public Health, 102*(7), 1267–1273. https://doi.org/10.2105/AJPH.2012.300750

Byne, W., Bradley, S. J., Coleman, E., Eyler, A. E., Green, R., Menvielle, E. J., Meyer-Bahlburg, H. F. L., Pleak, R. R., Tompkins, D. A., & the American Psychiatric Association Task Force on Treatment of Gender Identity Disorder. (2012). Report of the American Psychiatric Association task force on the treatment of gender identity disorder. *Archives of Sexual Behavior, 41*(4), 759–796. https://doi.org/10.1007/s10508-012-9975-x

Chang, S. C., Singh, A. A., & dickey, l. m. (2018). *A clinician's guide to gender affirming care: Working with transgender & gender nonconforming clients.* New Harbinger Publications.

Chen, D., Hidalgo, M. A., Leibowitz, S., Leininger, J., Simons, L., Finlayson, C., & Garofalo, R. (2016). Multidisciplinary care for gender-diverse youth: A narrative review and unique model of gender-affirming care. *Transgender Health, 1*(1), 117–123. https://doi.org/10.1089/trgh.2016.0009

Coleman, E., Radix, A. E., Bouman, W. P., Brown, G. R., de Vries, A. L. C., Deutsch, M. B., Ettner, R., Fraser, L., Goodman, M., Green, J., Hancock, A. B., Johnson, T. W., Karasic, D. H., Knudson, G. A., Leibowitz, S. F., Meyer-Bahlburg, H. F. L., Monstrey, S. J., Motmans, J., Nahata, L., . . . Arcelus, J. (2022). Standards of care for the health of transgender and gender diverse people, version 8. *International Journal of Transgender Health, 23*(Suppl. 1), S1-259. https://doi.org/10.1080/26895269.2022.2100644

Collins, P. H. (1991). *Black feminist thought: Knowledge, consciousness, and the politics of empowerment*. Routledge.

Counseling Compact. (2023). *Compact map*. https://counselingcompact.org/map/

Coyne, C. A., Yuodsnukis, B. T., & Chen, D. (2023). Gender dysphoria: Optimizing healthcare for transgender and gender diverse youth with a multidisciplinary approach. *Neuropsychiatric Disease and Treatment, 19*, 479–493. https://doi.org/10.2147/NDT.S359979

Crenshaw, K. W. (1991). Mapping the margins: Intersectionality, identity politics, and violence against women of color. *Stanford Law Review, 43*(6), 1241–1299. https://www.jstor.org/stable/1229039. https://doi.org/10.2307/1229039

Denaro, A., Pflugeisen, C. M., Colglazier, T., DeWine, D., & Thompson, B. (2023). Lessons from grassroots efforts to increase gender-affirming medical care for transgender and gender diverse youth in the community health care setting. *Transgender Health, 8*(3), 207–212. https://doi.org/10.1089/trgh.2021.0092

Deutsch, M. B. (2012). Use of the informed consent model in provision of cross-sex hormone therapy: A survey of the practices of selected clinics. *International Journal of Transgenderism, 13*(3), 140–146. https://doi.org/10.1080/15532739.2011.675233

dickey, l. m., Ducheny, K., & Ehrbar, R. D. (2016). Family creation options for transgender and gender nonconforming people. *Psychology of Sexual Orientation and Gender Diversity, 3*(2), 173–179. https://doi.org/10.1037/sgd0000178

Ducheny, K., Hardacker, C. T., Claybren, K. T., & Parker, C. (2019). The essentials: Foundational knowledge to support affirmative care for transgender and gender nonconforming (TGNC) older adults. In C. Hardacker, K. Ducheny, & M. Houlberg (Eds.), *Transgender and gender nonconforming health and aging* (pp. 1–20). Springer. https://doi.org/10.1007/978-3-319-95031-0

Ehrensaft, D. (2020). Treatment paradigms for prepubertal children. In M. Forcier, G. Van Schalkwyk, & J. L. Turban (Eds.), *Pediatric gender identity: Gender-affirming care for transgender and gender diverse youth* (pp. 171–185). Springer. https://doi.org/10.1007/978-3-030-38909-3_13

Erickson-Schroth, L. (Ed.). (2022). *Trans bodies, trans selves: A resource by and for transgender communities*. Oxford University Press.

Gay, Lesbian and Straight Education Network. (n.d.). *Model district policy for transgender and gender nonconforming students*. Retrieved from http://glsen.org/article/transgender-model-district-policy

Glassgold, J. M., & Ryan, C. (2022). The role of families in efforts to change, support, and affirm sexual orientation, gender identity, and expression in children and youth. In D. C. Haldeman (Ed.), *The case against conversion "therapy": Evidence, ethics, and alternatives* (pp. 89–107). American Psychological Association. https://doi.org/10.1037/0000266-005

Golden, R. L., & Oransky, M. (2019). An intersectional approach to therapy with transgender adolescents and their families. *Archives of Sexual Behavior, 48*(7), 2011–2025. https://doi.org/10.1007/s10508-018-1354-9

Hembree, W. C., Cohen-Kettenis, P., Delemarre-van de Waal, H. A., Gooren, L. J., Meyer, W. J., III, Spack, N. P., Tangpricha, V., Montori, V. M., & the Endocrine Society. (2009). Endocrine treatment of transsexual persons: An Endocrine Society clinical practice guideline. *The Journal of Clinical Endocrinology and Metabolism, 94*(9), 3132–3154. https://doi.org/10.1210/jc.2009-0345

Hendricks, M. L., & Testa, R. J. (2012). A conceptual framework for clinical work with transgender and gender nonconforming clients: An adaptation of the minority stress model. *Professional Psychology: Research and Practice, 43*(5), 460–467. https://doi.org/10.1037/a0029597

Imrie, S., Zadeh, S., Wylie, K., & Golombok, S. (2020). Children with trans parents: Parent–child relationship quality and psychological well-being. *Parenting: Science and Practice, 21*(3), 185–215. https://doi.org/10.1080/15295192.2020.1792194

James, S. E., Herman, J. L., Durso, L. E., & Heng-Lehtinen, R. (2024). *Early insights: A report of the 2022 U.S. transgender survey.* National Center for Transgender Equality. Retrieved from https://transequality.org/sites/default/files/2024-02/2022%20USTS%20Early%20Insights%20Report_FINAL.pdf

Keo-Meier, C., Ducheny, K., & Hendricks, M. L. (2018). Identity and support letters. In M. R. Kauth & J. C. Shipherd (Eds.), *Adult transgender care: An interdisciplinary approach for training mental health professionals* (pp. 194–207). Routledge.

Keo-Meier, C., & Ehrensaft, D. (Eds.). (2018). *The gender affirmative model: An interdisciplinary approach to supporting transgender and gender expansive children.* American Psychological Association. https://doi.org/10.1037/0000095-007

Keo-Meier, C. L., Herman, L. I., Reisner, S. L., Pardo, S. T., Sharp, C., & Babcock, J. C. (2015). Testosterone treatment and MMPI-2 improvement in transgender men: A prospective controlled study. *Journal of Consulting and Clinical Psychology, 83*(1), 143–156. https://doi.org/10.1037/a0037599

Koehler, A., Strauss, B., Briken, P., Szuecs, D., & Nieder, T. O. (2021). Centralized and decentralized delivery of transgender health care services: A systematic review and global expert survey in 39 countries. *Frontiers in Endocrinology, 12*, 717914. https://doi.org/10.3389/fendo.2021.717914

Kuper, L. E., Cooper, M. B., & Mooney, M. A. (2022). Supporting and advocating for transgender and gender diverse youth and their families within the sociopolitical context of widespread discriminatory legislation and policies. *Clinical Practice in Pediatric Psychology, 10*(3), 336–345. https://doi.org/10.1037/cpp0000456

Kuvalanka, K. A., Bellis, C., Goldberg, A. E., & McGuire, J. K. (2019). An exploratory study of custody challenges experienced by affirming mothers of transgender and gender-nonconforming children. *Family Court Review, 57*(1), 54–71. https://doi.org/10.1111/fcre.12387

Lee, J. L., Huffman, M., Rattray, N. A., Carnahan, J. L., Fortenberry, J. D., Fogel, J. M., Weiner, M., & Matthias, M. S. (2022). "I don't want to spend the rest of my life only going to a gender wellness clinic": Healthcare experiences of patients of a comprehensive transgender clinic. *Journal of General Internal Medicine, 37*(13), 3396–3403. https://doi.org/10.1007/s11606-022-07408-5

Mabel, H., Altinay, M., & Ferrando, C. A. (2019). The role of the ethicist in an interdisciplinary transgender health care team. *Transgender Health, 4*(1), 136–142. https://doi.org/10.1089/trgh.2018.0058

Magalhães, C., Sprott, R., & Rider, G. N. (Eds.). (2023). *Mental health practice with LGBTQ+ children, adolescents, and emerging adults in multiple systems of care.* Rowman & Littlefield.

Majid, S., Rasool, A., Rasool, A., & Zafar, A. (2023). Social exclusion of transgender (hijra): A case study in Lahore (Pakistan). *Pakistan Journal of Humanities and Social Sciences, 11*(2), 814–824. https://doi.org/10.52131/pjhss.2023.1102.0393

McIntosh, C. A. (2016). Interdisciplinary care for transgender patients. In K. Eckstrand & J. Ehrenfeld (Eds.), *Lesbian, gay, bisexual, and transgender healthcare: A clinical guide to preventive, primary, and specialist care* (pp. 339–349). Springer. https://doi.org/10.1007/978-3-319-19752-4_18

Meyerowitz, J. (2004). *How sex changed: A history of transsexuality in the United States.* Harvard University Press. https://doi.org/10.2307/j.ctv1c7zfrv

National Association of Social Workers. (2023). *Interstate licensure compact.* Retrieved June 11, 2023, from https://www.socialworkers.org/Advocacy/Interstate-Licensure-Compact-for-Social-Work

National LGBTQIA+ Health Education Center. (n.d.). *Project ECHO.* Retrieved from https://www.lgbtqiahealtheducation.org/project-echo/trans-echo/

Nieder, T. O., Renner, J., Zapf, A., Sehner, S., Hot, A., König, H.-H., Dams, J., Grochtdreis, T., Briken, P., & Dekker, A. (2022). Interdisciplinary, internet-based trans health care (i2TransHealth): Study protocol for a randomised controlled trial. *BMJ Open, 12*(2), e045980. https://doi.org/10.1136/bmjopen-2020-045980

Panchal, Z., Piper, C., Whitmore, C., & Davies, R. D. (2022). Providing supportive transgender mental health care: A systemized narrative review of patient experiences, preferences, and outcomes. *Journal of Gay & Lesbian Mental Health, 26*(3), 228–264. https://doi.org/10.1080/19359705.2021.1899094

Reisner, S. L., Bradford, J., Hopwood, R., Gonzalez, A., Makadon, H., Todisco, D., Cavanaugh, T., VanDerwarker, R., Grasso, C., Zaslow, S., Boswell, S. L., & Mayer, K. (2015). Comprehensive transgender healthcare: The gender affirming clinical and public health model of Fenway Health. *Journal of Urban Health, 92*(3), 584–592. https://doi.org/10.1007/s11524-015-9947-2

Renner, J., Blaszcyk, W., Täuber, L., Dekker, A., Briken, P., & Nieder, T. O. (2021). Barriers to accessing health care in rural regions by transgender, non-binary, and gender diverse people: A case-based scoping review. *Frontiers in Endocrinology, 12*, 717821. https://doi.org/10.3389/fendo.2021.717821

Rodriguez-Wallberg, K., Obedin-Maliver, J., Taylor, B., Van Mello, N., Tilleman, K., & Nahata, L. (2022). Reproductive health in transgender and gender diverse individuals: A narrative review to guide clinical care and international guidelines. *International Journal of Transgender Health, 24*(1), 7–25. https://doi.org/10.1080/26895269.2022.2035883

Schechter, L. S., & Schechter, R. B. (2018). Pursuing gender transition surgeries. In M. R. Kauth & J. C. Shipherd (Eds.), *Adult transgender care: An interdisciplinary approach for training mental health professionals* (pp. 140–160). Routledge.

Shipherd, J. C., Kauth, M. R., Firek, A. F., Garcia, R., Mejia, S., Laski, S., Walden, B., Perez-Padilla, S., Lindsay, J. A., Brown, G., Roybal, L., Keo-Meier, C. L., Knapp, H., Johnson, L., Reese, R. L., & Byne, W. (2016). Interdisciplinary transgender veteran care: Development of a core curriculum for VHA providers. *Transgender Health, 1*(1), 54–62. https://doi.org/10.1089/trgh.2015.0004

Shipherd, J. C., Kauth, M. R., & Matza, A. (2016). Nationwide interdisciplinary e-consultation on transgender care in the veterans health administration. *Telemedicine and e-Health, 22*(12), 1008–1012. https://doi.org/10.1089/tmj.2016.0013

Simmons, J., Hartman, S., Tanabe, K. O., & Hayden, M. E. (2025). Gender-diverse health on campus: Developing a comprehensive, multidisciplinary gender-diverse care team. *Journal of American College Health, 73*(1), 10–13. https://doi.org/10.1080/07448481.2023.2168545

Soled, K. R. S., Dimant, O. E., Tanguay, J., Mukerjee, R., & Poteat, T. (2022). Interdisciplinary clinicians' attitudes, challenges, and success strategies in providing care to transgender people: A qualitative descriptive study. *BMC Health Services Research, 22*(1134), 1–15. https://doi.org/10.1186/s12913-022-08517-x

Stroumsa, D. (2014). The state of transgender health care: Policy, law, and medical frameworks. *American Journal of Public Health, 104*(3), e31–e38. https://doi.org/10.2105/AJPH.2013.301789

Torrence, N. D., Mueller, A. E., Ilem, A. A., Renn, B. N., DeSantis, B., & Segal, D. L. (2014). Medical provider attitudes about behavioral health consultants in integrated primary care: A preliminary study. *Families, Systems, & Health, 32*(4), 426–432. https://doi.org/10.1037/fsh0000078

Unger, C. A. (2014). Care of the transgender patient: The role of the gynecologist. *American Journal of Obstetrics and Gynecology, 210*(1), 16–26. https://doi.org/10.1016/j.ajog.2013.05.035

Wagner, L. D., & Armstrong, E. (2020). Families in transition: The lived experience of parenting a transgender child. *Journal of Family Nursing, 26*(4), 337–345. https://doi.org/10.1177/1074840720945340

Warwick, R. M., & Shumer, D. E. (2023). Gender-affirming multidisciplinary care for transgender and non-binary children and adolescents. *Children's Health Care, 52*(1), 91–115. https://doi.org/10.1080/02739615.2021.2004146

Wesp, L. M., Malcoe, L. H., Elliott, A., & Poteat, T. (2019). Intersectionality research for transgender health justice: A theory-driven conceptual framework for structural analysis of transgender health inequities. *Transgender Health, 4*(1), 287–296. https://doi.org/10.1089/trgh.2019.0039

Wiegand, A. (2021). Barred from transition: The gatekeeping of gender-affirming care during the gender clinic era. *Intersect: The Stanford Journal of Science, Technology, and Society, 15*(1).

World Professional Association for Transgender Health. (2015). *WPATH statement on legal recognition of gender identity*. http://www.wpath.org/uploaded_files/140/files/WPATH%20Statement%20on%20Legal%20Recognition%20of%20Gender%20Identity%201-19-15.pdf

5

DEBUNKING BAD SCIENCE WITH TRANS AND NONBINARY COMMUNITIES

DOUGLAS KNUTSON, BEK URBAN, AND AARON S. BRESLOW

Bad science is a big problem. On the surface, a chapter on bad science may look out of place in a book on affirmative counseling and psychological practice with trans and nonbinary (TNB) communities, but this chapter is deeply relevant. Science serves as the foundation for effective intervention (Myers, 2007), and when flawed science underlies mental health practice, we run the risk of inefficacy and outright harm. Therefore, it is crucial to examine scientific literature related to TNB life and health. In this chapter, we aim to guide readers in debunking bad science by providing its history and tools to identify literature that is biased against TNB people, employs flawed methodologies, and pathologizes or denies TNB humanity.

Additionally, we seek to elevate "good" science: empirical and theoretical work that strives to accurately understand and address TNB health. While acknowledging the limitations inherent in any study—and naming that the majority of TNB research has been an enterprise belonging to White cisgender men (Stryker, 2020)—we assert that most contemporary research on TNB mental health is conducted with the intent to generate evidence for more precise and effective interventions in support of TNB communities. We must not overlook the value of this work amidst our critiques, meant to unmask anti-TNB bias, and the limitations we discuss.

---

https://doi.org/10.1037/0000471-006
Affirmative Counseling and Psychological Practice With Trans and Nonbinary Clients, Second Edition, A. Singh and R. McCullough (Editors)
Copyright © 2026 by the American Psychological Association. All rights reserved.

However, there is a preponderance of bad science about TNB life. This can be attributed, in part, to three interrelated ideologies: *cissexism*, which upholds differential power systems favoring cisgender people; *cisnormativity*, which biases cisgender people as normal and portrays TNB people as mentally ill; and *gender essentialism*, which assumes gender roles and expression are determined by inherent, immutable biological traits. These oppressive ideologies manifest in harmful ways, influencing even seemingly robust research design, recruitment procedures, data analysis methods, and interpretation of results.

We encourage mental health providers to evaluate the influence of cissexism, cisnormativity, and gender essentialism when encountering bad science and, by extension, in their own work. We also urge our colleagues to center the voices of gender diverse people, particularly TNB scholars, when reading or producing scientific literature. Although many cisgender authors, including some coauthors of this chapter, have a history of conducting scientifically rigorous gender-affirming studies, they should not do so in isolation. When TNB people are excluded from the production of gender-focused research, even well-intentioned research design can have negative consequences. Hence, we describe a process-oriented approach to TNB health research (Tebbe & Budge, 2016) that prioritizes the material and psychological needs of diverse TNB communities and invites mental health providers to consider connections to their own practice settings.

Approaching this chapter with humility and an awareness of the insidious impact of cissexism, our aim is to enhance clinical practice through a critical review of the science on gender identity and expression. The need for this critical, gender-affirming approach could not be more important. At the time of writing, American legislators have introduced at least 26 anti-TNB bills at the national level and over 500 others in state-level legislative bodies (Trans Legislation Tracker, n.d.). Many of these bills specifically target TNB youth by criminalizing gender-affirming medical care or deny TNB people access to sports and single-gender public spaces. The proliferation of such measures, even when not codified into law, contributes to a hostile sociopolitical environment that detrimentally affects the mental health and livelihood of all TNB people (Horne et al., 2022).

To address these issues and their impact on mental health practice, we will first discuss bad science in the context of cissexism, with a focus on history, funding, and the role of social media. We will then explore approaches to evaluating scientific methods and findings based on models endorsed by TNB scholars and national scientific organizations. Furthermore, we will provide an overview of misleading conclusions found in current research on autism, rapid onset gender dysphoria (ROGD), health care, and sports. Finally, we summarize key takeaways and offer recommendations for practice.

BAD SCIENCE IN THE CONTEXT OF CISSEXISM

Bad science related to TNB life does not occur in a vacuum. Rather, the intersecting ideologies of cissexism, cisnormativity, and gender essentialism form the underlying basis for the generation and interpretation of bad science targeting TNB people (Berger & Ansara, 2021). This phenomenon is not a recent development but rather has persisted throughout the history of psychological and medical inquiries regarding gender (Ansara & Hegarty, 2012). The influence of cissexism on bad science has manifested in various ways, affecting every stage of the research process, from disparities in funding availability to the formulation of conceptual models, research questions, hypotheses, variables of interest, data analysis, and dissemination. In other words, cissexism impacts bad science from start to finish.

Cissexism is structurally embedded in research, exemplified by the lack of national funding in the United States for transgender health research outside the context of HIV risk. A 2014 systematic review of national funding, for example, found that when excluding studies with HIV as the primary focus, only 0.1% of National Institutes of Health-funded studies focused on health in people with marginalized sexual orientations and gender identities. Of that 0.1%, merely 6.8% addressed transgender health (Coulter et al., 2014). The inadequate allocation of research funding, coupled with the systemic exclusion of TNB people from leadership positions within scientific institutions (Cech & Waidzunas, 2021), significantly impacts the support and understanding of TNB people's needs. Indeed, research in the 1990s (or the first century of scientific research focused on TNB people) was taken up and led almost exclusively by White, Western European and European American cisgender men. In this section, we will examine how cissexism has shaped the production, funding, and distribution of flawed science.

History of Bad Science and Its Relationship to Cissexism

Throughout history, psychiatric and medical fields have played a mixed, though primarily pernicious, role in the scientific assessment, diagnosis, and health care of TNB people. For more than a century, researchers and clinicians have explored various explanations, including biological, genetic, psychological, and sociocultural factors, to understand the etiology of TNB identity and expression. The field of psychiatry has played a significant role in medicalizing and pathologizing TNB people, defining gender diversity as gender dysphoria and classifying it as a symptom of psychological illness (Johnson, 2019).

The misperception that TNB people are disordered dates back centuries and was initially introduced into scientific literature in the 1800s, primarily by psychiatric scholars. One example is Austro-German Psychiatrist Dr. Richer Freiherr von Krafft-Ebing, who propagated unscientific beliefs about TNB individuals. In his work, most famously his 1886 book *Psychopathia Sexualis* (translated as *Psychopathy of Sex*), Krafft-Ebing extensively discussed homosexuality and gender deviance, attributing them to a mental disease caused by degenerate heredity. A subsequent generation of American psychiatrists in the early-to-mid 1900s advocated for harmful treatments to "fix" queer and TNB people. Scientifically validated interventions at the time included abstinence from masturbation, hydrotherapy, electroshock therapy, and even lobotomy.

These problematic theories and treatment approaches permeated other scientific disciplines in the United States during the same period. For example, American Psychoanalyst Charles Hughes wrote extensively about patients we would describe today as queer or TNB. Hughes aimed to explain sexual and gender "deviance" or prevision, framing different expressions of queerness and gender diversity as either a disease, criminal and moral flaw, or simply an intrapsychic consequence of perversion in a child's psychosexual development (Hughes, 1893). Hughes and colleagues pathologized gender diversity and contributed to further criminalization and harmful psychiatric interventions.

Moreover, early American scientists at the turn of the twentieth century, including Hughes, often intertwined their discussions of queerness and TNB identity within racist White supremacist ideologies. Hughes, for example, described early American queer and TNB life in proximity to Blackness and urbanity, using anti-Black tropes and racialized fetishization when discussing the emergence of urban spaces for queer and TNB people. In response to his 1893 paper, for example, Hughes described a social event for cross-dressing and feminine-presenting queer and TNB Black men. Hughes (1893) described "men lasciviously dressed in womanly attire" and wrote in explicit terms about the genitals of attendees. This racialized fear of and fascination with creative gender expression was a common reaction in medical sciences at this time to the emergence of mixed-race queer and TNB life in urban settings.

Bad science related to TNB identity evolved throughout the 1900s, with emerging theories suggesting TNB identity developed as a result of bad parenting, perversions in psychosexual development, and unhealthy family systems. One prominent figure in the mid-twentieth century was Psychiatrist Robert Stoller (1968), who published *Sex and Gender: The Transsexual Experiment*. Stoller proposed a commonly accepted theoretical model suggesting that the development of "transsexual identity" early in life occurred when a particularly attractive, feminine boy received excessive attention from his mother, further feminizing him and causing a disorder in his gender identity. Stoller argued for psychiatric treatment to correct "transsexual illness" which included resolving the *Oedipal complex*; this is the idea that a person is sexually attracted to the parent with a gender identity least like theirs and is in competition with the parent who holds a gender identity most similar to their own.

These theories were tested in empirical studies at major universities. Studies from as recently as 1993 exemplify the absurdity and danger of bad science. For instance, at the University of Toronto, Fridell and colleagues (1993) conducted a study that exemplifies the absurdity and danger of bad science. Using Stoller's theory as a conceptual model, they took color photographs of young TNB girls and young cisgender girls. They then presented them to university students, who were asked to rate the attractiveness of the children in the photographs without context. Participants would rate the girls on Likert-type scales in terms of how "attractive," "beautiful," "cute," "pretty," and "ugly" they were. The study, published in *Archives of Sexual Behavior*, employed quantitative statistical analyses and met criteria at the time for scientific rigor, yet the research approach explicitly objectified young girls and dehumanized TNB people in the process. The results were interpreted using a causal model of bad parenting causing pathological femininity in young boys, leading to exaggerated and harmful claims about the causes of gender dysphoria.

Though absurd by today's standards, this study and many other historical examples are clear demonstrations of bad science. Despite meeting certain criteria for scientific rigor, bad science objectifies, devalues, and criminalizes TNB people. It leads to erroneous and harmful conclusions that inform public policy and clinical practice in pernicious, systematic ways.

THE ROLE OF SOCIAL MEDIA IN THE DISTRIBUTION OF SCIENCE

Since the publication of Krafft-Ebing's (1886) manifesto, both bad and good science related to TNB communities have evolved, and social media now plays a significant role in how research is shared and interpreted. Social media platforms have become a rapid and extensive means to disseminate scientific information quickly (Dijkstra et al., 2018). However, they have also perpetuated and amplified negative messages about TNB communities. Recent studies suggest people often share content on social media without fully reading it, relying instead on summaries or statements written by others who also may not have read the primary source (Ward et al., 2023). Furthermore, character limits and the desire for digestible and appealing information can lead to the distortion of study results.

Consequently, rapid sharing without fidelity to the actual study can result in overgeneralizations and incorrect assumptions. Studies have shown that articles shared on social media may garner higher engagement and attention, as indicated by higher Altmetric scores, but the actual full-text readership did not significantly differ from articles that were not shared (Thoma et al., 2018). This suggests that although research shared on social media may receive more public attention, there may be a cost; the initial claims or widely shared statements may be believed by those who consume the media without referring to the original article to verify the accuracy of claims. For example, if a study indicates higher rates of depression and suicidality within the TNB community, without proper context, these increased odds may be attributed to TNB identity itself rather than the impact of social stigma and discrimination. Such a misunderstanding of results reinforces the notion that TNB identity is symptomatic of mental illness and pathologizes the experiences of many TNB people.

Although misrepresentations of findings can occur even without social media, its unique nature amplifies the impact of such mischaracterizations. The rapid distribution and broad reach of information, combined with the lack of context, create an environment where bad science and misinformation spread rapidly with far reaching consequences. Social media has been used to spread bad science in other health domains, including anti-vaccine sentiments and COVID-19 pandemic denials (Muhammed T & Mathew, 2022). Perhaps the most well-known example of social media colliding with bad science is the spread of misinformation about so-called ROGD, which will be discussed in detail later in the chapter.

EVALUATING ACCURATE SCIENTIFIC FINDINGS

Filtering out the mischaracterizations of TNB people in mainstream media, social media, and other scientific outlets can be challenging. Affirming mental health providers (MHPs) who work with TNB clients require tools and training to discern the myths and inaccuracies of bad science in order to provide effective evidence-based care. In this section, we present frameworks that can assist in evaluating research, including ethical research models, motivations behind research production, and limitations associated with different methods and approaches.

Frameworks Used to Evaluate Bad Science

Professional ethics codes endorsed by national organizations such as the American Psychological Association (APA; 2017) prohibit mental health researchers from making false or misleading statements about their research findings. Scholars in mental health fields are expected to adhere to these ethical guidelines, which discourage fabricating data or knowingly disseminating erroneous results. However, it can be challenging to detect intentional deception, as not all instances of bad science are based on falsified data or nefarious intentions. Strong biases against TNB people can subtly influence the questions asked, sample recruitment methods, and data interpretation.

To illustrate this, we present a hypothetical study conducted by two researchers, Researcher A and Researcher B. Researcher A is a counseling professor conducting research with a nonbinary graduate student who is interested in attitudes among cisgender people toward TNB people's use of public bathrooms. Researcher B is a psychologist working for a conservative think-tank focused on identifying what motivates adults to vote to restrict bathroom access for TNB people. Despite both researchers designing mixed-method, survey-based studies on bathroom access, their hypotheses, sample recruitment methods, and interpretation of results lead to vastly different outcomes. They both recruit samples of cisgender adults and administer standardized measures of disgust, anger, fear, religiosity, political affiliation, and support for restrictive bathroom legislation. Both include open-ended questions about voting patterns and motivations, yet there are clear differences likely resulting from their perspectives.

Researcher A begins by reviewing the literature and discovers that researchers have not yet investigated the role of disgust in voting patterns, but that disgust is a likely motivator because it is the focus of current political ads circulated by politicians who oppose the rights of TNB people. Based on their literature review, they forward the hypothesis, "Disgust will be the strongest predictor of support for restrictive bathroom legislation after controlling for other commonly researched variables." For their study, they

- recruit cisgender adults using a participant panel that promises to provide an unbiased, representative sample;
- design broad open-ended questions that ask things like, "How do you feel when you watch political advertisements about access to public bathrooms for TNB people;"
- randomize the order in which their measures are presented to reduce response order bias and present the open-ended question at the end of their survey;
- delete invalid responses based on set criteria such as participants who dropped out halfway through the survey;
- run their proposed analyses, focused on the role of disgust and controlling for the other variables in the study; and
- frame results within current literature and discuss implications for TNB peoples' health.

Researcher B begins by thinking about which findings will have the biggest impact on future voting patterns among cisgender adults.

Based on their goals, they forward the hypotheses: "Godliness and commitment to religion will be associated with higher levels of disgust, anger, and fear. Disgust, anger, and fear will be linked to higher levels of support for restrictive bathroom legislation." For their study, they

- recruit cisgender adults from conservative churches across the United States;
- design open-ended questions that ask things like, "How would you feel if you knew about a man in a dress using a women's bathroom;"
- place the open-ended questions before the disgust, anger and fear measures to ensure that participants are focused on bathroom use while they are completing the scales;
- delete responses from participants who endorse low levels of disgust, anger, and fear because they are outliers in the data;
- run their analyses, exploring any significant associations with religiosity to discover as much as possible about motivations for religious people; and
- frame their results within the context of religion by claiming that people with stronger faith in God have valid, appropriately negative reactions to unrestricted bathroom access.

In both cases, the researchers are guided by hypotheses, recruit samples, conduct analyses, and frame their results. However, the outcomes and the impact of the research are very different. Researcher A suggests that reducing disgust and pushing back against current political messaging may increase affirmation and support for TNB people. Researcher B suggests that inclusion of TNB people is a phenomenon that occurs in people who lack faith and that a stronger belief in God is the way to get more adults to vote in favor of restrictive bathroom legislation. We realize that these examples may seem a bit extreme, but they are not far off base. Cissexism can impact sampling techniques, data interpretation, interpretation of results, and the format and content of the questions posed to research subjects.

Given the potential for bias in gender research, professional and scientific organizations have developed guidelines to critically evaluate the validity and reliability of research findings. Two widely used frameworks include the Journal Article Reporting Standards (JARS) and the Preferred Reporting Items for Systematic Reviews and Meta-Analyses (PRISMA).

Journal Article Reporting Standards

The JARS, formulated by the APA (2024), provides standards for the presentation of quantitative, qualitative, and mixed-method studies, as well as standards for discussing race, ethnicity, and culture in the field of psychology.

They outline what should be included in a scientifically conducted and reliable study, including a review of the key literature supporting the study's design and hypotheses (Appelbaum et al., 2018). For example, the JARS for quantitative studies call on authors to provide a summary review of key literature that supports the design of the study and gives rise to its hypotheses. MHPs can use the JARS criteria to assess the rationale and biases of a given study, comparing it to the guidelines outlined in the APA *Publication Manual* (2020).

Preferred Reporting Items for Systematic Reviews and Meta-Analyses
The PRISMA checklist (Page et al., 2021) assists scholars in reporting complex and statistical reviews, such as meta-analyses and systematic reviews that extrapolate findings from multiple research studies. The checklist can be used much like the JARS to evaluate and engage with meta-analyses and systematic reviews of gender research. MHPs engaging with these types of reviews can use the PRISMA checklist to evaluate potential biases and inaccuracies. For example, the PRISMA checklist encourages scholars to explicate how they decided to include and exclude studies from their reviews, thus making clear how their selection procedures may have influenced the outcomes and findings of a meta-analysis.

Politically and Values-Motivated Research
So far, we have alluded to the impact of bias, particularly anti-TNB bias, on gender research. Our examples of studies conducted by Researcher A and Researcher B hint at the values-based motivations that may underlie gender research, but it is important for us to make those connections more explicit. Indeed, gender research is often driven by researchers' motivations, values, and convictions. We suggest that gender researchers who work with TNB populations typically fall into two categories: (a) those who aim to create more affirming environments for TNB people and (b) those who seek to maintain current social gender norms and fear the breakdown of those norms. Although we argue all TNB research is values-motivated to some extent, this does not necessarily imply biased research is inherently bad. Bias is present in all research, but its impact can be understood, managed, and minimized.

MHPs must critically analyze individual research studies while considering the underlying motivations behind the research. It is important to ask questions such as, "What motivated this research in the first place?" Strong bias, whether positive or negative, can lead to bad science when a nefarious end goal of the study (e.g., political impact, profitability) overshadows the study itself. In the next section, we will review studies that are heavily motivated by anti-TNB politics and values.

Issues and Limitations for Qualitative and Qualitative Methods and Neuroscience

In addition to the broader issues described previously, there are limitations and issues that are common in qualitative and quantitative research, as well as biased assumptions about biology that are prevalent in neuroscientific studies. Researchers who use these methods will be familiar with the common critiques of TNB research, but they are worth revisiting because they impact the ways that scholars, practitioners, and the public approach TNB people. In other words, the limitations of qualitative, quantitative, and neuroscientific research often influence the assumptions people make about TNB populations. We also look at secondary data sources as one possible solution to overcome these limitations.

Qualitative Research. Qualitative studies produce rich, deep, impactful data that often foreground quotes from TNB research participants. However, many qualitative studies include a limited number of participants (12–15) and that makes it difficult to apply to entire populations of TNB people. Health care providers may view qualitative results as less impactful or useful because they represent experiences of a small subset of the TNB population. Some studies analyze larger data sets (150–200) of responses to open-ended questions in broader surveys, but the value of such results is also regularly questioned because narrative responses to survey questions can vary widely in quality and completeness. One- or two-word answers to open-ended questions are common and difficult to interpret.

There are also differences in some experiences and challenges that trans men and women face as compared to nonbinary people. Qualitative studies that claim to represent TNB experiences that oversample nonbinary people, for example, should be interpreted with caution when they are applied to trans people who do not identify as nonbinary. Furthermore, qualitative studies can be subject to bias when questions that are presented to participants are skewed or designed to hunt for specific answers or acknowledge the impact of the research team on the study outcomes (through a reflexivity or similar section in a manuscript). Consumers of qualitative TNB research should closely attend to the questions participants were asked, potential biases that could have improperly shaped the analytic plan, or obvious misinterpretations of the findings. We suggest qualitative researchers (and others) include positionality statements to describe how their lived experiences may have contributed to assumptions about methods and interpretation of results.

A third concern about bad science in qualitative research is *tokenism*, where individual clinical cases or qualitative study participants tend to overrepresent people with similar identities. For example, for a long time, scholars have used individual case studies to make troubling arguments aimed at delaying or limiting gender-affirming interventions (e.g., Shore, 1984) and that practice persists even now. While qualitative studies are perhaps less susceptible to tokenism given safeguards such as positionality statements, case studies are more likely to be overinterpreted despite small sample sizes. These case studies have contributed historically to overdrawn conclusions and bad clinical practice.

Quantitative Research. Quantitative research, like qualitative studies, can suffer from issues related to sampling and generalization. Quantitative studies are notorious for oversampling White TNB participants and generalizing results to all TNB people, regardless of race. In addition, quantitative studies that offer incentives, such as a drawing for a gift card, may attract fake participants (i.e., bots, scam artists) who do not identify as TNB but access the survey for the incentive. Researchers are constructing more robust ways of detecting nefarious or false responders, but reducing their impact is a constant focus for online researchers.

TNB participants can be hard to reach and recruit for survey participation in large numbers. Some researchers collect convenience samples at their clinic, through their academic networks, and so on. However, the data offered by participants from convenience samples often reflect the pool from which they were drawn. For example, a sample drawn from a clinic is going to yield data that speak to issues facing clinical (e.g., depressed, anxious, physically ill, and so on) populations. Samples collected by conservative groups are likewise likely to reflect the networks through which they were accessed and will therefore support some of the assumptions in the study for which they were recruited. Wherever possible, it is a good idea for researchers to collect representative samples with sufficient representation of TNB people of color when answering general research questions about TNB populations. Participant panels, purposive sampling, stakeholder advisory boards, and partnerships with organizations that serve TNB people with multiple marginalized identities can assist with recruiting more balanced samples.

Neuroscience. Neuroscience research has traditionally employed a strict, binary understanding of sex categories, focusing on sex-based differences in behavior (Jordan-Young & Rumiati, 2012). This approach is informed by gender essentialism and disregards sexes and genders outside of the traditional man and woman or male and female binaries. These studies often seek to understand so-called "innate" differences despite limited and relatively inconsequential differences between female and male brains and behaviors (see Hines, 2020).

Some researchers in the field of neuroscience have begun exploring gender as a distinct construct from sex; however, many prominent studies still rely on binary approaches to sex assumed at birth and attempt to identify potential differences in brain structure or chemistry to identify innate differences based on sex and gender. Unfortunately, the incomplete understanding of sex and gender often limits research on TNB individuals, leading to studies that try to provide a reason or etymology for transness (Kiyar et al., 2020). These studies may focus on the brain structures and functions of TNB individuals, seeking to determine if they align with what is expected for their gender identity or sex assumed at birth, to validate one's gender identity. Researchers suggest that such studies empower TNB people by attempting to provide a scientifically sound basis for their existence, but they also essentialize TNB identities and discredit identities that lack a known biological basis.

This line of research has the potential to cause extensive harm to TNB communities. By emphasizing binary understandings of sex and gender, it erases the experiences of genderfluid, nonbinary, and other gender-expansive people. Simultaneously, the pursuit of biological differences between TNB and cis individuals perpetuates harmful beliefs about assumed differences. Additionally, the limited sample sizes and challenges with generalizability further complicate neuroscience research related to gender due to cost and time constraints, as well as other practical limitations (Kiyar et al., 2020).

The current focus on finding differences in or sources of TNB identity in neuroscience research has resulted in a narrow, pathologizing understanding of TNB people. It hinders the application of such research in ways that may benefit the community. Instead, there is a growing call for neuroscience research to shift its focus toward understanding the impacts of marginalization and oppression faced by TNB people (Edmiston & Juster, 2022). Approaches to neuroscience research based on limited biological assumptions, deliberate or not, are an extension of systems of power that have sought to control and surveil identities of individuals whose very existence challenges societal structures based on cisnormativity.

Secondary Data Analyses. In recent years, there has been a push to increase the size, diversity, and geographic representativeness of samples in TNB research. To address this need for larger samples, researchers have increasingly turned to secondary data sources, or datasets collected by other investigators. This approach allows researchers to utilize existing data to study TNB health and well-being. The National Institutes of Health recognized the importance of expanding TNB research samples, even issuing a special program announcement in 2018 calling for novel sampling methods in TNB health research. This announcement encouraged researchers to explore new ways to access and analyze existing datasets to better understand TNB people's concern (Department of Health and Human Services, 2017). Using secondary data sources offers several advantages. It allows researchers to access larger and more diverse samples than would be feasible with primary data collection alone. This is especially important for studying relatively small and marginalized populations like TNB individuals. By leveraging existing datasets, researchers can increase the statistical power and generalizability of their findings. However, there are also important limitations to consider.

There are many secondary data sources available online. We provide a brief overview of three of the most commonly used data sets: (a) nationally representative samples, (b) large community surveys, and (c) hospital-based data warehouses. We provide common data sources under each category and briefly discuss benefits and limitations associated with use of each data type.

Nationally Representative Samples. Many researchers use nationally "representative" surveys sponsored by governmental groups. These surveys are often conducted at the national level and aim to provide insights into various aspects of the population's health and well-being that may include modules asking about sex assigned at birth and gender identity. Examples of such surveys include the National Health Interview Survey in the United States and the General Social Survey in Canada. A key example is the Behavioral Risk Factor Surveillance System, led by the Centers for Disease Control and Prevention (CDC). In 2014, the CDC included an optional pilot set of questions called the Sexual Orientation and Gender Identity Module to assess gender identity that states could opt into. Through phone surveys, participants in multiple states could self-report their gender identities by answering the following questions: "Do you consider yourself to be transgender? If yes . . . Do you consider yourself to be (a) male-to-female, (b) female-to-male, or (c) gender nonconforming?" (CDC, n.d., p. 2).

There are multiple limitations to this approach. First, only certain states, in certain years, asked these questions, thus limiting generalizability. A primary limitation of the use of secondary national survey data is that the samples are, ironically, not nationally representative. Some scholars have been critiqued for making causal claims from data from two years or two states, which may not be appropriate or accurate methodologically. Second, the phrasing of the question and response options is limiting for people with diverse gender identities and experiences. Third, there is a consistent discrepancy in findings between probability and nonprobability samples, thus scholars recommend using secondary national datasets and community samples in tandem.

These methodological concerns emerged particularly in response to an article using data from the 2017–2019 Youth Risk Behavior Surveillance System (Turban et al., 2022). In a large sample of TNB people living in 16 states, researchers measured the ratio between having been assigned female versus male at birth and associated this with bullying, victimization, and suicidality. The purported goal of the study was to debunk the transphobic theory posited by literature on ROGD (described in a later section) that young girls are highly vulnerable to "social contagion" and are influenced to identify as TNB. Though the mission of this study was likely to find alternative hypotheses, the study was widely critiqued as taking a poor methodological approach, assuming generalizability, and using trans-antagonistic theory (or working from the assumption that TNB people are disordered) to inform the research questions. In response to the article, a group of mostly TNB researchers argued the paper lacked methodological rigor and was complicit with the practices and design of bad science (Lett et al., 2022). They argued the use of data from a limited subset of states and years was misinterpreted in ways that would in fact be harmful to TNB people, rather than liberatory.

Large Community Surveys. Researchers reanalyze data from large community surveys supported by national non-profits and other organizations. The United States Transgender Survey (USTS) is one of the most-used large community surveys in TNB research. It collects self-reported data from a large number of TNB people in the United States, providing valuable information about experiences with stigma, health outcomes, and barriers to care. Similar to surveillance samples, scholars may also use community surveys to analyze secondary data. The most cited example is the USTS. The USTS likely contains the largest sample of TNB adults to date given that the current report sampled 92,329 participants from all 50 states (Rastogi et al., 2025). The report describing this sample was published in 2016 and has been cited over 5,645 times (James et al., 2016). It is clear researchers are heavily reliant on these data, and issues related to causality and generalizability must be considered. For example, USTS is a convenience sample that likely overrepresents urban populations where samples of TNB people are easier to access. If USTS data and other large community surveys are assumed to be representative of entire populations because of their large sample sizes, the experiences of rural populations may be overlooked.

Hospital-Based Data Warehouses. These data sources contain information from electronic health records, administrative records, or insurance claims collected in health care settings. They can provide insights into the health and health care experiences of TNB people by providing details about health services utilization as well as clinical outcomes, using procedural and diagnostic codes. To identify a likely TNB sample in a hospital or insurance claim records, researchers have started to use a validated algorithm to identify patients in two ways. First, they will search for any patients who have received a gender identity–related diagnostic code in the past by searching for specific International Classification of Diseases codes that indicate a likely TNB identity. Second, they search for patients who have had any procedures that may indicate having pursued a medical step to gender affirmation by searching for relevant Current Procedural Terminology codes. Some researchers also search clinician-entered free text data in patients' charts for commonly used terminology to describe a patient's TNB identity (e.g., transmasculine or transfeminine, gender-affirming care, etc.), or they read through a selection of a patient's chart to manually verify if they are likely TNB.

This type of research has many benefits. Using an algorithm is helpful as it allows researchers to replicate methods across studies and sites. For example, using the same identification procedures other researchers have used allows researchers to compare outcomes across different subsamples, hospitals, cities, and insurance coverages. It enables researchers to study health care utilization, including disparities in health care coverage and services used.

However, this approach has many drawbacks. First, using an identification algorithm on electronic health record data will only identify TNB people if they (a) have health care access and (b) have received a diagnosis or procedure that indicates TNB identity. This skews samples to TNB people who are utilizing health care or have health insurance. Additionally, it reinforces *transmedicalism*, whereby TNB identity is only conferred or measured when someone is diagnosed with an "illness." This top-down method has been critiqued by TNB community advisory boards for reinforcing a narrow definition of TNB and creating a medicalizing or pathologizing picture of TNB people. Community advisory boards are interested in engaging in an ongoing and dynamic relationship with researchers.

MISLEADING CONCLUSIONS IN RESEARCH

The biases, politics, and motivations we discussed in the previous sections show up in specific areas of gender research. The ways that bad research has impacted several areas of inquiry are unique and profound enough to merit a special focus. Findings related to autism, medical affirmation, sport, and so on impact policies, politics, and laws—but they also impact the care that MHPs offer TNB people. Here, we attempt to dispel some misnomers, challenge inaccurate findings, and add clarity regarding specific topics in gender research. We are unable to provide a comprehensive analysis of each topic, but we hope these discussions serve as a starting point for further explorations for readers of this chapter.

Misconceptions About Autism and Gender Dysphoria

There is a common and growing belief among scholars that gender diversity and autism co-occur (van der Miesen et al., 2018). Researchers of clinical (Pasterski et al., 2014) and nonclinical (Kristensen & Broome, 2015) populations suggest that gender dysphoria and autism diagnoses are positively associated, suggesting the presence of one diagnosis is likely to be accompanied by the other. The regularity with which elevated levels of autism are reportedly detected in TNB people may make the proposed connection seem established beyond a doubt, but that is not at all the case. Even though autism research for TNB people has been conducted for more than two decades (see Landén & Rasmussen, 1997), more remains unknown than known in this area of the field. Several red flags show up in this research that make it hard to state definitive claims.

For one thing, researchers have failed to detect consistent levels of autism in TNB samples. For example, one study may find elevations of autism symptoms in trans women relative to trans men (Kristensen & Broome, 2015), whereas another study might find that trans men and trans women exhibit similar symptom frequencies (Pasterski et al., 2014). Furthermore, the use of self-reported measures of autism generally produces unreliable results (Thrower et al., 2020). Autism diagnoses generally require direct, methodical diagnostic processes. Also, gender dysphoria is rather difficult to measure and a complex construct (Goldbach & Knutson, 2021). The way that gender dysphoria associates with other variables tends to be somewhat unstable (e.g., van der Miesen et al., 2016).

Moreover, similar elevated rates of autism diagnoses are found in other populations at psychiatry clinics (Thrower et al., 2020), indicating that the general focus on people with preexisting diagnoses (e.g., gender dysphoria, clinical anxiety and depression) may skew results. Collectively, evidence depicting elevations of autism in TNB populations remains low quality, and theories related to this phenomenon lack considerable empirical support (Thrower et al., 2020; Wattel et al., 2024). The emerging nature of this research should be carefully considered and evaluated by MHPs. It is possible that imprecise measurement approaches to gender dysphoria and autism pathologize social behaviors that develop as a response to social stress, interpersonal deprivation, as well as peer and family rejection (Nobili et al., 2018; Turban, 2018). It remains unclear how autism and gender dysphoria interact. Compound stress may be one reason autistic TNB adults are more likely to experience further elevations in depression and anxiety relative to other TNB adults (Murphy et al., 2020). It is important for MHPs not to become so focused on prevalence rates and their reinforcement of cissexist and ableist narratives that they lose sight of the actual needs and experiences of autistic TNB people (Moore, 2022).

Rapid Onset Gender Dysphoria

Another growing line of bad science surrounds the purported phenomenon of ROGD—a sudden experience of gender incongruence that results from social pressure, a desire to follow a trend, or a desire to fit in. This concept was first popularized by Littman (2019) in a study (now republished) that claimed to have found evidence for a rapid rise in adolescents who were assumed female at birth reporting sudden gender dysphoria during and after puberty. The literature on ROGD has generated significant controversy in recent years and the concept is hotly contested by most researchers (e.g., Bauer et al., 2022). ROGD is not a medical diagnosis, does not appear in any diagnostic manuals, and is not recognized by any major medical society.

When Littman's (2019) paper was published there was immediate criticism from the scientific and TNB communities about methodological concerns, study framing, and the conclusions drawn from the findings. Nevertheless, the idea that some reports of gender dysphoria among adolescent girls were due to a combination of other mental illnesses and social contagion was widely shared on social media and conservative news outlets (Boskey, 2021). Due to the extensive reach of social media and news coverage, the concept of ROGD and challenges to TNB individuals' identities reached a wide audience who may not have otherwise encountered this example of bad science. Unfortunately, this misinformation contributed to anti-TNB rhetoric and dangerous efforts to restrict minors from accessing gender-affirming care.

ROGD literature is widely considered to be bad science by researchers and major medical societies for two primary reasons. First, its underlying theoretical frame is overtly transphobic. The theory relies on a pathologizing understanding of TNB identity, explicitly framing gender dysphoria and the emergence of TNB personhood as a mental illness stemming from social contagion. Second, the methodological approaches used to capture evidence for ROGD are flawed. In the first empirical study related to ROGD, Littman (2019) interviewed parents who were concerned about their children and adolescents who were influenced by TNB-affirming online message boards. Although the study is widely cited, there are myriads of theoretical and methodological issues described by Restar (2020) in a published response.

First, Restar argues the framework and premise are flawed because they frame the identity of a historically marginalized community as diseased and seek to find a core reason for this perceived defect. Second, Restar critiques the consent process used which informed participants up front that the study intended to measure something called social and peer contagion. This created a priming effect, leading to selection bias (as parents concerned about ROGD would be more likely to enroll as participants) and likely influencing parent-respondent data. Restar also critiqued the enrollment, selection and sampling processes, methods, and analyses.

Conversion Therapy and Gender Identity Change Efforts

Similar flawed and tenuous conclusions have been drawn from research of conversion therapy, also described as sexual orientation and gender identity change efforts. Conversion therapists use abusive interventions to encourage TNB patients to be or act cisgender. Although myriad research studies purport to demonstrate its effectiveness, conversion therapy is widely criticized by all major medical societies such as the American Psychological Association (2009; 2021), the American Psychiatric Association (2018), and the U.S. Substance Abuse and Mental Health Services Administration (2015). Each organization has denounced efforts to change individuals' sexual orientation or gender, refuted claims of pathology as the source of noncis and nonheterosexual identities, and affirmed the validity of queer and trans people.

Despite contemporary repudiation of the practice, the use of conversion therapy proliferated in the late twentieth century in part due to bad science. Perhaps the most pernicious example was a 1979 paper by behavioral psychologist David Barlow and colleagues in *JAMA Psychiatry*, a leading journal in the medical field. In this paper, Barlow argues for psychotherapy as an alternative to surgical treatments for TNB people. Specifically, he discusses case material from work with an adolescent "transsexual" that resulted in alleged modifications in behaviors and arousal patterns. He describes methods of the treatment, creating a blueprint for future providers to change patients' sexual orientation and gender identity.

This foundational paper touched off decades of research studies that contributed to the development and use of supposedly empirically validated interventions that were used to abuse TNB adolescents. Notably, the Association for Behavioral and Cognitive Therapies (2022) issued an apology statement for its contributions to the field of conversion therapy. Many members critiqued the apology, arguing it was defensive and insincere (Flaherty, 2022). The Association continues to contend publicly with its historical and contemporary contributions to bad science.

Flawed Science Behind Gender-Based Sport Participation

The exclusion of TNB people from sport is a complex issue that requires nuanced understanding of the science and politics involved. Traditionally, sports have been divided into men's and women's teams based on supposed physiological or performance advantages (e.g., speed, strength) that men may hold in many sports. Dividing athletes solely based on binary sex categories poses issues for TNB and cis athletes. This approach does not capture the full range of variance among humans, regardless of their sex or gender (Wahlert & Fiester, 2012) or actually bolster fairness and equity (Ivy & Conrad, 2018). Indeed, humans are biologically and phenomenologically diverse in terms of primary and secondary sex characteristics. Splitting athletes into separate male and female competitive pools is not like sorting ones and zeros. Rather, it is akin to trying to discern the boundaries between different shades of orange in a sunset.

Physiological variability poses little threat to men's sports (due to our assumptions of masculinity and high testosterone among people assigned male at birth), but it poses challenges when determining who can compete in women's sports, especially when a person is intersex. The debate about fairness in women's athletics has become the focal point of policy discussions surrounding the inclusion of TNB athletes (Ingram & Thomas, 2019). One common approach (adopted by World Athletics and others) has been to ban people from women's sports who have a testosterone level higher than 5 nmol/L (World Athletics, 2019).

Despite social movements to increase sex and gender diversity in sports, advocates for binary male and female competitive athletics continue to cite bad science as a rationale for excluding TNB people and people born with intersex traits. In particular, scholars have dedicated significant funding and time to operationalize womanhood based on physiological characteristics. It is crucial to recognize that anyone claiming to have a definitive and fair method for determining eligibility in women's sports is misleading the public (Buzuvis, 2011). The science surrounding gender and sport is in flux and the premise that humans can be categorized into strict and discreet gender categories is fundamentally flawed.

A comprehensive overview of the flawed arguments surrounding gender-based sport participation is beyond the scope of this chapter, but when debunking the bad science behind those arguments, it is important to consider their implications. One obvious implication is the suggestion that all trans men and all trans women are the same, with the same anatomy, experiences, transition journeys, and physiological responses to hormones. This is simply not true. A person's body is shaped by the gendered context in which they grew up, their genes, the puberty they experience, their body's unique response to hormones, and so on (Torres et al., 2022). For example, some scholars try to use case examples like Renee Richards and her assertions about her performance advantages as a reason that all trans women should not be able to participate in women's sports (West-Sell et al., 2019). However, such case examples draw the focus toward cultural arguments by suggesting that the experience of one person stands for an entire population and away from the more complex, individualized factors at play at the intersection of psychological and physiological science.

Much of the debate around sport participation focuses on specific aspects of physiology, such as hormone levels. In general, the presence of a certain level of testosterone in a body (either presently or in the past) is believed to give a person an advantage over individuals with lower levels of testosterone in their system. However, there is ongoing debate about the developmental advantages women who have had elevated levels may hold over women who have not (Hilton & Lundberg, 2021). Mounting evidence suggests the differences are limited with increased duration of hormone therapy (Harper et al., 2021; Luigi et al., 2023). Such arguments likely gain so much traction because they mirror arguments against the use of illicit substances or drugs to gain a performance advantage (Devine, 2019). In the case of debates concerning sport access, testosterone is framed as the illicit performance enhancing substance. See Chapter 15 for further discussion of TNB participation in sports.

Bans on Gender-Affirming Health Care

Rhetoric encouraging bans on gender-affirming health care, including access to hormone therapy and gender-affirming surgeries, has been spreading across multiple states. Such services are often lifesaving and greatly improve quality of life for TNB individuals who can access them. State-wide bans on the provision of such care have largely focused on health care for TNB minors, but some states have extended bills regarding this matter to individuals under 21-years-old (OK HB1011), with calls for bans up to age 26 (such as the Millstone Act, OK SB129, filed by Oklahoma State Senator Bullard). These bans, while overt efforts to exert control over TNB bodies, are intimately tied to bad research or ignorance of research entirely.

Bans on TNB health care heavily rely on poorly conducted studies that suggest individuals later regret medical transition and ignore the fact that most

TNB individuals under 18 do not receive gender-affirming surgeries. Anti-TNB hate groups point to studies that claim most children whose genders do not align with their sex assigned at birth do not grow up to be adults who are TNB (Skinner et al., 2021). However, studies used to limit the rights of TNB people are rife with methodological concerns such as inconsistent use of terminology, recruitment issues, and design limitations (Skinner et al., 2023).

TNB individuals who may, throughout their life, change their expression or understanding of their gender are often labeled as desisters or detransitioners (Expósito-Campos, 2021). Due to a lack of scientific consensus and widespread use in popular culture, however, these terms may be used in different ways in different settings. Experiences of such individuals are also often used by anti-TNB hate groups who sensationalize these cases and paint a picture of individuals who have been "tricked" into surgery or other gender-affirming care (Hildebrand-Chupp, 2020). Although it is possible for TNB folks to be unhappy with the results of a surgery or to regret surgical decisions, as can be the case with any surgical procedure, very few TNB people do. In fact, a meta-analysis of regret after gender-affirming surgery found the rate of regret as low as 1% across studies included in analysis (Bustos et al., 2021). Furthermore, out of the small number of people who decide to stop their gender transition and once again identify as their gender assigned at birth, a majority report doing so as a result of social pressure and not a sizeable shift in their gender identity.

Researchers who completed qualitative interviews with young adults who had discontinued transition or detransitioned found that the process of transitioning and detransitioning is nonlinear, involves complex emotions, and does not necessarily result in individuals returning to a cisgender identity (Pullen Sansfaçon et al., 2023). If an individual's relationship with their gender changes, however, their experience is often written off by individuals who support bans on gender-affirming heath care (review Dr. Kinnon MacKinnon's scholarship in this area for more discussion and nuance). As such, there is a paucity of research about how to best support TNB individuals and those whose understanding of their gender changes throughout or after a transition process (Hildebrand-Chupp, 2020).

RECOMMENDATIONS FOR RESEARCH-BASED PRACTICE

To avoid contributing to bad science, investigators can follow practices that are TNB-affirming, methodologically rigorous, and center diverse TNB communities. We specifically recommend two frameworks to guide future studies that are relevant for researchers and research-informed clinicians to consider.

First, we recommend adopting the process-oriented approach to TNB research and assessment, proposed by Tebbe and Budge (2016). This approach provides a philosophical and methodological framework that prioritizes the needs, wisdom, and leadership of TNB people throughout the research process. Tebbe and Budge (2016) recommend incorporating participatory action research, community-based participatory research, and community participatory action research approaches that center stakeholder input and leadership and recognize TNB people's ownership of content and data. Researchers can critically consider two questions when designing a study: "Who benefits in this situation?" and "How do power and privilege shape what we see and the decisions we make?"

When recruiting TNB participants and clients, it is critical to build trust and acknowledge legacies of extraction and lack of mutuality between academia and community. Use effective, affirming, and locally created language. Consider the specific gender, racial, and cultural norms of recruitment venues and engage in purposive sampling to ensure intentional representation of TNB people of color and with other marginalized identities.

Select a methodological or clinical approach that directly relates to community-generated research questions and presenting concerns and affirms diverse TNB experiences. Exercise caution when using gender-binary psychometric measurement tools and when choosing gendered cutoff scores. Furthermore, ensure your approach to publishing and distributing data has a direct, positive impact on the needs of TNB people. Engage study participants by communicating study results, even during the analysis phase, to solicit community feedback and promote co-ownership of knowledge.

Second, we recommend scientists and practitioners expand the language used in gender research to more comprehensively and humanistically capture the diversity of gendered experiences. In a recent Nature essay, TNB scholars Ashley and colleagues (2024) recommend expanding gender terminology in research to move beyond the male or female and transgender or cisgender binaries. Instead, they suggest that scientists capture a participant's *gender modality*, or the nuanced experiences by which they relate over time to the gender they were assigned at birth. Many people who would be included within the broad umbrella of TNB may not identify as transgender, despite having a gender identity incongruent with what may be expected by their gender assigned at birth. As such, we recommend scholars capture the complexity of people's gender modalities by including possibilities beyond cisgender and transgender, as well as capturing how gender modalities may evolve throughout the lifespan.

Third, we recommend following guidance by TNB scholars that meaningful work must center TNB people with lived experience. TNB stakeholders should hold positions of empirical, clinical, administrative, and public leadership.

Given the proliferation of experts entering the field, we argue there is no excuse for an all-cisgender authorship list on a contemporary manuscript about TNB health. Rather, we echo the argument from a recent commentary in *The Lancet* (Restar & Opcrario, 2019) that it is critical to advance TNB representation in undergraduate and graduate education, clinical training, and research faculty positions (Matsuno et al., 2022). Advancing TNB leadership is a pivotal goal of advancing gender-based equity in science. We as a field must strive to ensure the scientific methods we use—with participants, colleagues, and community—are rigorous and rooted in TNB liberation.

CHAPTER SUMMARY

In this chapter, we addressed the critical need for TNB-affirming scholars and practitioners to mitigate the adverse impact of bad science. We discussed the influence of oppressive ideologies such as cissexism and cisnormativity on the production and interpretation of scientific literature and emphasized the need to critically evaluate their impact. We highlighted the importance of centering the voices of gender diverse individuals in research and advocated for a process-oriented approach that prioritizes the material and psychological needs of diverse TNB communities. We then explored misleading conclusions in current research on autism, health care, and sports. The chapter concluded with key takeaways and recommendations.

REFERENCES

American Psychiatric Association. (2018). *Position statement on conversion therapy and LGBTQ patients*. https://www.psychiatry.org/getattachment/3d23f2f4-1497-4537-b4de-fe32fe8761bf/Position-Conversion-Therapy.pdf

American Psychological Association. (2009). *Resolution on appropriate affirmative responses to sexual orientation distress and change efforts*. https://www.apa.org/about/policy/sexual-orientation

American Psychological Association. (2017). *Ethical principles of psychologists and code of conduct* (2002, amended effective June 1, 2010, and January 1, 2017). https://www.apa.org/ethics/code

American Psychological Association. (2020). *Publication manual of the American Psychological Association* (7th ed.). https://doi.org/10.1037/0000165-000

American Psychological Association. (2024). *Journal article reporting standards*. https://apastyle.apa.org/jars

American Psychological Association. (2025). Resolution on gender identity change efforts. https://www.apa.org/about/policy/resolution-gender-identity-change-efforts.pdf

Ansara, Y. G., & Hegarty, P. (2012). Cisgenderism in psychology: Pathologising and misgendering children from 1999 to 2008. *Psychology and Sexuality, 3*(2), 137–160. https://doi.org/10.1080/19419899.2011.576696

Appelbaum, M., Cooper, H., Kline, R. B., Mayo-Wilson, E., Nezu, A. M., & Rao, S. M. (2018). Journal article reporting standards for quantitative research in psychology: The APA Publications and Communications Board task force report. *American Psychologist, 73*(1), 3–25. Advance online publication. https://doi.org/10.1037/amp0000191

Ashley, F., Brightly-Brown, S., & Rider, G. N. (2024). Beyond the trans/cis binary: Introducing new terms will enrich gender research. *Nature, 630*(8016), 293–295. https://doi.org/10.1038/d41586-024-01719-9

Association for Behavioral and Cognitive Therapies. (2022). *ABCT apology for behavior therapy's contribution to the development and practice of sexual orientation and gender identity and expression change efforts: History and next steps.* https://www.abct.org/wp-content/uploads/2022/06/Untitled-document-6.pdf

Bauer, G. R., Lawson, M. L., Metzger, D. L., & the Trans Youth CAN! Research Team. (2022). Do clinical data from transgender adolescents support the phenomenon of "Rapid Onset Gender Dysphoria"? *The Journal of Pediatrics, 243*, 224–227.e2. https://doi.org/10.1016/j.jpeds.2021.11.020

Berger, I., & Ansara, Y. G. (2021). Cisnormativity. In A. Goldberg (Ed.), *The SAGE Encyclopedia of Trans Studies* (Vol. 2, pp. 122–125). SAGE Publications. https://doi.org/10.4135/9781544393858

Boskey, E. (2021). *The rapid onset gender dysphoria controversy.* Verywell Health. https://www.verywellhealth.com/rapid-onset-gender-dysphoria-4685597

Bustos, V. P., Bustos, S. S., Mascaro, A., Del Corral, G., Forte, A. J., Ciudad, P., Kim, E. A., Langstein, H. N., & Manrique, O. J. (2021). Regret after gender-affirmation surgery: A systematic review and meta-analysis of prevalence. *Plastic and Reconstructive Surgery—Global Open, 9*(3), e3477. https://doi.org/10.1097/GOX.0000000000003477

Buzuvis, E. E. (2011). Transgender student-athletes and sex-segregated sport: Developing policies of inclusion for intercollegiate and interscholastic athletics. *Seton Hall Journal of Sports and Entertainment Law, 21*(1), 1–60. https://ssrn.com/abstract=1646059

Cech, E. A., & Waidzunas, T. J. (2021). Systemic inequalities for LGBTQ professionals in STEM. *Science Advances, 7*(3), eabe0933. https://doi.org/10.1126/sciadv.abe0933

Centers for Disease Control. (n.d.). *Statistical brief: Using sexual orientation, gender identity, sex, and sex-at-birth variables in analysis.* https://www.cdc.gov/brfss/data_documentation/pdf/BRFSS-SOGI-Stat-Brief-508.pdf

Coulter, R. W., Kenst, K. S., Bowen, D. J., & Scout (2014). Research funded by the National Institutes of Health on the health of lesbian, gay, bisexual, and transgender populations. *American Journal of Public Health, 104*(2), e105–e112. https://doi.org/10.2105/AJPH.2013.301501

Department of Health and Human Services. (2017). *Research on the health of transgender and gender nonconforming populations (R01).* https://grants.nih.gov/grants/guide/pa-files/PA-17-478.html

Devine, J. W. (2019). Gender, steroids, and fairness in sport. *Sport, Ethics and Philosophy, 13*(2), 161–169. https://doi.org/10.1080/17511321.2017.1404627

Dijkstra, S., Kok, G., Ledford, J. G., Sandalova, E., & Stevelink, R. (2018). Possibilities and pitfalls of social media for translational medicine. *Frontiers in Medicine, 5*, 345. Advance online publication. https://doi.org/10.3389/fmed.2018.00345

Di Luigi, L., Greco, E. A., Fossati, C., Aversa, A., Sgrò, P., & Antinozzi, C. (2023). Clinical concerns on sex steroids variability in cisgender and transgender women athletes. *International Journal of Sports Medicine, 44*(2), 81–94. Advance online publication. https://doi.org/10.1055/a-1909-1196

Edmiston, E. K., & Juster, R. P. (2022). Refining research and representation of sexual and gender diversity in neuroscience. *Biological Psychiatry: Cognitive Neuroscience and Neuroimaging, 7*(12), 1251–1257. https://doi.org/10.1016/j.bpsc.2022.07.007

Expósito-Campos, P. (2021). A typology of gender detransition and its implications for healthcare providers. *Journal of Sex & Marital Therapy, 47*(3), 270–280. Advance online publication. https://doi.org/10.1080/0092623X.2020.1869126

Flaherty, C. (2022). 'Beliefs change.' Inside Higher Ed. https://www.insidehighered.com/news/2022/06/14/conversion-therapy-apology-statement-raises-questions

Fridell, S. R., Zucker, K. J., Bradley, S. J., Maing, D. M. (1996). Physical attractiveness of girls with gender identity disorder. *Archives of Sexual Behavior, 25*, 17–31. https://doi.org/10.1007/BF02437905

Goldbach, C., & Knutson, D. (2023). Gender-related minority stress and gender dysphoria: Development and initial validation of the Gender Dysphoria Triggers Scale (GDTS). *Psychology of Sexual Orientation and Gender Diversity, 10*(3), 383–396. https://doi.org/10.1037/sgd0000548

Harper, J., O'Donnell, E., Sorouri Khorashad, B., McDermott, H., & Witcomb, G. L. (2021). How does hormone transition in transgender women change body composition, muscle strength and haemoglobin? Systematic review with a focus on the implications for sport participation. *British Journal of Sports Medicine, 55*(15), 865–872. https://doi.org/10.1136/bjsports-2020-103106

Hildebrand-Chupp, R. (2020). More than 'canaries in the gender coal mine': A transfeminist approach to research on detransition. *The Sociological Review, 68*(4), 800–816. https://doi.org/10.1177/0038026120934694

Hilton, E. N., & Lundberg, T. R. (2021). Transgender women in the female category of sport: Perspectives on testosterone suppression and performance advantage. *Sports Medicine, 51*(2), 199–214. https://doi.org/10.1007/s40279-020-01389-3

Hines, M. (2020). Human gender development. *Neuroscience and Biobehavioral Reviews, 118*, 89–96. https://doi.org/10.1016/j.neubiorev.2020.07.018

Horne, S. G., McGinley, M., Yel, N., & Maroney, M. R. (2022). The stench of bathroom bills and anti-transgender legislation: Anxiety and depression among transgender, nonbinary, and cisgender LGBQ people during a state referendum. *Journal of Counseling Psychology, 69*(1), 1–13. https://doi.org/10.1037/cou0000558

Hughes, C. H. (1893). Erotopathia—Morbid erotism. *Alienist and Neurologist, 14*, 531–578.

Ingram, B. J., & Thomas, C. L. (2019). Transgender policy in sport, a review of current policy and commentary of the challenges of policy creation. *Current Sports Medicine Reports, 18*(6), 239–247. Advance online publication. https://doi.org/10.1249/JSR.0000000000000605

Ivy, V., & Conrad, A. (2018). Including trans women athletes in competitive sport: Analyzing the science, law, and principles and policies of fairness in competition. *Philosophical Topics, 46*(2), 103–140. https://doi.org/10.5840/philtopics201846215

James, S., Herman, J., Rankin, S., Keisling, M., Mottet, L., & Anafi, M. A. (2016). *The report of the 2015 US transgender survey*. National Center for Transgender Equality. https://transequality.org/sites/default/files/docs/usts/USTS-Full-Report-Dec17.pdf

Johnson, A. H. (2019). Rejecting, reframing, and reintroducing: Trans people's strategic engagement with the medicalisation of gender dysphoria. *Sociology of Health & Illness, 41*(3), 517–532. https://doi.org/10.1111/1467-9566.12829

Jordan-Young, R., & Rumiati, R. I. (2012). Hardwired for sexism? Approaches to sex/gender in neuroscience. *Neuroethics, 5*, 305–315. https://doi.org/10.1007/s12152-011-9134-4

Kiyar, M., Collet, S., T'Sjoen, G. & Mueller, S. (2020). Neuroscience in transgender people: An update. *Neuroforum, 26*(2), 85–92. https://doi.org/10.1515/nf-2020-0007

Kristensen, Z. E., & Broome, M. R. (2015). Autistic traits in an internet sample of gender variant UK adults. *International Journal of Transgenderism, 16*(4), 234–245. https://doi.org/10.1080/15532739.2015.1094436

Landén, M., & Rasmussen, P. (1997). Gender identity disorder in a girl with autism—A case report. *European Child & Adolescent Psychiatry, 6*(3), 170–173. https://doi.org/10.1007/BF00538990

Lett, E., Everhart, A., Streed, C., & Restar, A. (2022). Science and public health as a tool for social justice requires methodological rigor. *Pediatrics, 150*(6). https://doi.org/10.1542/peds.2022-059680A

Littman, L. (2019). Correction: Parent reports of adolescents and young adults perceived to show signs of a rapid onset of gender dysphoria. *PLOS One, 14*(3), e0214157. https://doi.org/10.1371/journal.pone.0214157

Matsuno, E., Bricker, N., Collazo, E. N., & Mohr, R. (2022). "The default is just going to be getting misgendered": Minority stress experiences among nonbinary adults. *Psychology of Sexual Orientation and Gender Diversity, 11*(2), 202–214. https://www.researchgate.net/publication/364571308_The_default_is_just_going_to_be_getting_misgendered_Minority_stress_experiences_among_nonbinary_adults

Moore, F. (2022). Autism and transgender identity. *Murmurations: Journal of Transformative Systemic Practice, 4*(2), 1–9. https://doi.org/10.28963/4.2.2

Muhammed T, S., & Mathew, S. K. (2022). The disaster of misinformation: A review of research in social media. *International Journal of Data Science and Analytics, 13*(4), 271–285. https://doi.org/10.1007/s41060-022-00311-6

Murphy, J., Prentice, F., Walsh, R., Catmur, C., & Bird, G. (2020). Autism and transgender identity: Implications for depression and anxiety. *Research in Autism Spectrum Disorders, 69*, 101466. Advance online publication. https://doi.org/10.1016/j.rasd.2019.101466

Myers, D. (2007). Implication of the scientist-practitioner model in counseling psychology training and practice. *American Behavioral Scientist, 50*(6), 789–796. https://doi.org/10.1177/0002764206296457

Nobili, A., Glazebrook, C., Bouman, W. P., Glidden, D., Baron-Cohen, S., Allison, C., Smith, P., & Arcelus, J. (2018). Autistic traits in treatment-seeking transgender adults. *Journal of Autism and Developmental Disorders, 48*(12), 3984–3994. https://doi.org/10.1007/s10803-018-3557-2

Pasterski, V., Zucker, K. J., Hindmarsh, P. C., Hughes, I. A., Acerini, C., Spencer, D., Neufeld, S., & Hines, M. (2015). Increased cross-gender identification independent of gender role behavior in girls with congenital adrenal hyperplasia: Results from a standardized assessment of 4- to 11-year-old children. *Archives of Sexual Behavior, 44*(5), 1363–1375. https://doi.org/10.1007/s10508-014-0385-0

Pullen Sansfaçon, A., Gelly, M. A., Gravel, R., Medico, D., Baril, A., Susset, F., & Paradis, A. (2023). A nuanced look into youth journeys of gender transition and detransition. *Infant and Child Development, 32*(2), e2402. https://doi.org/10.1002/icd.2402

Rastogi, A., Menard, L., Miller, G. H., Cole, W., Laurison, D., Caballero, J. R., Murano-Kinney, S., & Heng-Lehtinen, R. (2025, June). *Health and wellbeing: A report of the 2022 U.S. Transgender Survey.* Advocates for Transgender Equality. https://ustranssurvey.org/download-reports/

Restar, A. J. (2020). Methodological critique of Littman's (2018) parental-respondents accounts of "rapid-onset gender dysphoria." *Archives of Sexual Behavior, 49*(1), 61–66. https://doi.org/10.1007/s10508-019-1453-2

Restar, A. J., & Operario, D. (2019). The missing trans women of science, medicine, and global health. *The Lancet, 393*(10171), 506–508. https://doi.org/10.1016/S0140-6736(18)32423-1

Shore, E. R. (1984). The former transsexual: A case study. *Archives of Sexual Behavior, 13*(3), 277–285. https://doi.org/10.1007/BF01541654

Skinner, S. R., McLamore, Q., Donaghy, O., Stathis, S., Moore, J. K., Nguyen, T., Rayner, C., Tait, R., Anderson, J., & Pang, K. C. (2023). Recognizing and responding to misleading trans health research. *International Journal of Transgender Health, 25*(1), 1–9. https://doi.org/10.1080/26895269.2024.2289318

Stoller, R. (1968). *Sex and gender: The transsexual experiment* (Vol. 2). Hogarth.

Stryker, S. (2020). Introduction: Trans* studies now. *Transgender Studies Quarterly, 7*(3), 299–305. https://doi.org/10.1215/23289252-8552908

Substance Abuse and Mental Health Services Administration. (2015). *Ending conversion therapy: Supporting and affirming LGBTQ youth.* https://www.freestatesocialwork.com/articles/endingconversiontherapy_course_readings.pdf

Tebbe, E. A., & Budge, S. L. (2016). Research with trans communities: Applying a process-oriented approach to methodological considerations and research recommendations. *The Counseling Psychologist, 44*(7), 996–1024. https://doi.org/10.1177/0011000015609045

Thoma, B., Murray, H., Huang, S. Y. M., Milne, W. K., Martin, L. J., Bond, C. M., Mohindra, R., Chin, A., Yeh, C. H., Sanderson, W. B., & Chan, T. M. (2018). The impact of social media promotion with infographics and podcasts on research dissemination and readership. *Canadian Journal of Emergency Medical Care, 20*(2), 300–306. https://doi.org/10.1017/cem.2017.394

Thrower, E., Bretherton, I., Pang, K. C., Zajac, J. D., & Cheung, A. S. (2020). Prevalence of autism spectrum disorder and attention-deficit hyperactivity disorder amongst individuals with gender dysphoria: A systematic review. *Journal of Autism and Developmental Disorders, 50*(3), 695–706. https://doi.org/10.1007/s10803-019-04298-1

Torres, C. R., Lopez Frias, F. J., & Patiño, M. J. M. (2022). Beyond physiology: Embodied experience, embodied advantage, and the inclusion of transgender athletes in competitive sport. *Sport, Ethics and Philosophy, 16*(1), 33–49. https://doi.org/10.1080/17511321.2020.1856915

Trans Legislation Tracker. (n.d.). *Anti-trans bills: Trans legislation tracker.* Retrieved June 13, 2023, from https://translegislation.com

Turban, J. L. (2018). Potentially reversible social deficits among transgender youth. *Journal of Autism and Developmental Disorders, 48*(12), 4007–4009. https://doi.org/10.1007/s10803-018-3603-0

Turban, J. L., Dolotina, B., King, D., & Keuroghlian, A. S. (2022). Sex assigned at birth ratio among transgender and gender diverse adolescents in the United States. *Pediatrics, 150*(3), e2022056567. Advance online publication. https://doi.org/10.1542/peds.2022-056567

van der Miesen, A. I. R., Hurley, H., Bal, A. M., & de Vries, A. L. C. (2018). Prevalence of the wish to be of the opposite gender in adolescents and adults with autism spectrum disorder. *Archives of Sexual Behavior, 47*(8), 2307–2317. https://doi.org/10.1007/s10508-018-1218-3

van der Miesen, A. I. R., Hurley, H., & de Vries, A. L. C. (2016). Gender dysphoria and autism spectrum disorder: A narrative review. *International Review of Psychiatry, 28*(1), 70–80. https://doi.org/10.3109/09540261.2015.1111199

von Krafft-Ebing, R. F. (1886). *Psychopathia sexualis: Eine klinisch-forensische studie* [Sexual psychopathy: A clinical-forensic study]. Stuttgart.

Wahlert, L., & Fiester, A. (2012). Gender transports: Privileging the "natural" in gender testing debates for intersex and transgender athletes. *The American Journal of Bioethics, 12*(7), 19–21. https://doi.org/10.1080/15265161.2012.683750

Ward, A. F., Zheng, J., & Broniarczyk, S. M. (2023). I share, therefore I know? Sharing online content—even without reading it—inflates subjective knowledge. *Journal of Consumer Psychology, 33*(3), 469–488. https://doi.org/10.1002/jcpy.1321

Wattel, L. L., Walsh, R. J., & Krabbendam, L. (2024). Theories on the link between autism spectrum conditions and trans gender modality: A systematic review. *Review Journal of Autism and Developmental Disorders, 11*(2), 275-295. https://doi.org/10.1007/s40489-022-00338-2

West-Sell, S. A., Van Ness, J. M., & Ciccolella, M. E. (2019). Law, policy, and physiology as determinants of fairness for transgender athletes. *Professionalization of Exercise Psychology Online, 22*(2), 1–10.

World Athletics. (2019). *Eligibility regulations for the female classification.* https://worldathletics.org/about-iaaf/documents/book-of-rules

PART II
WORKING WITH DIVERSE CLIENT IDENTITIES AND LIFE STAGES

6

TRANS AND NONBINARY PEOPLE AND COMMUNITIES OF COLOR

Resilience, Resistance, and Liberation

ANNELIESE SINGH, SEL J. HWAHNG, TOCHUKWU AWACHIE, ALÉX BASSI, TRAE BROWN, AND HEIDI BREAUX

Research with trans and nonbinary (TNB) communities of color has increased over the past two decades (Arora et al., 2022; Hwahng, 2021; Singh & McKleroy, 2011), and still there is little attention to counseling competency with this group. Much of this research has focused on the multiplicative harm and violence that TNB communities of color experience as a result of racist, sexist, and heterosexist discrimination (Farvid et al., 2021; Flores et al., 2016). Scholars and practitioners have continuously called for increased work in this area, attending to the power and privilege that mental health providers (MHPs) have to create more affirming environments for these communities (Erby & White, 2020; McCullough et al., 2017; Singh & McKleroy, 2011). In addition, studies examining the use of counseling found that TNB clients used more sessions than their cisgender peers, and that TNB people of color (POCs) had higher levels of distress than their White TNB and cis counterparts (Lefevor et al., 2019).

In this chapter, we review the important research examining the experiences of intersectional systemic oppressions (e.g., racism, anti-TNB bias, classism) that impact the lives and well-being of TNB POCs in counseling. We also describe important sources of mutual aid that TNB communities of color access,

---

https://doi.org/10.1037/0000471-007
Affirmative Counseling and Psychological Practice With Trans and Nonbinary Clients, Second Edition, A. Singh and R. McCullough (Editors)
Copyright © 2026 by the American Psychological Association. All rights reserved.

including a case study from one of our authors. Finally, we examine counseling approaches that can be helpful with TNB POCs, as well as crucial advocacy strategies and training that promote wellness for TNB people and communities of color, thriving, and liberation.

COMPOUNDED RACIAL AND GENDER INEQUITIES EXPERIENCED BY TRANS AND NONBINARY COMMUNITIES OF COLOR

TNB POC experience compounded racialized and gendered inequities and, consequently, higher psychological stress than individuals holding one or no minoritized statuses (Farvid et al., 2021; Galupo & Orphanidys, 2022; Millar & Brooks, 2021). These multilayered oppressions infiltrate various aspects of life. For instance, health care biases against POC and LGBTQ+ patients lead to less effective treatment methods and poorer health outcomes than for White and non-LGBTQ+ patients (Angelino et al., 2020; Apodaca et al., 2022). In addition, experiences of health care bias toward TNB POCs are higher than White TNB patients (Agénor et al., 2022; Mazon et al., 2024). Studies also show that TNB POCs experience microaggressions, discrimination, and the dismissal of minoritization experiences—all of which can show up in therapeutic dynamics with MHPs (Compton & Morgan, 2022). In academic spaces such as K–12 and higher education, racism and cissexism undermine the educational opportunities, potential for affirming relationships, and overall safety of TNB people and POCs in educational settings (Barrita et al., 2023). Racial and gender discrimination in professional environments can limit the safety, satisfaction, and success of employed TNB POCs (Goates et al., 2024; Holloway, Gottlieb, & Cason, 2023; McEntarfer & Rice, 2023). TNB POCs who are perceived to deviate from gendered cultural norms often experience stigmatization and consequent deprivation of cultural resources (e.g., use of their native language and access to their spiritual communities; Abreu et al., 2021; Etengolf & Rodriguez, 2022; Thai et al., 2021).

It is important to note that the interlocking oppressions of White supremacy and cisheteropatriarchy foster high rates of interpersonal and institutional violence for TNB communities of color (Takahashi et al., 2020). For example, transmisogyny and gender binarism can fuel abuse in intimate partner relationships and can create obstacles for help-seekers when victim advocates are not competent about queer and TNB identities or relationship dynamics. In addition to physical and sexual abuse, TNB young POCs impacted by foster care systems often face intentional misgendering and sex-based segregation, being labeled as difficult or undesirable by foster guardians or potential adoptive parents. Additionally, they can experience police targeting due to their race and gender, often leading to a pipeline of further abuse within juvenile detention (Roberts-Sampson, 2023). Many researchers have adopted deficit-based approaches to health research in TNB communities of color that focus on discrimination and violence as risk factors and emphasize outcomes such as suicidality (Millar & Brooks, 2021). However, TNB communities of color have expressed the need for research to prioritize health-promoting factors (e.g., sexual health resources, positive health outcomes such as recovery from substance dependency) to better reflect the complexities experienced by TNB communities of color and how they cultivate full and meaningful lives (LeBlanc et al., 2022).

Within the field of psychology, there are three realms of inquiry that can support MHPs in providing gender-affirming care to TNB communities of color: (a) identity development and pride, (b) resilience as resistance to oppression, and (c) attention to liberation approaches. While the field of psychology upholds long-standing constructs of human development, identity development milestones may be differently timed in POCs, nonbinary and genderqueer people, and other communities facing higher levels of systemic oppression (Doyle, 2022). These constructs contribute to the broader understanding that mainstream psychology's models of development are narrowed by White cisheteronormativity, and thus insufficient references for the developmental trajectories of TNB communities of color (Dunham & Olson, 2018; Lindley et al., 2021; Restar et al., 2019). In light of this, it is important to have more inclusive theories of identity development for TNB POCs, recognizing how various forms of marginalization affect developmental processes and psychological functioning (Meca et al., 2023; Singh, 2013).

Identity Development and Pride

One realm of inquiry MHPs can be mindful of when providing gender-affirming care to TNB POCs includes supporting clients in exploring both their racial and gender identities in tandem while also acknowledging the impact of interlocking racial and gender oppressive systems (Galupo & Orphanydys, 2020; Singh, 2013; Singh & McKleroy, 2011). MHPs can support TNB clients of color by encouraging gender and racial self-expression to affirm identity and build TNB POC community in the absence of broader societal representation (Dolan & Garvey, 2024). MHPs can also support TNB clients of color to explore gender exploration and ways of adorning, labeling, and expressing themselves authentically, including conversations in supportive relationships that allow both critical and compassionate self-discovery of gender and racial identity development and pride (Nordmarken, 2023). Helping TNB clients of color develop pride in their gender and racial identity can occur through explorations of how they may define their gender and racial identities with their own words, while also identifying specific ways having pride in their identities can increase their well-being (Coburn et al., 2023; Poquiz et al., 2022; Thai et al., 2021). For TNB communities of color targeted by multiple systemic oppressions, developing both gender and racial pride in their identities often includes internal and external processes for reckoning with and rejecting the emotional, intellectual, physical, and sociopolitical violence or racism, as well as anti-trans prejudice, heterosexism, and other oppressive systems. Resilience as a form of resistance promotes positive outcomes for TNB POCs, which we discuss next.

Resilience as Resistance to Oppression

As defined by a cohort of young LGBTQ+ POCs, *resilience* is the cultivation of individual and community awareness, self-sufficiency, rebelliousness, and logistics for survival (Williams et al., 2022). A gerontology storytelling project centering voices from ethnically diverse, gender expansive, and other historically neglected communities illustrated resilience as resisting, unlearning, and healing from White, cisheteronormative notions of self, relationships, and longevity (Chazan & Baldwin, 2021). These community-generated definitions displace individualistic, trait-based definitions of resilience that minimize or erase the impacts of oppression and the labors of surviving it. Bolstering resilience factors such as affective generative resources (Edwards et al., 2023), intersectional identity affirmation (Papa & Parmenter, 2025), and agency (Austin et al., 2023) may enhance the capacity that TNB POCs have for healing from and resisting oppressive systems. In defense against multilevel racism and cissexism, these resilience factors can be strengthened at individual, interpersonal, and societal levels (Ramos & Marr, 2023).

While much of the broader resilience literature focuses on individual resilience, social relationships and social capital are deeply intertwined with the resilience of TNB communities of color (Stone et al., 2020). For some TNB POCs who have safe and supportive families of origin, resilience is modeled by communities of older relatives, often maternal figures, whose guidance aids navigation of webs of trauma and marginalization (Stone et al., 2020). A study conducted among trans Asian Americans found that family support was associated with lower reports of verbal harassment, perhaps by facilitating greater safety in public settings (Lerner & Lee, 2022). Black LGBTQ+ youth without familial support often develop bespoke kinship networks whose support may directly impact their resilience (Hailey et al., 2020). TNB Latinx individuals also cultivate resilience through community support—which aids in overcoming systemic barriers to immigration processes—and promoting mental health, access to medical services, and other wellness-related factors (Lee et al., 2023). Indigenous LGBTQ+ communities practice resilience and nurture well-being through resistance to the intergenerational, cultural, and institutional oppressions of settler colonialism (Soldatic et al., 2022). These findings demonstrate the powerful resilience processes of TNB communities of color and support the position of resilience as integral to healing and liberation (Singh & Awachie, 2025).

Attention to Liberation Approaches

Liberation can be understood as the unraveling of conditions, or conditioning, that restrict authentic ways of being and cultivation of critical consciousness in order to act upon and transform those conditions (Singh, 2020). These oppressive conditions operate through internalized oppressive, hegemonic cultural norms facilitated by collective participation, and are sustained through institutions designed to silence, harm, and eliminate those without systemic power (Domínguez & Noriega, 2022; Duran, 2019). Actualizing liberation for TNB communities of color requires that MHPs wield the privileges of their systemic authority to repair this harm. As evidenced by the work of Martín-Baró (1996), Runswick-Cole & Goodley (2013), Singh (2020), Leach & Zeineddine (2022), and other scholars, the impetus of resilience, resistance, and liberation research has been growing for decades within the field of psychology. Although TNB affirming approaches for people and communities of color are clearly needed, there have been calls to move from affirming to liberatory therapeutic approaches (Singh, 2016; Singh & Awachie, 2025). Liberation psychology tenets can increase MHP awareness and the use of critical consciousness and mutual aid efforts (e.g., recovering historical memory, concientización [or consciousness-raising], problematización [or problematizing], deideologizing [or demystifying psychology]) when supporting TNB POCs. This work must further expand to deepen sociopolitical advocacy and societal transformation (Singh, 2016, 2020). Working against systems of injustice requires creativity and collaboration, both of which are possessed by TNB communities of color; these communities are known to carry a vital blueprint for mutual aid.

RESEARCH, MUTUAL AID, AND ANECDOTAL EVIDENCE ON RESISTANCE BY TRANS AND NONBINARY PEOPLE AND COMMUNITIES OF COLOR

Mutual aid can be described as cooperation for the common good, in which members of a community gather to support one another. This is crucial for MHPs who are working with TNB communities of color to understand how they have accessed support TNB mutual aid networks. Mutual aid communities are often characterized by horizontal modes of organization in which there are little to no hierarchies. Official state bodies or governmental resources are not the central focus within mutual aid and often are not accessible or available (Solidarity Economy Association, 2023). There has been a long history of mutual aid in communities of color—including TNB people of color—with increased recent focus on mutual aid in activism and community organizing (Spade, 2020).

There is also a long tradition of communities of color and immigrant communities engaging in mutual aid practices that also inform mutual aid practices for TNB communities of color, including political organizations for and by POCs that provide food, housing, legal, and advocacy assistance. Examples include the Black Panther Party, Fraternal and African American Mutual Aid Societies, Sociedades Mutualistas, the Young Lords Party, United Farmworkers, and the seminal organization called Street Transvestite Action Revolutionaries led by Marsha P. Johnson and Sylvia Rivera (Holloway, Hostetter, et al., 2023; Kenworthy et al., 2023; Nelson, 2011).

Examples of mutual aid in TNB medical and health literature include utilizing queer and trans kinship to navigate medical systems when dealing with medical trauma; serving as emergency contacts; coordinating health care visits, transportation, and home-based care; offering emotional support; and partaking in the sharing of meals (Jackson Levin et al., 2020). Some TNB people have even engaged in do-it-yourself hormone replacement therapy, which is community-driven and incorporates online forums and mutual aid practices that not only include information sharing but also emotional and social support (August-Rae et al., 2024).

Alternative Kinship Structures and Thick Trust Capital

Researchers have discussed the intersectional and compounding stressors that TNB POCs experience, resulting in negative health outcomes (Hwahng & Nuttbrock, 2007, 2014; Levitt et al., 2017). In this section, mutual aid among TNB communities of color will be examined through the lenses of alternative kinship structures and thick trust capital. *Alternative kinship structures* refer to a network of people who form close emotional, psychological, and social bonds with one another, often taking on the role of surrogate family members (Hwahng et al., 2019). Alternative kinship structures have been referred to as fictive kin, chosen family, houses, gay family, family networks, and framily in TNB communities (Horne et al., 2015; Huynh, 2023; Hwahng & Nuttbrock, 2007; Jackson Levin et al., 2020; Levitt et al., 2017). Social creativity is considered intrinsic to the formation of alternative kinship structures and is itself considered a type of resilience (Hwahng et al., 2019).

In one study among trans and Latina immigrants in New York City, ages 22–50 years old, Hwahng and colleagues (2019) found a strong alternative kinship structure that first existed as part of a peer-delivered syringe exchange program for gender-affirming hormone therapy injections in Queens, New York. When a weekly TNB support group was subsequently set up by a harm reduction program in Queens, this alternative kinship structure extended the members' capacity to include other forms of health care and legal support or provision, provide gender-transition affirmation, improve educational access and skills training, and reduce substance use.

In a related study, researchers examined two low-income Black (African American and Afro-Caribbean) and Latina and trans immigrant communities in New York City, ages 22–50, who were a part of trans support groups offered by two harm-reduction programs in Brooklyn and Queens, New York (Hwahng et al., 2021). In this study, thick trust capital was identified as foundational to the functioning of both these communities. *Thick trust capital* is considered a subset of bonding capital, and *bonding capital* is defined by linkages formed between those who have shared demographic characteristics, often between family members, close friends, and neighbors (Putnam, 2000). Thick trust capital, as the heart of bonding social capital, is also a relational capital in which risk and vulnerability are implicit—thus, when trusters take a risk and their expectations are met or exceeded, the result is a cultivation of deep or "thick" trust. This type of relational capital occurs within networks in which close and intimate ties have been formed.

Therefore, MHPs can consider how thick trust can be supportive of TNB clients of color. In another study (Hwahng et al., 2021) of the types of thick trust that were operating within TNB people of color support groups, scholars found that group members experienced psychological and emotional safety when diversity of experiences and opinions and cross-generational support networks were shared. Outside of the support groups, TNB people of color in this study shared that they experienced thick trust in their romantic partnerships, when transporting other group members to state-level advocacy conferences, and when cultivating stronger ties with biological family members. The study authors also found that thick trust capital fosters greater *thin trust capital*, defined as "a component of bridging or linking social capital . . . directed at a 'generalized other'" (p. 216), which can aid communities with new perspectives, information, and assets. This thin trust allowed trans support group members to link across communities and groups, accessing a variety of medical, mental health, housing, substance use, educational, and vocational resources with greater efficacy.

MHPs can also be mindful of the research base examining other types of kinship structures TNB communities of color create in their mutual aid networks. For instance, Levitt et al. (2017) found two types of alternative kinship structures in a study with mostly Black and Latinx young people who belonged to gay family networks, which were also called "houses" by participants to indicate their strong relationship to them. Both alternative kinship structures were built upon traditional Black values of respect for elders and responsibility to other family networks. These structures served as sites of resistance in the face of social, familial, and economic stressors. Gay family networks and houses that promoted building relationships and had strong (fictive kin) parental leadership and kinship bonds were associated with increasing knowledge of HIV transmission, practicing safer sex, and engaging in HIV testing. Gay family networks and houses provided support specific to the needs of members that families of origin could not provide, acting as refuge from discrimination and stigmatization and addressing the intersectional challenges particular to the experiences of gay, bisexual, and TNB POCs. Trans women of color experienced the highest levels of resiliency within families that were exclusively trans women of color.

A study based in the Los Angeles area found that all forms of family networks are crucial for LGBTQ+ communities of color as well as for health resiliency (Huynh, 2023). Conducted through Viet Rainbow of Orange County (VROC), a community-based organization, participants ranged from 18 to 65 years old and considered the fostering of family-of-choice bonds central to creating a safe and affirming environment for queer and trans Vietnamese Americans. Because of this emphasis on creating familial intimacy—which included socializing, sharing meals, and expressing vulnerability—VROC was an alternative kinship structure in which thick trust capital was generated. Intergenerational relationality was encouraged, and so was the incorporation of cisgender heterosexual female members who served in motherly roles to support the LGBTQ+ people in VROC. Several members emphasized the importance of mental health or experienced improved mental health outcomes from participating in VROC. In this next section, one of the coauthors of this chapter provides a case study of TNB mutual aid in New Orleans.

Mutual Aid in New Orleans: A Personal Sharing From Trae Brown

The following description of how mutual aid networks in New Orleans supported Trae Brown (author on this chapter) as a Black, nonbinary person provides an important example of the role mutual aid organizations can play in both culture and society. Trae's story illustrates the wide-reaching benefits of mutual aid for TNB POCs that can help mitigate the harm of everyday racial and gender inequities across multiple domains of society (e.g., housing, education, finances, natural disasters).

My mother, whom we affectionately called Peaches, taught me about the significance of benevolent societies and social aid and pleasure clubs (SAPCs). These were mutual aid organizations that had been around since the 1800s. During a time when things like health and death insurance were not available, especially for Black people in New Orleans, the Black members of these groups depended on these organizations to pay for expenses. These organizations have not disappeared, and today there are over 70 SAPCs. Most people may only know the elaborate second lines put on after church on Sunday, but these groups still provide care for their members and communities through food drives, fundraisers, and various forms of mutual aid. The tie these organizations have to the music of New Orleans is steeped in activism and mutual aid, and they continue to bring joy to their communities through second line performances. For example, the Zulu parade, loved by so many locals and tourists alike in New Orleans, is an SAPC that has supported members in paying for expenses. Beyond these organizations, mutual aid is found throughout the city and in our current history.

New Orleans is home to several inspiring organizations that are making a positive impact on their communities. From House of Tulip, which provides much-needed support to TNB communities of color, to Feed the Second Line, which started during the pandemic to feed community elders and those in need, and the Bvlbancha Collective, a network of indigenous people who are providing education and mutual aid to their community. These organizations and many others in New Orleans are engaging in mutual aid and making a meaningful difference in people's lives. I have benefited from and engaged in mutual aid efforts for my community. During Hurricane Ida, when many people from New Orleans were displaced, I was working as a community MHP and at a therapeutic day program. When Ida hit, the city had no power, and it was not safe for individuals to return for a period of time. During this time, I was offered support by a network of individuals from my community. I requested instead that we fundraise for displaced families. Together, we raised $25,000 and provided these families with room and board and lost wages.

During this time, I also drove back to New Orleans, knowing that community support would be needed for those unable to leave the city. I checked on families, handed out water, and delivered gasoline to people who needed it. As I did this, various individuals and groups began to set up food and supply stations for people in the community; this included anything from free food giveaways at local cafes to people giving away the food in their own fridges. In my recent past, I was forced to rely on mutual aid to get through a tough time. The year was 2023, and I had to leave my childhood home due to domestic violence and transphobia. As a graduate student, my life had become an uphill battle. I was struggling to survive and find a way to rebuild my life. Fortunately, mutual aid played a crucial role in helping me find a new home, put food on my table, and slowly regain my footing. Without this support, I would not have been able to pick up the pieces and move on from the traumatic experience.

For these reasons, I believe mutual aid is such an essential aspect of care for TNB communities of color that MHPs must not only be aware of it but must also know how to support and expand as they work within our communities. It is heartening to know that there are communities and organizations that value compassion, empathy, and solidarity over individualism and profit. Through mutual aid, we can build a more equitable and just society where everyone has access to the resources and support they need to thrive. It is my hope that we can all contribute to this effort and create a better world for ourselves and future generations.

COUNSELING APPROACHES WITH TRANS AND NONBINARY COMMUNITIES OF COLOR

As we have discussed earlier, TNB communities of color face multiple forms of oppression at the intersection of race and gender, which can negatively impact both physical and mental health (Agénor et al., 2022). Compared to their cisgender counterparts, TNB POCs may experience higher rates of poverty, discrimination, and unemployment (McCullough et al., 2017; Singh & dickey, 2017). Additionally, they may lack traditional support networks such as biological family ties, which can limit access to resources that support thriving (Huynh, 2023; Jackson Levin et al., 2020). When seeking support through mental health care, TNB POCs may encounter a paucity of MHPs who affirm or share their racial, ethnic, or gender identities, which often leads to harmful therapeutic dynamics (Lefevor et al., 2019; McCullough et al., 2017). Within the counseling field, competent care for TNB POCs must be informed by the complex systemic conditions that threaten their mental health as well as how those conditions infiltrate the therapy space, rendering it unsafe and ineffective. Liberatory counseling approaches with TNB communities of color must support the healthy development of intersecting identities, awaken critical consciousness about those identities within broader social and historical contexts, foster and cultivate resistance, and advocate for a transformed world. In this section, we will discuss priorities for a strong foundation for counseling with TNB POCs, then describe liberatory counseling approaches across three categories: (a) navigating minority stressors and the injustices of marginalization, (b) racial and gender identity development and pride, and (c) cultivating resilience as resistance.

An essential first step for MHPs working with TNB POCs in counseling is to build a strong and collaborative therapeutic alliance to help foster positive health outcomes (Li et al., 2024). This requires intentional rejection of White supremacy, cissexism, heteropatriarchy, and other oppressive constructs that can lead to the minimization of TNB POCs experiences in counseling sessions (Arora et al., 2022). As minority stress among LGBTQ+ communities is associated with emotional dysregulation, mental distress, and substance use, MHPs working with TNB POCs who present with any of these concerns must address them as rooted in structural oppressions (e.g., racism, heterosexism, antitrans prejudice) as opposed to inherent to the individual (Hendricks & Testa, 2012; Meyer, 2003, 2015; Singh & Awachie, 2025).

In addition, the multidimensional model of broaching behavior offers strategies for MHPs to communicate about client concerns in light of identity, power dynamics, and other culturally-relevant topics (Day-Vines et al., 2018). This model emphasizes counselor self-awareness, client worldview, and counseling relationship dynamics (Ratts et al., 2016), all of which influence counselor credibility, depth of client disclosure, and client satisfaction. While some MHPs avoid broaching dissimilar identities and perspectives, Erby and White (2020) illustrate that doing so is crucial for client safety and healing, through their experiences broaching partially shared identities. Models of minority stress and broaching behavior create a strong foundation for liberatory counseling with TNB communities of color by divesting from societal systems of oppression and suppression.

Navigating Minority Stressors and the Injustices of Marginalization

To navigate minority stressors and the injustices of marginalization for TNB POCs in therapy spaces, MHPs can use affirming, intersectional therapy techniques from a strengths-based perspective to help recognize the strengths of TNB POCs (Golden & Oransky, 2019). Clinical methods that are specific to and supportive of ethnically diverse and gender expansive identities must replace those that would pathologize or dismiss them. Affirming, intersectional therapy techniques are a necessary priority as they create space for the strengths and triumphs of TNB POCs (Golden & Oransky, 2019).

Antiracist adaptations of manualized therapies such as dialectical behavior therapy (DBT) can correct biases that arise when failure to acknowledge racism decontextualizes client behaviors (Pierson et al., 2022). Within DBT skills training, MHPs working with POCs must acknowledge the role of racism and racial trauma in client behaviors that may otherwise be considered skill deficits. For example, a Black client navigating the chronically oppressive atmosphere of White supremacy may display emotional dysregulation related to racist encounters or struggle with interpersonal effectiveness when engaging with White people. Rather than simply emphasizing the relevant DBT skills, MHPs should identify unjustified versus justified emotion, maladaptive versus adaptive coping, and the stakes of assertiveness in a society that punishes Black vocality. Further, MHPs working with Black clients must commit to deepening awareness of their own racial identity and racial perspectives while recognizing a client's internalized racism as an obstacle to self-efficacy that results from a chronically invalidating environment. Ultimately, MHPs practicing antiracist DBT must recognize presenting behaviors of POCs as informed by multiple oppressive systems, practice curiosity about typically pathologized behaviors that may function as survival strategies amidst injustice, and incorporate problematization of the social world into clinical work and antiracist advocacy.

While empirically-tested applications of cognitive behavioral therapy (CBT) for TNB communities of color do not exist, scholars have offered case vignettes to demonstrate the efficacy of culturally tailored cognitive and behavioral strategies that acknowledge the minoritized experiences of clients (Berke et al., 2022). For example, during a client assessment, an MHP may begin with a discussion about choosing an affirming name, pronouns, and gender identity to use with the client, as well as determine whether the client consents to these being documented in their medical record. In addition, use of measures that assess forms of oppression (e.g., Gender Minority Stress and Resilience Measure, Race-Based Traumatic Stress Symptom Scale, scales of acculturative stress, etc.) can create a comprehensive picture of the client's exposure to traumatic stressors.

Diagnostic conceptualization should be mindful of the discrimination and violence that a TNB client of color may have experienced based on their race, gender, sexual orientation, or other identity. For instance, the diagnostic criteria for anxiety and depression should be applied with understanding of how TNB clients of color might be avoiding relationships and not accessing support due to fears of anticipated harm. These fears might be functional for client survival while also being detrimental to their mental health because of a lack of connection to social support. In addition, consideration of a gender dysphoria diagnosis should be thoroughly discussed with a client, including its history, limitations, and utility in accessing gender-affirming care. This diagnosis can be complicated for a variety of reasons, such as a client not personally identifying with this medicalized term; a client needing this in their record in order to obtain preauthorization or insurance coverage for gender-affirming medical treatments and interventions; a client not wanting this in their chart out of fear of state specific laws, lack of insurance coverage, or safety concerns; or even generally rejecting the pathologizing of their life's experience by placing a label based on criteria from mental health diagnoses, therein implying that gender dysphoria or TNB identities are a mental disorder or psychological issue. This is especially true when, for some, society is the "problem." This can be characterized most recently by the many ways a gender dysphoria diagnosis may help or hinder TNB clients based on constantly changing legislation in their states. This also differs for TNB adults versus adolescents, especially regarding legislative impacts (Kraschel et al., 2022).

Treatment plans should support clients' agency by prioritizing their own concerns and helping them make informed decisions about treatment methods. The MHP must also invest in strengthening the therapeutic alliance with special attention to areas of cultural mistrust and gender and sexuality biases. With liberation in mind, the therapeutic goals should not be for a client to habituate to the traumas of oppression. Rather, clinical work should strengthen client strategies to navigate oppression and engage with the emotions oppression generates. Some considerations to include in treatment plans with TNB POCs in counseling may be questions such as the following:

- What messages about gender, gender identity, and expression were you given, shown, told as a child? Where and whom did these messages come from? How have those shifted over time for you?
- What, if any, short-term and long-term goals do you have for your social gender identity and presentation? Are there any you are considering but aren't sure yet? Why or why not? What barriers are preventing you from achieving your goals? What kind of support do you have that will help with these barriers?
- Are all of your basic needs met: stable housing, safety, nutritious food, affirming clothing, consistent health care and affirming exams, steady employment or school (when applicable), and a stable support network? If any of these are not met, how can we work to achieve these goals together?

- What degree of connection do you have to other TNB community members, other TNB communities of color, community groups, and safe spaces? What would connecting more with "community" look like for you and would it be beneficial?
- What life goals do you have in general, not related to your gender identity and expression? What barriers are preventing you from achieving your goals? What kind of support system do you have to help with these barriers?
- What are your biggest fears about affirming your true gender identity? What steps can you take to overcome them (when possible)?
- If you experience feeling overwhelmed, needing support, or an unwillingness to go on with life, who can you reach out to for support? How likely are they to help? What are alternate resources you would also consider even if it was not your primary plan?

Broadly, clinical work with TNB POCs can be rooted in ecological theory to work with clients holistically, which identifies micro (individual), mezzo (social), and macro (institutional) points of intervention to promote affirmation and liberation of TNB people and communities of color (Matsuno, 2019). As mentioned previously, extricating one's sense of self from the conditioning of oppressive societies and institutions is integral to liberation (Singh, 2020) and is well within the purview of MHPs working with minoritized clients. At this first level of intervention, an MHP should support TNB POCs in distinguishing the distresses of oppression from their self-concept and developing it into a holistic, integrated, and positive one. One method is by fostering racial and gender identity and pride.

Fostering Racial and Gender Identity and Pride

The second category of liberatory approaches to counseling with TNB communities of color is fostering racial and gender identity development and pride. As a micro (individual) point of intervention, this category involves creating safe space for exploration and celebration of clients' multifaceted identities while disentangling those identities from multiple forms of marginalization. MHPs and clients alike will benefit from a decolonial psychotherapy approach, which addresses the psychological, physical, and spiritual wellness of populations harmed by European colonial domination (Comas-Díaz & Jacobsen, 2024). Decolonial practices comprise client narration of their experience of intersecting oppressions, exploration of spiritual traditions, social justice action, nurturing positive emotions, and other pluriversal methods of healing colonial, intergenerational, and racial or ethnic traumas. In addition, MHPs can practice the five steps of developing cultural awareness to enhance their cultural sensitivity and, thus, the therapeutic alliance: (a) acknowledge personal biases and faulty assumptions that may lead to culturally inequitable treatment, (b) acknowledge that a client's cultural identity and worldview may differ from their own, (c) acknowledge and embrace the vastness of cultural diversity, (d) make efforts to develop diverse cultural knowledge and relationships, and (e) develop a capacity to navigate novel encounters with ethnic minority communities (Parker et al., 2021). Within such frameworks, TNB POCs can deconstruct conceptualizations of self that are shaped by colonial assertions of White supremacy, binary and sex-essentialist gender, and heteropatriarchy in order to (re)construct selves emboldened by their ancestral, communal, and individual strengths.

As previously discussed, identity pride, self-definition, self-determination, and authenticity support well-being for communities who experience identity-based oppressions (Coburn et al., 2023). MHPs can support identity pride in TNB people and communities of color by applying an intersectional lens to conversations about adversity and processes of navigating it (Galupo & Orphanidys, 2022). For example, one group therapy intervention for TNB adolescents and young adults of color used educational activities, skills training, and discussion to explore the cumulative effects of race and gender related stressors, the complexities of navigating multiple social group memberships, and coping with oppression through activism (e.g., the Black Lives Matter movement; Poquiz et al., 2022). Participants reported appreciation of a supportive space to process discrimination with peers with similar identities and challenges, such as navigating racist and antitrans content on social media. An intersectional lens can also add important nuance to cognitive behavioral therapy approaches for TNB POCs. CBT has been adapted to affirm TNB populations and has been used to transform negative emotions (e.g., shame) and maladaptive behaviors (e.g., excessive substance use) that arise from internalized transprejudice (Austin et al., 2017). Specifically, gender-affirming CBT is rooted in unconditional positive regard for all gender expressions and preliminary assessment of a client includes exploration of early gender experiences, as these can establish core beliefs about the validity and value of their gender identity (Austin et al., 2017). For TNB POCs in counseling, culturally-attuned CBT techniques include developing cultural self-awareness (e.g., exploring ancestry, racial and ethnic privileges, cultural beliefs, etc.), building upon cultural strengths (e.g., ethnic pride, spiritual empowerment, etc.), and coping strategies for acculturative stress (e.g., behavioral activation for client engagement in identity-affirming activities, social skills training to develop responses to discrimination; Parker et al., 2021).

Cultivating Resilience as Resistance
The third category of liberatory approaches to counseling with TNB communities of color is cultivation of *resilience as resistance*. MHPs can invest in resilience as resistance for TNB people and communities of color to account for the environmental and relational circumstances the client navigates at the intersection of their race and gender. Defining resilience as a process impacted by societal conditions and communal resources more accurately reflects the lived experiences of systemically marginalized individuals than defining resilience as an innate individual trait (Singh, 2016). However, TNB POCs may face obstacles to resources that contribute to community resilience, such as a sense of belonging, due to racial and gender discrimination even within LGBTQ+ or TNB spaces (Parmenter & Galliher, 2024; Stone et al., 2020). Within clinical practice, MHPs must account both for the value of communal resources in resilience processes and the barriers that TNB POCs may face in accessing them. For example, while positive associations have been found between religiosity and TNB POCs' psychological well-being, rather than simply encouraging participation in religious traditions that may be culturally significant, MHPs can uplift a client's priorities for their spiritual life while supporting recovery from any religious trauma (Coburn et al., 2023). It is the identification of such resources, especially those that may not be easily accessible, and the agentic use of them that establishes resilience as a practice of resistance. MHPs can support TNB POCs in developing resilience as resistance by acknowledging the barriers marginalization creates and leaning into opportunities for empowerment and liberation. We have outlined seven points of therapeutic intervention that can foster resilience as resistance with TNB POCs.

First, MHPs can affirm the intersectional identities of TNB people in counseling by embracing the complex interplay of identity factors such as race, gender, and sexuality as well as internalized prejudices, all of which can impact a client's presenting concerns and the most effective courses of treatment (Chang & Singh, 2016). This can contribute to the development of resilience as resistance when providers engage in a collaborative process with TNB people, honoring their lived experiences and expertise and allowing that wisdom to be influential in ways that may not be possible outside of the counseling office. Second, MHPs can aid TNB POCs in counseling and embodying radical, decolonial self-care by inviting into the counseling space the strengths, beliefs, and healing practices of their communities, particularly those that counter oppressive social restrictions and prescriptions (Ansloos et al., 2021). These can include discussing ancestral spiritualities, languages, forms of self-adornment, and culinary and medicinal recipes. Third, MHPs can support clients in finding accessible and fulfilling forms of social justice activism to channel emotions related to oppression into action, develop skills for self-advocacy, and deepen a sense of community solidarity. However, MHPs must be attentive to the impacts of these efforts and be prepared to care for negative aspects such as fatigue, emotional distress, and experiences of violence (Sostre et al., 2024). Fourth, MHPs can support TNB POCs who hold spiritual beliefs or are undergoing spiritual development in order to strengthen spiritual wisdom, coping skills, and empowerment (Ford, 2021). Specifically, MHPs can help TNB POCs in counseling explore religious histories of both trauma and transcendence, deconstruct discriminatory religious dogma, cultivate meaningful religious practices, and discover affirming community spaces. Our fifth point of therapeutic intervention is community connections, which include kinship networks as mentioned earlier (Hwahng et al., 2019). Enhancing community connectedness can include investing in TNB POC's interpersonal effectiveness skills, as well as helping clients access group therapy programs, peer support groups, opportunities to become a peer support specialist, or community organizing spaces. The sixth point is critical consciousness, as awareness of systems of oppression can help TNB POCs develop more complex perspectives and more assertive approaches to their realities while expanding their range of responses to oppressive conditions. To nourish critical consciousness within the therapy space, MHPs can incorporate sociopolitical education, reflexive practice, and multilevel analysis (ex. micro, mezzo, macro) of client concerns during sessions. The seventh point of intervention we offer is advocacy, which can strengthen a TNB POC's ability to identify loci of support in their environment and form strategies to mobilize that support (Lockett et al., 2023). A client's methods of self and community advocacy can be developed through skills training, role-playing exercises, study of the advocacy efforts of elders or other members of the client's communities, and identification of resources and organizations that can be leveraged for social change. For providers and clients alike, community advocacy is a macro (institutional) level intervention that must be implemented outside of the therapy space. In the following section, we will discuss advocacy approaches for MHPs who are working for the liberation of TNB communities of color.

ADVOCACY APPROACHES WITH TRANS AND NONBINARY COMMUNITIES OF COLOR

Advocacy is an important aspect of providing culturally responsive counseling with TNB POCs. Throughout this chapter, we have discussed the ways in which TNB people are continuing to be discriminated against, marginalized, and oppressed (see Chapter 3, this volume, for further discussion of MHP advocacy with TNB clients). For example, there has been an increasing influx of anti-TNB bills on the rise in recent years. When the intersectional identity of also being a part of communities of color is present, there is an even greater risk of facing discrimination, marginalization, and oppression. For instance, in 2023 at least 33 TNB people's lives were taken in a violent manner, of whom 84% of the individuals were identified as POCs (Human Rights Campaign Foundation, 2023). Though these examples are related to policies and violence, it is an important grounding in why MHP advocacy is integral in TNB POC-affirming counseling.

MHPs have an ethical duty to incorporate advocacy into our work, not only with clients, but also in communities to promote and support systemic change (American Counseling Association, 2014; Funk et al., 2003; Ratts et al., 2016). Due to the expansive environments that MHPs may occupy, advocacy may appear in different ways. For example, a school counselor may engage in daily community and institutional advocacy by calling other students and staff in when misgendering TNB students of color, while an MHP in private practice may have to be more intentional about engaging in their advocacy with TNB POCs outside of the intrapersonal level. In addition to the intrapersonal level, the *Multicultural and Social Justice Cultural Competencies* indicate MHPs can collaborate and discuss interventions at the interpersonal, institutional, community, public policy, international, and global levels with clients (McLeroy et al., 1988; Ratts et al., 2016).

When engaging in interpersonal advocacy, these interventions will likely involve working with the TNB families of color, friends, colleagues, or others in their social network (McLeroy et al., 1988; Ratts et al., 2016). For example, when working with TNB young POCs, it is important not only to work with the youth's family, but also to create a space where encouragement, family acceptance, and resilience can be cultivated (Parker-Barnes et al., 2022; Toomey, 2021). In order to foster a working relationship with TNB families of color, friends, and others in their social network, MHPs are advised to approach intrapersonal relationships with cultural humility to develop strong working alliances (Hook et al., 2013). With these strong working alliances developed, MHPs and social networks for TNB POCs may better engage in conversations to better support TNB POCs. Katz-Wise et al. (2018) indicated that the more a young TNB person felt supported by their families, the better their health outcomes were. With MHPs, families, friends, and other social networks working in alliance and engaging in discussion around advocacy, all parties will be able to tackle advocacy at the institutional level.

MHPs will also need to address issues affecting TNB POCs from institutions—including but not limited to schools, the justice system, religious organizations, and the medical system (McLeroy et al., 1988; Ratts et al., 2016).

One example of advocacy in institutions is advocating for TNB POCs with their doctors, as well as their insurance company. As Yarbrough (2018) notes, there are many insurance companies that are not only confusing and vague, but also have policies that are discriminatory. In a system that is already difficult to navigate, MHPs must understand the necessity of advocacy within the health care system (Yarbrough, 2018). MHPs must also recognize that the role we are often positioned in could be considered as a "gatekeeper" in TNB health care. In some countries, a diagnosis is required for TNB individuals to gain access to gender-affirming care (Coleman et al., 2022). As "gatekeepers," MHPs must educate themselves on how to advocate and support TNB POCs in clinical and medical settings, their gender-affirming care, and their intersectional identities when navigating institutions such as the medical system. MHPs of all professions as "gatekeepers" are tasked with reducing barriers to care and advocating equally for all clients, including marginalized identities. This often results in MHPs having to educate interdisciplinary providers or examine their own internal policies in order for their clients to gain access and not become traumatized by lack of competence or systemic oppression. One common way MHPs "gatekeep" TNB POCs is by not immediately providing them letters for gender-affirming care—including surgery—making clients attend a certain number of sessions to "earn" their letter, or letting a client know they are not "emotionally ready" to receive their letter for treatment. Another example may be calling the police or 911 or LGBTQ+ emergency hotlines that redirect to 911 if a TNB POC is having a mental health emergency, rather than providing crisis counseling, resources such as Trans Lifeline (https://translifeline.org/), or a local affirming crisis intervention that does not rely on law enforcement involvement. These gatekeeping practices anecdotally are known to cause far more harm and trauma to TNB POCs in clinical settings rather than protect them. Our own cultural competency goes hand in hand with advocating for TNB clients of color (Doughty Shaine et al., 2021; McCullough et al., 2017; Ratts et al., 2016; Yarbrough, 2018).

Cultural competency of MHPs assists with all levels of advocacy, but especially within the community level. In this level, MHPs will address the community's norms and values (McLeroy et al., 1988; Ratts et al., 2016). When the MHP is able to address their own self-awareness, their support can extend out into advocacy (Ratts et al., 2016). MHPs can then listen, make space, uplift, amplify, and share the voices of TNB POCs that will provide others with the knowledge to dismantle false narratives that may exist, bringing about structural and systemic change within the community (Lacombe-Duncan et al., 2022; Singh et al., 2013). Though in recent years the effects of a high number of anti-TNB bills have led to increased feelings of hopelessness (Tebbe et al.,

2022), continued advocacy work which promotes trans-affirming norms and values in the community may in turn lead to systemic change in public policy within the local laws and policies (Lacombe-Duncan et al., 2022; McLeroy et al., 1988; Ratts et al., 2016). Continuing the ripple effect of advocacy, the more systemic change there is within local laws and policies, the more likely there is going to be change in state, federal, and international laws and policies (Lacombe-Duncan et al., 2022; McLeroy et al., 1988; Ratts et al., 2016).

Community care, alternative kinship structures, and thick trust capital—discussed in an earlier section of this chapter—are all different ways in which TNB POCs engage in community advocacy. In a study conducted with LGBTQ+ communities of color in New York City, many of the participants described their advocacy as being more than just interpersonal advocacy moving towards community advocacy, but rather as advocacy that could embrace multiple levels of advocacy at once (Hudson & Romanelli, 2020). Clients, however, may face barriers accessing these community supports; this is where MHPs may have opportunities to engage in advocacy with TNB people and communities of color.

Let us use the following case study as an example about employed TNB POCs with limited social supports: Mariel is a 27-year-old, bilingual, trans woman who moved into town about 7 months ago.[1] She originally began services with an MHP seeking support in adapting to life in a new environment. Mariel enjoys her job, has built some friendships, and is financially secure enough to pay for necessities and have a small emergency fund. Mariel, however, is finding it difficult to find a community that can understand her lived experiences as a TNB POC, especially as someone who lived out of the country for most of her life. Mariel is running low on hormone therapy medication and having difficulty finding a bilingual doctor who is open to new patients. What are some first steps that MHPs may take to be able to engage in advocacy with Mariel?

The answers may differ depending on the resources available to certain MHPs. For example, if there is a local LGBTQ+ Center in town, an MHP could find information on whether they offer affinity groups for TNB POCs in order to help Mariel potentially find a community with shared lived experiences. If there is no LGBTQ+ Center nearby, and the MHP knows that there is a need for TNB POCs to find a community space, the MHP may engage in advocacy by starting their own affinity group for TNB POCs. Depending on Mariel's preferences in regard to telehealth, perhaps even an online affinity group might be an option. Advocating for Mariel's medical care may look like providing a list of bilingual doctors open to new patients, providing resources to local mutual aid

---

[1] This is a fictional case example based on a composite sketch of multiple clients.

communities, or any other resources available remotely. By engaging in advocacy, the hope is to assist in providing Mariel with opportunities to build community care, alternative kinship structures, and thick trust capital.

Advocacy can look many different ways, some of which will be more visible than others, but all forms equally as important. Some examples include, but are not limited to, an email signature including pronouns in both English and other languages the MHP speaks, working with TNB POCs as a TNB MHP of color, lists of local inclusive resources for TNB communities of color, attending workshops on advocating for TNB POCs, and voting for legal rights. The list is ever growing, and we all have the capability to advocate for TNB communities of color.

CHAPTER SUMMARY

In this chapter, we discussed the evolving landscape of counseling and psychological practice with TNB communities of color. We have outlined some instances of the history of harm done in the counseling environment to TNB communities of color and provided examples to support the importance of understanding intersectional oppression for TNB POCs. MHPs increasing their working knowledge of mutual aid practices and how to effectively utilize the three realms of inquiry provide clinically oriented frameworks toward building an anti-oppressive practice. We have also described examples of counseling approaches and liberatory practices, however this information only functions successfully when MHPs are fully dedicated to continuous growth, examining their own identities, advocating, and promoting anti-racist liberatory practices in all areas of their work. Nothing less will accomplish these goals. Our greatest hope is that MHPs, and those who train them, understand that the escalating attacks on TNB people will always land disproportionately on TNB communities of color, so there is simultaneously an opportunity to reimagine what we consider to be affirming mental health care with TNB communities of color while uplifting and deepening mutual aid networks for TNB people.

REFERENCES

Abreu, R. L., Sostre, J. P., Gonzalez, K. A., Lockett, G., Matsuno, E., & Mosley, D. V. (2022). Impact of gender-affirming care bans on transgender and gender diverse youth: Parental figures' perspective. *Journal of Family Psychology, 36*(5), 643–652. https://doi.org/10.1037/fam0000987

Agénor, M., Geffen, S. R., Zubizarreta, D., Jones, R., Giraldo, S., McGuirk, A., Caballero, M., & Gordon, A. R. (2022). Experiences of and resistance to multiple discrimination in health care settings among transmasculine people of color. *BMC Health Services Research, 22*(1), 369. https://doi.org/10.1186/s12913-022-07729-5

American Counseling Association. (2014). *ACA Code of Ethics.* https://www.counseling.org/docs/default-source/default-document-library/ethics/2014-aca-code-of-ethics.pdf

Angelino, A. C., Bell, S., Roxby, A., Thomas, M., Leston, J., Coker, T. R., & Crouch, J. M. (2020). Developing resources for American Indian/Alaska Native transgender and two-spirit youth, their relatives, and healthcare providers. *Progress in Community Health Partnerships, 14*(4), 509–516. https://doi.org/10.1353/cpr.2020.0056

Ansloos, J., Zantingh, D., Ward, K., McCormick, S., & Bloom Siriwattakanon, C. (2021). Radical care and decolonial futures: Conversations on identity, health, and spirituality with Indigenous queer, trans, and two-spirit youth. *International Journal of Child, Youth & Family Studies, 12*(3–4), 74–103. https://doi.org/10.18357/ijcyfs123-4202120340

Apodaca, C., Casanova-Perez, R., Bascom, E., Mohanraj, D., Lane, C., Vidyarthi, D., Beneteau, E., Sabin, J., Pratt, W., Weibel, N., & Hartzler, A. L. (2022). Maybe they had a bad day: How LGBTQ and BIPOC patients react to bias in healthcare and struggle to speak out. *Journal of the American Medical Informatics Association, 29*(12), 2075–2082. https://doi.org/10.1093/jamia/ocac142

Arora, S., Gonzalez, K. A., Abreu, R. L., & Gloster, C. (2022). "Therapy can be restorative, but can also be really harmful": Therapy experiences of QTBIPOC clients. *Psychotherapy, 59*(4), 498–510. https://doi.org/10.1037/pst0000443

August-Rae, B. C., Baker, J. T., & Buzzanell, P. M. (2024). "Not just rebellious, it's revolutionary": Do-it-yourself hormone replacement therapy as liberatory harm reduction. *Social Science & Medicine, 345*, 116681. https://doi.org/10.1016/j.socscimed.2024.116681

Austin, A., Craig, S. L., & Alessi, E. J. (2017). Affirmative cognitive behavior therapy with transgender and gender nonconforming adults. *The Psychiatric Clinics of North America, 40*(1), 141–156. https://doi.org/10.1016/j.psc.2016.10.003

Austin, A., Dentato, M. P., Holzworth, J., Ast, R., Verdino, A. P., Alessi, E. J., Eaton, A., & Craig, S. L. (2023). Artistic expression as a source of resilience for transgender and gender diverse young people. *Journal of LGBT Youth, 20*(2), 301–325. https://doi.org/10.1080/19361653.2021.2009080

Barrita, A., Hixson, K., Kachen, A., Wong-Padoongpatt, G., & Krishen, A. (2023). Centering the margins: A moderation study examining cisgender privilege among LGBTQ+ BIPoC college students facing intersectional microaggressions. *Psychology of Sexual Orientation and Gender Diversity, 11*(4), 563–573. https://doi.org/10.1037/sgd0000636

Berke, D. S., Liautaud, M. M., Chen, D., & Sloan, C. A. (2022). Applying cognitive behavioral principles to promote health in transgender and gender diverse individuals. *Cognitive and Behavioral Practice.* Advance online publication. https://doi.org/10.1016/j.cbpra.2022.05.002

Chang, S. C., & Singh, A. A. (2016). Affirming psychological practice with transgender and gender nonconforming people of color. *Psychology of Sexual Orientation and Gender Diversity, 3*(2), 140–147. https://doi.org/10.1037/sgd0000153

Chazan, M., & Baldwin, M. (2021). Queering generativity and futurity: LGBTQ2IA+ stories of resistance, resurgence, and resilience. *International Journal of Ageing and Later Life, 15*(1), 73–102. https://doi.org/10.3384/ijal.1652-8670.1574

Coburn, K. O., Vennum, A., McGeorge, C. R., Stafford Markham, M., & Spencer, C. M. (2023). "It's like a happy little affirmation circle": A grounded theory study of nonbinary peoples' internal processes for navigating binary gender norms. *International Journal of Transgender Health, 25*(4), 751–769. https://doi.org/10.1080/26895269.2023.2268052

Coleman, E., Radix, A. E., Bouman, W. P., Brown, G. R., de Vries, A. L. C., Deutsch, M. B., Ettner, R., Fraser, L., Goodman, M., Green, J., Hancock, A. B., Johnson, T. W., Karasic, D. H., Knudson, G. A., Leibowitz, S. F., Meyer-Bahlburg, H. F. L., Monstrey, S. J., Motmans, J., Nahata, L., ... Arcelus, J. (2022). Standards of care for the health of transgender and gender diverse people, version 8. *International Journal of Transgender Health, 23*(Suppl. 1), S1–S259. https://doi.org/10.1080/26895269.2022.2100644

Comas-Díaz, L., & Jacobsen, F. M. (2024). Decolonial psychotherapy: Joining the circle, healing the wound. In L. Comas-Díaz, H. Y. Adames, & N. Y. Chavez-Dueñas (Eds.), *Decolonial psychology: Toward anticolonial theories, research, training, and practice* (pp. 295–320). American Psychological Association. https://doi.org/10.1037/0000376-013

Compton, E., & Morgan, G. (2022). The experiences of psychological therapy amongst people who identify as transgender or gender non-conforming: A systematic review of qualitative research. *Journal of Feminist Family Therapy, 34*(3–4), 225–248. https://doi.org/10.1080/08952833.2022.2068843

Day-Vines, N. L., Booker Ammah, B., Steen, S., & Arnold, K. M. (2018). Getting comfortable with discomfort: Preparing counselor trainees to broach racial, ethnic, and cultural factors with clients during counseling. *International Journal for the Advancement of Counseling, 40*(2), 89–104. https://doi.org/10.1007/s10447-017-9308-9

Dolan, C. V., & Garvey, J. C. (2024). Dismantling gender binaries: An emergent model for nonbinary identity development. *Journal of Women and Gender in Higher Education, 17*(3), 167–185. https://doi.org/10.1080/26379112.2024.2306850

Domínguez, D. G., & Noriega, M. (2022). Testimonios in the mouth of the dragon: A call for Black liberation in psychology. *Journal of Counseling Psychology, 69*(2), 146–156. https://doi.org/10.1037/cou0000577

Doyle, D. M. (2022). Transgender identity: Development, management and affirmation. *Current Opinion in Psychology, 48*, 101467. https://doi.org/10.1016/j.copsyc.2022.101467

Dunham, Y., & Olson, K. R. (2018). Beyond discrete categories: Studying multiracial, intersex, and transgender children will strengthen basic developmental science. *Journal of Cognition and Development, 17*(4), 642–665. https://doi.org/10.1080/15248372.2016.1195388

Duran, E. (2019). *Healing the soul wound: Trauma-informed counseling for Indigenous communities*. Teachers College Press.

Edwards, O. W., Lev, E., Obedin-Maliver, J., Lunn, M. R., Lubensky, M. E., Capriotti, M. R., Garrett-Walker, J. J., & Flentje, A. (2023). Our pride, our joy: An intersectional constructivist grounded theory analysis of resources that promote resilience in SGM communities. *PLOS One, 18*(2), e0280787. Advance online publication. https://doi.org/10.1371/journal.pone.0280787

Erby, A. N., & White, M. E. (2020). Broaching partially-shared identities: Critically interrogating power and intragroup dynamics in counseling practice with trans people of Color. *International Journal of Transgender Health, 23*(1–2), 122–132. https://doi.org/10.1080/26895269.2020.1838389

Etengoff, C., & Rodriguez, E. M. (2022). "At its core, Islam is about standing with the oppressed": Exploring transgender Muslims' religious resilience. *Psychology of Religion and Spirituality, 14*(4), 480–492. https://doi.org/10.1037/rel0000325

Farvid, P., Vance, T. A., Klein, S. L., Nikiforova, Y., Rubin, L. R., & Lopez, F. G. (2021). The health and wellbeing of transgender and gender non-conforming people of colour in the United States: A systematic literature search and review. *Journal of Community & Applied Social Psychology, 31*(6), 703–731. https://doi.org/10.1002/casp.2555

Flores, A. R., Brown, T. N. T., & Herman, J. L. (2016). *Race and ethnicity of adults who identify as transgender in the United States*. The Williams Institute.

Ford, D. (2021). The salve and the sting of religion/spirituality in queer and transgender BIPOC. In K. L. Nadal & M. Scharrón-del Río (Eds.), *Queer psychology: Intersectional perspectives* (pp. 275–290). Springer.

Funk, M., Saraceno, B., Minoletti, A., & World Health Organization. (2003). *Advocacy for mental health: Mental health policy and service guidance package*. World Health Organization.

Galupo, M. P., & Orphanidys, J. C. (2022). Transgender Black, Indigenous, and people of color: Intersections of oppression. *International Journal of Transgender Health, 23*(1-2), 1–4. https://doi.org/10.1080/26895269.2022.2020035

Goates, J. D., Szymanski, D. M., Pulice-Farrow, L., & Gonzalez, K. A. (2024). "Me being myself isn't a barrier": Identity and praxis of nonbinary psychotherapists. *Journal of Counseling Psychology, 71*(1), 48–62. https://doi.org/10.1037/cou0000718

Golden, R. L., & Oransky, M. (2019). An intersectional approach to therapy with transgender adolescents and their families. *Archives of Sexual Behavior, 48*(7), 2011–2025. https://doi.org/10.1007/s10508-018-1354-9

Hailey, J., Burton, W., & Arscott, J. (2020). We are family: Chosen and created families as a protective factor against racialized trauma and anti-LGBTQ oppression among African American sexual and gender minority youth. *Journal of GLBT Family Studies, 16*(2), 176–191. https://doi.org/10.1080/1550428X.2020.1724133

Hendricks, M. L., & Testa, R. J. (2012). A conceptual framework for clinical work with transgender and gender nonconforming clients: An adaptation of the Minority Stress Model. *Professional Psychology: Research and Practice, 43*(5), 460–467. https://doi.org/10.1037/a0029597

Holloway, B. T., Gottlieb, K. G., & Cason, A. R. (2023). Exploring the experiences of transgender & nonbinary individuals working on cisgender-led research projects. *Affilia, 38*(2), 175–189. https://doi.org/10.1177/08861099221134724

Holloway, B. T., Hostetter, C. R., Morris, K., Kynn, J., & Kilby, M. (2023). "We're all we have": Envisioning the future of mutual aid from queer and trans perspectives. *Journal of Sociology and Social Welfare, 50*(1), 155. https://doi.org/10.15453/0191-5096.4693

Hook, J. N., Davis, D. E., Owen, J., Worthington, E. L., Jr., & Utsey, S. O. (2013). Cultural humility: Measuring openness to culturally diverse clients. *Journal of Counseling Psychology, 60*(3), 353–366. https://doi.org/10.1037/a0032595

Horne, S. G., Levitt, H. M., Sweeney, K. K., Puckett, J. A., & Hampton, M. L. (2015). African American gay family networks: An entry point for HIV prevention. *Journal of Sex Research, 52*(7), 807–820. https://doi.org/10.1080/00224499.2014.901285

Hudson, K. D., & Romanelli, M. (2020, July). "We are powerful people": Health-promoting strengths of LGBTQ communities of color. *Qualitative Health Research, 30*(8), 1156–1170. https://doi.org/10.1177/1049732319837572

Human Rights Campaign Foundation. (2023, November 20). *The epidemic of violence against the transgender and gender non-conforming community in the United States.* HRC Digital Reports. https://reports.hrc.org/an-epidemic-of-violence-2023

Huynh, J. (2023). "Family is the beginning but not the end": Intergenerational LGBTQ chosen family, social support, and health in a Vietnamese American community organization. *Journal of Homosexuality, 70*(7), 1240–1262. https://doi.org/10.1080/00918369.2021.2018879

Hwahng, S. J., Allen, B., Zadoretzky, C., Barber, H., McKnight, C., & Des Jarlais, D. (2019). Alternative kinship structures, resilience and social support among immigrant trans Latinas in the USA. *Culture, Health & Sexuality, 21*(1), 1–15. https://doi.org/10.1080/13691058.2018.1440323

Hwahng, S. J., Allen, B., Zadoretzky, C., Barber Doucet, H., McKnight, C., & Des Jarlais, D. (2021). Thick trust, thin trust, social capital, and health outcomes among trans women of color in New York City. *International Journal of Transgender Health, 23*(1–2), 214–231. https://doi.org/10.1080/26895269.2021.1889427

Hwahng, S. J., & Nuttbrock, L. (2007). Sex workers, fem queens, and cross-dressers: Differential marginalizations and HIV vulnerabilities among three ethnocultural male-to-female transgender communities in New York City. *Sexuality Research & Social Policy, 4*(4), 36–59. https://doi.org/10.1525/srsp.2007.4.4.36

Hwahng, S. J., & Nuttbrock, L. (2014). Adolescent gender-related abuse, androphilia, and HIV risk among transfeminine people of color in New York City. *Journal of Homosexuality, 61*(5), 691–713. https://doi.org/10.1080/00918369.2014.870439

Jackson Levin, N., Kattari, S. K., Piellusch, E. K., & Watson, E. (2020). "We just take care of each other": Navigating 'chosen family' in the context of health, illness, and the mutual provision of care amongst queer and transgender young adults. *International Journal of Environmental Research and Public Health, 17*(19), 7346. Advance online publication. https://doi.org/10.3390/ijerph17197346

Katz-Wise, S. L., Ehrensaft, D., Vetters, R., Forcier, M., & Austin, S. B. (2018). Family functioning and mental health of transgender and gender-nonconforming youth in the trans teen and family narratives project. *Journal of Sex Research, 55*(4–5), 582–590. https://doi.org/10.1080/00224499.2017.1415291

Kenworthy, N., Hops, E., & Hagopian, A. (2023). Mutual aid praxis aligns principles and practice in grassroots COVID-19 responses across the US. *Kennedy Institute of Ethics Journal, 33*(2), 115–144. https://doi.org/10.1353/ken.2023.a904080

Kraschel, K. L., Chen, A., Turban, J. L., & Cohen, I. G. (2022). Legislation restricting gender-affirming care for transgender youth: Politics eclipse healthcare. *Cell Reports Medicine, 3*(8), 100719. https://doi.org/10.1016/j.xcrm.2022.100719

Lacombe-Duncan, A., Jadwin-Cakmak, L., Trammell, R., Burks, C., Rivera, B., Reyes, L., Abad, J., Ward, L., Harris, H., Harper, G. W., & Gamarel, K. E. (2022). "…Everybody else is more privileged. Then it's us…": A qualitative study exploring community responses to social determinants of health inequities and intersectional exclusion among trans women of color in Detroit, Michigan. *Sexuality Research & Social Policy, 19*, 1419–1439. https://doi.org/10.1007/s13178-021-00642-2

Leach, C. W., & Zeineddine, F. B. (2022). Sentiments of the dispossessed: Emotions of resilience and resistance. In C. Tileagă, M. Augoustinos, & K. Durrheim (Eds.), *The Routledge international handbook of discrimination, prejudice and stereotyping* (pp. 244–257). Taylor & Francis Group.

LeBlanc, M., Radix, A., Sava, L., Harris, A. B., Asquith, A., Pardee, D. J., & Reisner, S. L. (2022). "Focus more on what's right instead of what's wrong:" research priorities identified by a sample of transgender and gender diverse community health center patients. *BMC Public Health, 22*(1), 1741. https://doi.org/10.1186/s12889-022-14139-z

Lee, J. J., Leyva Vera, C. A., Ramirez, J., Munguia, L., Aguirre Herrera, J., Basualdo, G., Small, L., & Robles, G. (2023). 'They already hate us for being immigrants and now for being trans—we have double the fight': A qualitative study of barriers to health access among transgender Latinx immigrants in the United States. *Journal of Gay & Lesbian Mental Health, 27*(3), 319–339. https://doi.org/10.1080/19359705.2022.2067279

Lefevor, G. T., Janis, R. A., Franklin, A., & Stone, W. M. (2019). Distress and therapeutic outcomes among transgender and gender nonconforming people of color. *The Counseling Psychologist, 47*(1), 34–58. https://doi.org/10.1177/0011000019827210

Lerner, J. E., & Lee, J. J. (2022). Transgender and gender diverse (TGD) Asian Americans in the United States: Experiences of violence, discrimination, and family support. *Journal of Interpersonal Violence, 37*(21–22), NP21165–NP21188. https://doi.org/10.1177/08862605211056721

Levitt, H. M., Horne, S. G., Freeman-Coppadge, D., & Roberts, T. (2017). HIV prevention in gay family and house networks: Fostering self-determination and sexual safety. *AIDS and Behavior, 21*(10), 2973–2986. https://doi.org/10.1007/s10461-017-1774-x

Li, Y., Whiston, S., Wong, Y. J., & Gilman, L. (2024). Clients' race/ethnicity as a moderator of the relationship between the therapeutic alliance and treatment outcome. *International Journal for the Advancement of Counseling, 46*(2), 219–241. Advance online publication. https://doi.org/10.1007/s10447-024-09546-3

Lindley, L. M., Nagoshi, J. L., Nagoshi, C. T., Hess, R., III, & Boscia, A. (2021). An eco-developmental framework on the intersectionality of gender and sexual identities in transgender individuals. *Psychology and Sexuality, 12*(3), 261–278. https://doi.org/10.1080/19419899.2020.1713873

Lockett, G. M., Klein, K. G., Mike, J., Sostre, J. P., & Abreu, R. L. (2023). "To feel supported in your community is to feel loved": Cultivating community and support for Black transmasculine people navigating anti-Black racism, transphobia, and COVID-19 pandemic. *International Journal of Transgender Health, 24*(3), 263–280. https://doi.org/10.1080/26895269.2023.2204084

Martín-Baró, I. (1996). *Writings for a liberation psychology*. Harvard University Press.

Matsuno, E. (2019). Nonbinary-affirming psychological interventions. *Cognitive and Behavioral Practice, 26*(4), 617–628. https://doi.org/10.1016/j.cbpra.2018.09.003

Mazon, C., Badillo, C. B., Walters, F. P., & Gordon, A. R. (2024). "There's preconceived notions about what I'm experiencing": Experiences of racial and gender discrimination in sexual healthcare settings among transgender and nonbinary young adults of color. *The Journal of Adolescent Health, 74*(3), S56. Advance online publication. https://doi.org/10.1016/j.jadohealth.2023.11.303

McCullough, R., Dispenza, F., Parker, L. K., Viehl, C. J., Chang, C. Y., & Murphy, T. M. (2017). The counseling experiences of transgender and gender nonconforming clients. *Journal of Counseling and Development, 95*(4), 423–434. https://doi.org/10.1002/jcad.12157

McEntarfer, H. K., & Rice, M. D. (2023). Working within trans-affirmative, anti-trans, and cisnormative storylines: The experiences of transgender and non-binary teachers. *Teaching and Teacher Education, 135*, 104333. https://doi.org/10.1016/j.tate.2023.104333

McLeroy, K. R., Bibeau, D., Steckler, A., & Glanz, K. (1988). An ecological perspective on health promotion programs. *Health Education Quarterly, 15*(4), 351–377. https://doi.org/10.1177/109019818801500401

Meca, A., Allison, K. K., Passini, J., Veniegas, T., Cruz, B., Castillo, L. G., Schwartz, S. J., Zamboanga, B. L., Michikyan, M., Bessaha, M., Regan, P. C., Subrahmanyam, K., Bartholomew, J., Pina-Watson, B., Cano, M. A., & Martinez, C. R., Jr. (2023). Navigating identity uncertainty: Identity distress during the COVID-19 pandemic. *Emerging Adulthood, 11*(6), 1518–1534. https://doi.org/10.1177/21676968231203031

Meyer, I. H. (2003). Prejudice, social stress and mental health in lesbian, gay, and bisexual populations: Conceptual issues and research evidence. *Psychological Bulletin, 129*(5), 674–697. https://doi.org/10.1037/0033-2909.129.5.674

Meyer, I. H. (2015). Resilience in the study of minority stress and health of sexual and gender minorities. *Psychology of Sexual Orientation and Gender Diversity, 2*(3), 209–213. https://doi.org/10.1037/sgd0000132

Millar, K., & Brooks, C. V. (2021). Double jeopardy: Minority stress and the influence of transgender identity and race/ethnicity. *International Journal of Transgender Health, 23*(1–2), 133–148. https://doi.org/10.1080/26895269.2021.1890660

Nelson, A. (2011). *Body and soul: The Black Panther Party and the fight against medical discrimination.* University of Minnesota Press. https://doi.org/10.5749/minnesota/9780816676484.001.0001

Nordmarken, S. (2023). Coming into identity: How gender minorities experience identity formation. *Gender & Society, 37*(4), 584–613. https://doi.org/10.1177/08912432231172992

Papa, L. A., & Parmenter, J. G. (2025). At the intersection of intersectional identity and microaggressions: An examination of the experiences and identity of sexual and gender diverse BIPOC individuals. *Cultural Diversity & Ethnic Minority Psychology, 31*(1), 175–186. https://doi.org/10.1037/cdp0000624

Parker, J. S., Joyce-Beaulieu, D., & Zaboski, B. A. (2021). Culturally responsive mental health services. In D. Joyce-Beaulieu & B. A. Zaboski (Eds.), *Applied cognitive behavioral therapy in schools* (pp. 65–82). Oxford University Press. https://doi.org/10.1093/med-psych/9780197581384.003.0004

Parker-Barnes, L., McKillip, N., & Powell, C. (2022, July). Systemic advocacy for BIPOC LGBTQIA + clients and their families. *The Family Journal, 30*(3), 479–486. https://doi.org/10.1177/10664807221090947

Parmenter, J. G., & Galliher, R. V. (2024). Development and initial validation of the LGBTQ+ Community Resilience and Inequity Scale. *Psychology of Sexual Orientation and Gender Diversity, 11*(1), 56–68. https://doi.org/10.1037/sgd0000601

Peavy, K. M., Garrett, S., Doyle, S., & Donovan, D. (2017). A comparison of African American and Caucasian stimulant users in 12-step facilitation treatment. *Journal of Ethnicity in Substance Abuse, 16*(3), 380–399. https://doi.org/10.1080/15332640.2016.1185657

Pierson, A. M., Arunagiri, V., & Bond, D. M. (2022). "You didn't cause racism, and you have to solve it anyways": Antiracist adaptations to dialectical behavior therapy for White therapists. *Cognitive and Behavioral Practice, 29*(4), 796–815. https://doi.org/10.1016/j.cbpra.2021.11.001

Poquiz, J. L., Shrodes, A., Garofalo, R., Chen, D., & Coyne, C. A. (2022). Supporting pride, activism, resiliency, and community: A telemedicine-based group for youth with intersecting gender and racial minority identities. *Transgender Health, 7*(2), 179–184. https://doi.org/10.1089/trgh.2020.0152

Putnam, R. D. (2000). *Bowling alone: The collapse and revival of American community*. Simon & Schuster.

Ramos, N., & Marr, M. C. (2023). Traumatic stress and resilience among transgender and gender diverse youth. *Child and Adolescent Psychiatric Clinics of North America, 32*(4), 667–682. https://doi.org/10.1016/j.chc.2023.04.001

Ratts, M. J., Singh, A. A., Nassar-McMillan, S., Butler, S. K., & McCullough, J. R. (2016, January). Multicultural and Social Justice Counseling Competencies: Guidelines for the counseling profession. *Journal of Multicultural Counseling and Development, 44*(1), 28–48. https://doi.org/10.1002/jmcd.12035

Restar, A., Jin, H., Breslow, A. S., Surace, A., Antebi-Gruszka, N., Kuhns, L., Reisner, S.L., Garofalo, R., & Mimiaga, M. J. (2019). Developmental milestones in young transgender women in two American cities: Results from a racially and ethnically diverse sample. *Transgender Health, 4*(1), 162–167. https://doi.org/10.1089/trgh.2019.0008

Roberts-Sampson, T. (2023). Queer and trans foster youth of color: Mapping the margins of the child welfare system. *Dukeminier Awards: Best Sexual Orientation Law Review Articles, 22*.

Rodriguez-Seijas, C., McClendon, J., Wendt, D. C., Novacek, D. M., Ebalu, T., Hallion, L. S., Hassan, N. Y., Huson, K., Spielmans, G. I., Folk, J. B., Khazem, L. R., Neblett, E. W., Cunningham, T. J., Hampton-Anderson, J., Steinman, S. A., Hamilton, J. L., & Mekawi, Y. (2024). The next generation of clinical-psychological science: Moving toward anti-racism. *Clinical Psychological Science, 12*(3), 526–546. https://doi.org/10.1177/21677026231156545

Runswick-Cole, K., & Goodley, D. (2013). Resilience: A disability studies and community psychology approach. *Social and Personality Psychology Compass, 7*(2), 67–78. https://doi.org/10.1111/spc3.12012

Shaine, M. J. D., Cor, D. N., Campbell, A. J., & McAlister, A. L. (2021, July). Mental health care experiences of trans service members and veterans: A mixed-methods study. *Journal of Counseling and Development, 99*(3), 273–288. https://doi.org/10.1002/jcad.12374

Singh, A. A. (2013). Transgender youth of color and resilience: Negotiating oppression and finding support. *Sex Roles, 68*(11–12), 690–702. https://doi.org/10.1007/s11199-012-0149-z

Singh, A. A. (2016). Moving from affirmation to liberation in psychological practice with transgender and gender nonconforming clients. *American Psychologist, 71*(8), 755–762. https://doi.org/10.1037/amp0000106

Singh, A. A. (2020). Building a counseling psychology of liberation: The path behind us, under us, and before us. *The Counseling Psychologist, 48*(8), 1109–1130. https://doi.org/10.1177/0011000020959007

Singh, A., & Awachie, T. (2025). Black, indigenous, and people of color trans and nonbinary liberation: A transcestral journey of critical consciousness, reckoning, and healing. *American Psychologist, 80*(4), 618–629. https://doi.org/10.1037/amp0001388

Singh, A. A., & dickey, l. m. (Eds.). (2017). *Affirmative counseling and psychological practice with transgender and gender nonconforming clients*. American Psychological Association. https://doi.org/10.1037/14957-000

Singh, A. A., & McKleroy, V. S. (2011). "Just getting out of bed is a revolutionary act": The resilience of transgender people of color who have survived traumatic life events. *Traumatology, 17*(2), 34–44. https://doi.org/10.1177/1534765610369261

Singh, A. A., Meng, S., & Hansen, A. (2013). "It's already hard enough being a student": Developing affirming college environments for trans youth. *Journal of LGBT Youth, 10*(3), 208–223. https://doi.org/10.1080/19361653.2013.800770

Soldatic, K., Briskman, L., Trewlynn, W., Leha, J., & Spurway, K. (2022). Social and emotional wellbeing of indigenous gender and sexuality diverse youth: Mapping the evidence. *Culture, Health & Sexuality, 24*(4), 564–582. https://doi.org/10.32920/27956520.v1

Solidarity Economy Association. (2023). *What is mutual aid?* Retrieved from https://www.mutualaid.coop/what-is-mutual-aid/

Sostre, J. P., Abreu, R. L., Lockett, G. M., Vincent, D., & Mosley, D. V. (2024). "I'm going to be visible because . . . that's what's gonna help other people like me": Young Black trans and gender diverse people's experiences in activism work. *The Counseling Psychologist, 52*(4), 614–649. https://doi.org/10.1177/00110000241229232

Spade, D. (2020). *Mutual aid: Building solidarity during this crisis (and the next)*. Verso Books.

Stone, A. L., Nimmons, E. A., Salcido, R., Jr., & Schnarrs, P. W. (2020). Multiplicity, race, and resilience: Transgender and non-binary people building community. *Sociological Inquiry, 90*(2), 226–248. https://doi.org/10.1111/soin.12341

Takahashi, L. M., Tobin, K., Li, F. Y., Proff, A., & Candelario, J. (2020). Healing transgender women of color in Los Angeles: A transgender-centric delivery of seeking safety. *International Journal of Transgender Health, 23*(1–2), 232–242. https://doi.org/10.1080/15532739.2020.1819508

Tebbe, E. A., Simone, M., Wilson, E., & Hunsicker, M. (2022). A dangerous visibility: Moderating effects of antitrans legislative efforts on trans and gender-diverse mental health. *Psychology of Sexual Orientation and Gender Diversity, 9*(3), 259–271. https://doi.org/10.1037/sgd0000481

Thai, J. L., Budge, S. L., & McCubbin, L. D. (2021). Qualitative examination of transgender Asian Americans navigating and negotiating cultural identities and values. *Asian American Journal of Psychology, 12*(4), 301–316. https://doi.org/10.1037/aap0000239

Toomey, R. B. (2021). Advancing research on minority stress and resilience in trans children and adolescents in the 21st century. *Child Development Perspectives, 15*(2), 96–102. https://doi.org/10.1111/cdep.12405

Williams, R., Pride, C., Anaya, J., Nimmons, E., Salcido, R., Jr., & Stone, A. L. (2022). Centering the voices of queer youth in defining resilience. *Journal of Critical Thought and Praxis, 11*(3), Article 8. Advance online publication. https://doi.org/10.31274/jctp.12940

Yarbrough, E. (Ed.). (2018). *Transgender mental health*. American Psychiatric Association. https://doi.org/10.1176/appi.books.9781615378944

7. WORKING WITH NONBINARY COMMUNITIES

EM MATSUNO, JAY BETTERGARCIA, AND NAT L. BRICKER

In this chapter, we describe gender-affirming counseling and psychological practice with nonbinary communities. In doing so, we review the history of nonbinary communities and address societal myths commonly held about nonbinary people. We also describe some important areas mental health providers (MHPs) can explore with nonbinary clients (e.g., gender dysphoria vs. gender euphoria, societal barriers, individual and group resilience) that support nonbinary client well-being, and a case example is shared to bring to light gender-affirming MHP work with nonbinary communities.

USING AFFIRMING LANGUAGE WITH NONBINARY COMMUNITIES

Language related to TNB communities has always been evolving, with the meaning of various terms varying over time and across cultures. Therefore, the terms and definitions we provide in this chapter may differ from nonbinary person to person or may become outdated over time. We provide definitions for the most popular nonbinary gender identities and terminology at the time of writing but do not address all terminology, as there are hundreds of nonbinary gender identity labels and new language is constantly emerging

---

https://doi.org/10.1037/0000471-008
Affirmative Counseling and Psychological Practice With Trans and Nonbinary Clients, Second Edition, A. Singh and R. McCullough (Editors)
Copyright © 2026 by the American Psychological Association. All rights reserved.

to capture the nuanced and unique experiences of gender (Nonbinary Wiki, 2023). Becoming familiar with common nonbinary language and terms—while maintaining humility and acknowledgment of each client's unique experience of gender (Matsuno, 2019)—is a crucial aspect of gender-affirming work. It may be helpful for MHPs to check in with clients about their responses to different terminology.

Nonbinary is an umbrella term that refers to genders outside of the gender binary and refers to those who do not exclusively identify as a man or woman (Matsuno & Budge, 2017; Nonbinary Wiki, 2023). The term nonbinary can also be used as an identity label in addition to an umbrella term. People with nonbinary gender identities experience their gender in a number of ways including but not limited to not identifying with or relating to any gender (e.g., *agender, genderless*), identifying with multiple genders either simultaneously or at different times (e.g., *bigender, multigender*), experiencing fluidity within their gender identity or expression that changes over time (e.g., *genderfluid*), identifying with a different gender outside the binary of man and woman (e.g., *nonbinary, gender-neutral*), or identifying partially but not fully with a binary gender (e.g., *demi girl* or *demi woman, demi boy* or *demi man*; Matsuno, Webb, et al., 2021). The term *enby* comes from the phonetic version of the abbreviation of nonbinary (NB; Kassel, 2022). The acronym NB by itself is typically avoided as it is historically used to refer to people who are non-Black (e.g., NB person of color [POC]; Kassel, 2022), though it is acceptable as part of another acronym that offers additional context (e.g., TNB). Enby is used as a noun rather than an adjective (e.g., men, women, and enbies). Some nonbinary individuals intentionally indicate that their gender is transgressive or nonnormative through labels such as *genderqueer* or *genderfuck* (Nonbinary Wiki, 2023). Genderqueer emerged as a popular term in the 1990s and is sometimes used as an umbrella term similar to nonbinary (Tobia, 2018). The term *boi* emerged in African American cultures in the 1990s and similarly indicates a transgression of gender and is associated with masculinity (The Brown Boi Project, 2012). Other gender identity labels that may fall under the nonbinary umbrella include *genderflux*, which refers to people whose gender identity varies in intensity over time such as sometimes identifying as agender and other times identifying with one or more genders, and *neutrois*, referring to being gender-neutral and often associated with people who seek to remove the major physical signifiers that indicate gender to others (Nonbinary Wiki, 2023).

Some people use terms related to their gender expression to describe their gender such as gender nonconforming, trans feminine, trans masculine, femme, butch, etc. People who use these terms may or may not identify under the nonbinary umbrella. *Gender nonconforming* typically refers to those whose gender expression or appearance does not conform with expressions associated with one's gendered physical traits (e.g., someone with facial hair who wears makeup; Domínguez & Budge, 2021; Nonbinary Wiki, 2023). Gender nonconforming can also refer to people who defy stereotypical gender norms and roles. *Trans feminine* and *trans masculine* are terms that indicate that someone primarily identifies with femininity or masculinity and may or may not identify as a trans woman or trans man (Resnick, 2023); *butch* and *femme* typically refer to masculine or feminine gender expressions respectively (Herbitter & Levitt, 2016).

Pronoun Usage Among Nonbinary Communities

Pronouns are words used in place of a proper name and typically have a gendered meaning, such as she/her/hers or he/him/his. So, pronouns are often an important source of gender affirmation for TNB people. They are also a common and often chronic source of misgendering impacting TNB well-being. Many nonbinary people use gender-neutral pronouns or pronouns not associated with a binary gender, most commonly they/them/theirs (Gender Census, 2023). However, nonbinary people sometimes use other pronoun sets referred to as *neopronouns*. Examples include em/eir/eirs, fae/faer/faers, ne/nem/nirs, hir/hir/hirs, xe/xem/xyrs, and zie/zir(zim)/zirs. Most neopronouns are associated with genders outside of the binary, although some may connote masculinity or femininity (American Psychological Association, 2015).

Many nonbinary people (and people of other genders) use more than one pronoun set, such as using he/him and they/them pronouns (Conover et al., 2021). Some people are comfortable with any pronouns being used to refer to them, and others wish to not use any pronouns and only use a name. Some nonbinary people who use multiple pronoun sets prefer one pronoun, which is sometimes indicated by listing the preferred pronoun first (e.g., someone who lists pronouns as they/she may prefer they/them pronouns). However, others may like to have different sets of pronouns used interchangeably. In some cases (especially among genderfluid people), pronouns change depending on which gender the person is identifying with at a given time.

It is important to distinguish pronouns from gender identity. Many nonbinary people use she/her or he/him pronouns rather than they/them or other pronouns. Therefore, it is important not to assume someone's gender identity based on what pronouns they use and to not assume someone's pronouns based on their gender identity. According to the 2023 Gender Census Worldwide Report (an annual survey conducted with a large sample of nonbinary people worldwide, $N = 39,765$), over 75% of nonbinary people use they/them pronouns. Nonbinary people may experience stigma and discrimination when disclosing the use of they/them pronouns as others may struggle to use they/them pronouns and blame nonbinary people for their own feelings of discomfort, frustration, or shame (Dolan & Matsuno, 2023).

In a clinical context, it is important to provide an opportunity for clients to share their pronouns given that pronouns will be used in clinical documentation and consultation with others (Conover et al., 2021). Normalizing pronoun sharing by the MHP sharing their own pronouns, having pronoun pins, or listing pronouns within email signatures can provide an environment where clients feel more comfortable disclosing their pronouns. Asking for accurate names and pronouns on intake paperwork is a great opportunity to learn a client's pronouns and disrupts the cisnormative assumption that pronouns are evident based on someone's appearance. Further, if a client uses multiple pronouns, it can be helpful to ask nonbinary clients which pronoun set over another they would like, or if the MHP should use them interchangeably (Conover et al., 2021).

For clients who use pronouns that differ from the pronouns associated with their sex assigned at birth, it is important to be mindful of how pronouns can potentially "out" a client as TNB. In these situations, it is helpful to have a collaborative conversation with the client about what pronouns they would like to be used in clinical documentation and when consulting with others. For example, an adolescent may disclose using they/them pronouns but would prefer not to use those pronouns in their clinical documentation which their parents have legal access to. It can also be helpful for MHPs to acknowledge that pronouns change and let nonbinary clients know that they are open to using the pronouns and language most important to them at any point.

Finally, it is vital that MHPs use the pronouns that a client indicates and practice doing so if they are having difficulty. Using the correct pronouns not only affirms the client's gender, but it can also help the MHP accurately perceive the client as their affirmed gender. Unlearning binary gender assumptions takes time and practice but can make a significant difference in building a strong therapeutic bond with nonbinary clients. Nonbinary people can often recognize when they are truly being perceived and understood as their affirmed gender versus when others put them in a binary category (Matsuno et al., 2020). For this reason, we encourage MHPs to make it a consistent practice to recognize when cis binary assumptions are being made and to actively work towards deconstructing these assumptions. For example, notice when you are still perceiving a nonbinary person as a man or woman and then consciously use their correct pronouns in order to avoid automatically viewing someone's gender in a binary way.

HISTORY OF GENDERS OUTSIDE OF THE BINARY

The term *nonbinary* is relatively new with it first being used in the early 2000s and has become popularized within Western Eurocentric cultures since the mid-2010s (Monro, 2019). However, people have experienced gender outside of the genders of man and woman for as long as history has been recorded in all cultures. Most Indigenous cultures had, or still have, gender systems that do not reflect the binary gender categorization that is widespread today (Boag, 2011). For example, the Bugis people of Indonesia have divided their society into five genders including the gender *bissu*, a gender that includes all aspects of other genders combined (Ibrahim, 2019). Another example is the māhū (meaning "in the middle") which refers to people with a gender role outside of the Western concept of gender in the Kanaka Maoli (Hawaiian) and Maohi (Tahitian) cultures (Robertson, 1989).

In North America, hundreds of precolonial Native tribes recognized genders outside the Western gender binary. The term *two-spirit* was created in 1990 and is a pan-Indian umbrella term used by some Native Americans to describe people in their communities who fulfill a ceremonial and social role outside of male and female roles (Estrada, 2011). The term was created to replace the offensive terminology *berdache* used by colonizers and as a way for Native people to create their own terminology and conceptualizations of gender and sexual orientation. Various Native American and First Nations communities have their own terms for gender variant peoples in their communities and not all Native American people embrace the umbrella term two-spirit. Today, two-spirit people may or may not resonate with the non-Native term nonbinary. Historically, people who fall under the two-spirit umbrella were often highly respected members of their communities and given important ceremonial roles within their tribes (Estrada, 2011).

Reducing gender into two binary categories is not natural nor is it an inherent universal system, but rather was created by European Christian traditions (Binaohan, 2014). The gender binary system has been forcibly imposed on communities of color as a tactic of colonization and racial oppression (Schuller, 2018). In many Indigenous communities, the notion of "man" and "woman" did not exist prior to colonization. The invention of the sex and gender binary was used to create a social hierarchy that privileged White cisgender men and oppressed women, TNB people, and POCs (Akpome, 2021). In the 18th and 19th centuries, definitions of manhood and womanhood were exclusive to White people, and the gender binary system was used to dehumanize Black and Indigenous people and justify their captivity (Thomas, 2007). European scientists argued that White people were superior and more "civilized" due to having stronger contrasts between men and women, whereas POCs were considered sex "indistinguishable" (Schuller, 2018). Thus, the gender binary was used to justify racism and was also imposed on Indigenous communities in attempts to "civilize" Indigenous people. These acts have erased the history of gender diversity among Indigenous people and communities of color. See Chapter 14 for further discussion of the role of religion and spirituality with TNB communities.

Gender expansive and nonbinary people continued to be outcast and criminalized in the United States in the 19th and 20th centuries. In the late 1800s, anticrossdressing laws were introduced across the country banning wearing clothing of the "opposite sex" (Stryker, 2017). These laws allowed police to enforce gender norms and harass and arrest people with gender nonconforming gender expressions. In attempts to avoid police scrutiny, some lesbian, gay, bisexual, transgender, and queer (LGBTQ+) bars and organizations excluded and distanced themselves from TNB people (Stryker, 2017). Due to the criminalization of gender nonconformity and the formal and informal policing of binary gender norms, nonbinary people in the 20th century may have concealed their true identities and presentation and may be why nonbinary people lacked visibility until the early 2000s.

GENDER-AFFIRMING CARE WITH NONBINARY COMMUNITIES

MHPs should be mindful when providing gender-affirming care to nonbinary clients, including being aware of the external distal stressors (including gender-related prejudice, victimization, and societal myths) and internal proximal stressors (including internalized trans negativity) that this community faces. In addition, MHPs should be knowledgeable that nonbinary people are often considered a subgroup under the broader trans umbrella based on its definition—which includes anyone with a gender identity different from the gender associated with their sex assigned at birth. Based on the broad definition of trans, nonbinary people make up about a third of the broader trans community (James et al., 2016), and the number of people identifying with nonbinary labels is growing. For young adults, the portion nonbinary people within broader trans community is much higher. For example, a large survey of college students found that over three quarters of TNB students identified with at least one nonbinary label (Beemyn, 2022).

It is important to note that not all nonbinary people identify as trans (Matsuno & Budge, 2017) and several nonbinary people challenge the cis–trans binary (i.e., the assumption that cisgender and transgender identities exist as two opposite, nonoverlapping gender categories) and do not identify with or feel comfortable being labeled as either category (Darwin, 2020). To address the limitations of the cis–trans binary, scholars have pushed for new terminology such as *gender modality* which can capture a larger variety of gender experiences (Ashley et al., 2024). Gender modality refers to how a person's gender identity relates to the gender they were assigned at birth, whereas gender identity refers to a person's sense of gender at any given time (Ashley, 2022). Ashley and colleagues (2024) propose more gender modalities than just the most popular two (cisgender and transgender), such as agender, meaning not identifying with a gender.

Compared to the general population, nonbinary people are at heightened risk for psychological distress, generalized anxiety, social anxiety, depression, eating concerns, substance misuse, and suicidal ideation (Aparicio-García et al., 2018; Lefevor et al., 2019; Reisner & Hughto, 2019; Rimes et al., 2017). For example, 49% of nonbinary adults report experiencing serious psychological distress, a rate 10 times higher than the general population (James et al., 2016). These disparities are due to the minority stressors experienced by nonbinary people as described below.

MINORITY STRESS AMONG NONBINARY COMMUNITIES

Research on minority stress often explores experiences of trans men and trans women with nonbinary people either left out, combined with trans men and trans women, or included as an afterthought with little intentionality (Matsuno & Budge, 2017). Although there are important overlapping experiences, there are also distinctions in the lived experiences of nonbinary people and trans men or trans women (Matsuno, Bricker, Collazo, Huynh, et al., 2024). It is not simply the binary or nonbinary identities that may create distinctions in experiences of minority stress. Gender presentation, degree of visible gender nonconformity, and the types of structural and interpersonal stigma nonbinary people face contribute to minority stress experiences differences. Most extant research exploring minority stress and mental health does not distinguish trans women, trans men, and nonbinary groups, although some research has found that nonbinary people may experience greater rates of distal stressors and have worse mental health than trans men and trans women (e.g., Lefevor et al., 2019). Research has also suggested distal stressors have adverse effects on nonbinary people's mental health, contributing to depression, anxiety, and suicidality (Lefevor et al., 2019; Price-Feeney et al., 2021).

Distal Minority Stressors

Discrimination refers to systemic exclusion from resources or opportunities (Matsuno, Bricker, Collazo, Mohr, & Balsam, 2024). Like trans men and trans women, nonbinary people face discrimination when seeking employment and housing opportunities (Davidson, 2016; Kattari & Begun, 2017). Additionally, nonbinary people experience discrimination when they do not have access to all-gender restrooms or when they are denied access to gender-affirming medical care (Matsuno, Bricker, Collazo, Mohr, & Balsam, 2024; Puckett et al., 2018). Nonbinary people also experience *rejection* at both an interpersonal level (e.g., from friends, family members, or romantic partners) and a community level (e.g., religious communities, various LGBTQ+ communities; Matsuno, Bricker, Collazo, Mohr, & Balsam, 2024). Rejection has particularly negative consequences for nonbinary people's mental health as it deprives them of possible sources of social support. Family support, in particular, is a strong protective factor for nonbinary people's mental health, and conversely, the lack of family support is associated with poor mental health outcomes (Samrock et al., 2021; Valente et al., 2020).

Nonbinary people may experience *victimization* in several ways, such as through verbal, physical, or sexual harassment or violence (Matsuno, Bricker, Collazo, Mohr, & Balsam, 2024). Harassment may include when nonbinary people are asked invasive questions about their identity, body, or transition, as well as being made fun of for being nonbinary or gender nonconforming. Research has found that nonbinary people who are assigned male at birth or POCs may be more likely to experience overt sexual and physical violence than White nonbinary people assigned female at birth (Matsuno, Bricker, Collazo, Mohr, & Balsam, 2024; Shultz et al., 2023). Overall, nonbinary people may experience higher rates of harassment, sexual abuse, and trauma than trans men, trans women, and cisgender people (Lefevor et al., 2019).

Nonbinary people are also often subjected to several microaggressions (i.e., subtle, often unintentional, acts or comments that communicate negative messages to members of marginalized groups; Sue, 2010). One common type of microaggression is *misgendering*, meaning to refer to someone with incorrect pronouns (e.g., using she instead of they) or incorrect gendered language (e.g., ma'am or sir; Croteau & Morrison, 2022). Another nonbinary microaggression is *invalidation*, which refers to sentiments that nonbinary genders do not exist or that a specific nonbinary person is not "really" nonbinary (Johnson et al., 2020; Matsuno, Bricker, Collazo, Mohr, & Balsam, 2024). Experiences of invalidation can be internalized and lead nonbinary people to feel "not nonbinary enough" (Matsuno, Bricker, Collazo, Mohr, & Balsam, 2024). Nonbinary people are also often subjected to *burdening* or *educational burdening*—the expectation they should educate others about nonbinary identities while prioritizing the comfort of others in the process (Matsuno, Bricker, Collazo, Mohr, & Balsam, 2024; Mizock & Lundquist, 2016).

Common Misconceptions of Nonbinary People
The following sections explore common misconceptions that underlie these gender microaggressions.

Misconception 1: There Is No Such Thing as Being Nonbinary. There remains a pervasive idea in mainstream Western society that nonbinary genders are not real (Croteau & Morrison, 2022; Johnson et al., 2020). This results in nonbinary people being constantly told that nonbinary genders are not real, are made up, or are otherwise invalid (Johnson et al., 2020; Matsuno, Bricker, Collazo, Mohr, & Balsam, 2024). It is important to note that the subsequent misconceptions throughout the rest of this section ultimately stem from the core assumption in society that nonbinary genders are not as real or legitimate as other genders. Additionally, this invalidation of nonbinary genders is one manifestation of binary normativity. More broadly, *binary normativity* refers to systems that promote the idea that there are only two genders (Matsuno, Bricker, Collazo, Mohr, & Balsam, 2024). On a structural level, this often involves messages of omission, such as when there are only binary gender options on forms, no gender-neutral restrooms, and a lack of nonbinary people in the media—each of these reinforces the message that only two genders exist. Binary normativity is also related to the broader concept of *cisnormativity*, which is the societal expectation that people's gender identities "should" align with their sex assigned at birth and never change throughout their lives. Research has found a positive relationship between cisnormativity and stigma against nonbinary people, highlighting how cisnormativity and invalidation of nonbinary identities contribute to harmful stigma (Worthen, 2021).

Misconception 2: Nonbinary People Are Mentally Ill. All trans identities are subject to being pathologized. There are health care providers who believe that trans identities, and particularly nonbinary identities, are caused by a traumatic upbringing (Simms, 2020). Some MHPs also misidentify a nonbinary person's identity as identity confusion or an unstable sense of self—such as that seen in borderline personality disorder—resulting in overdiagnosis of borderline personality disorder among TNB people (Meyer-Bahlburg, 2010). Even when MHPs do not overtly pathologize nonbinary identity itself, there is often still a tendency to overly focus on clients' nonbinary identities in therapy, even if the client did not present to therapy with any gender-related concerns (Goldberg et al., 2019). Any form of pathologizing nonbinary identities may result in nonbinary clients feeling misunderstood by their MHP and not being able to focus on their actual goals in therapy.

Misconception 3: Nonbinary People Will Become Trans Men or Trans Women. Nonbinary identities are sometimes viewed as lesser or partial manifestations of trans men or trans women identities or as an intermediate identity one takes on before fully committing to identifying as a trans man or trans woman (Vincent, 2019). There are similarities between this stereotype and that of bisexuality as a temporary identity, with bisexual people pressured to "pick a side." Nonbinary people are also pressured to "pick a side" in terms of a binary gender and may be pressured to transition in a binary way. These notions stem from binary normativity as well as the transnormative narrative that all trans people will fully transition from one binary gender to the other (Bradford & Syed, 2019). While it is true that some people holding nonbinary identities will later come to identify as a trans man or trans woman, many nonbinary people continue identifying as nonbinary throughout their lives.

Misconception 4: There Is a "Right" Way to Be Nonbinary. As nonbinary identities have received greater recognition, stereotypes have emerged about what a nonbinary person looks and acts like. These stereotypes tend to perpetuate ideas of nonbinary people as being White, assigned female at birth, androgynous, young, thin, and able-bodied (Matsuno, Bricker, Collazo, Mohr, & Balsam, 2024). These stereotypes make it more difficult for nonbinary people who do not fit these categories to both develop confidence in their own nonbinary identity and to have their identity accepted by others. These stereotypes may also contribute to negative mental health, such as disordered eating and associated behaviors, for those struggling to attain this idealized nonbinary appearance (Cusack & Galupo, 2021).

Misconception 5: Nonbinary Genders Are a New Phenomenon. Another way that nonbinary genders are often invalidated is through the assertion that nonbinary genders are a new phenomenon. Nonbinary people are stereotyped as young people engaging in a new trend or fad, often attributed to participating on social media websites. However, genders outside the binary have existed throughout human history and the world (Stryker, 2017).

Misconception 6: Nonbinary People Are Taking the Easy Way Out. There are also stereotypes that nonbinary people have it "easier" than trans men and trans women. These stem from ideas that nonbinary people experience fewer minority stressors, fewer mental health challenges, and have less interest in medical transition than trans men and trans women. In fact, nonbinary people do experience minority stressors and negative mental health challenges, and they may face unique barriers to accessing gender-affirming medical care when they do seek transition. A growing body of research has found that nonbinary people may experience even worse mental health than trans men and trans women (Lefevor et al., 2019; Thorne et al., 2019), and there is a relationship between gender nonconformity and victimization (Hu et al., 2024). Nonbinary people may also experience both rejection from cisgender people as well as exclusion from trans communities (Croteau & Morrison, 2022). Thus, there is no evidence that nonbinary experiences are any "easier" than those of trans men or trans women.

Misconception 7: Singular "They" Is Not Grammatically Correct. Nonbinary people experience high rates of misgendering (Matsuno, Bricker, Collazo, Mohr, & Balsam, 2024). This stems from both the invalidation of nonbinary identities and misconceptions about gender-neutral pronouns, such as that singular "they" is not grammatically correct. However, usage of singular "they" dates back at least 600 years, and today there is increased recognition of singular they as a gender-neutral pronoun (Saguy & Williams, 2021). In addition, the *Publication Manual of the American Psychological Association, Seventh Edition*, explicitly calls for the use of singular they in academic writing (American Psychological Association, 2020, pp. 120–121). The argument against a singular "they" pronoun may be a way that people express their implicit negative attitudes and unconscious prejudice against nonbinary people.

Proximal Minority Stressors

The distal minority stressors described previously contribute to proximal (internal) minority stressors such as internalizing negative beliefs about one's gender, anticipating experiences of rejection, and feeling pressure to hide one's gender (Hendricks & Testa, 2012). Proximal stressors among nonbinary communities include internalized nonbinary stigma, anticipated minority stress, forced concealment, gender dysphoria, and mental and emotional labor (Matsuno, Bricker, Collazo, Mohr, & Balsam, 2024). In addition to the broad internalization that being nonbinary is "bad" or "wrong," nonbinary people may experience self-invalidation or find themselves not feeling nonbinary enough. For example, repeated exposure to invalidating messages and others challenging the validity of one's nonbinary identity may lead to feelings of self-doubt and impostor syndrome. Similarly, nonbinary people may internalize messages about their identities and pronouns being burdensome or an inconvenience to others (Matsuno, Bricker, Collazo, Mohr, & Balsam, 2024).

Additionally, nonbinary people may anticipate distal minority stressors such as negative interactions and rejection, which can lead nonbinary people to self-monitor their gender expression and behaviors and feel the need to be hypervigilant about possible threats to safety (Dolan & Matsuno, 2023; Matsuno, Bricker, Collazo, Mohr, & Balsam, 2024). For example, nonbinary people may struggle with decisions about whether to disclose their gender to others and how to present their gender. When nonbinary people disclose their gender, they are often burdened with educating others about nonbinary identities as well as being tasked with proving the validity of their gender (Dolan & Matsuno, 2023; Matsuno, Bricker, Collazo, Mohr, & Balsam, 2024). Forced concealment is another common stressor that refers to feeling the need to conceal one's gender identity or expression or compartmentalize one's gender to avoid judgment and mistreatment (Matsuno, Bricker, Collazo, Mohr, & Balsam, 2024). Altogether, nonbinary people experience an additional burden of mental and emotional energy used to educate others, manage possible threats to safety, and navigate disclosure.

ACCESS AND BARRIERS TO CARE FOR NONBINARY PEOPLE

Binary assumptions of gender exist across various systems and create barriers for nonbinary people to access health care. Across both physical and mental health settings, nonbinary people often must contend with binary expectations their providers have about their gender identity, expression, and transition-related goals (Bettergarcia & Israel, 2018). Nonbinary clients often are expected to educate their providers about nonbinary identities and have their identities dismissed or invalidated (Matsuno, 2019). Nonbinary clients can face some unique challenges when attempting to access gender-affirming health care due to widespread assumptions that medical transition involves "fully transitioning" from one binary gender to the other. Nonbinary people often report feeling misunderstood in their identities and pressured to conform to binary gender labels or expectations and modify their prescribed treatment to fit their gender goals (Lykens et al., 2018; Puckett et al., 2018). Thus, nonbinary people may be prevented from accessing gender-affirming interventions if they wish to transition in a more nonbinary way (e.g., low-dose hormone replacement therapy or top surgery without hormones). While not all nonbinary people desire medical transition, many do, and their transition goals may be different than trans men and trans women; so, it is critical for them to access affirmative medical interventions in line with their goals (Kennis et al., 2022).

GENDER DYSPHORIA AND GENDER EUPHORIA

Gender dysphoria as an experience (rather than the diagnosis) refers to the distress that people feel when their gender identity does not feel congruent with their body or appearance (Ashley, 2021). Gender dysphoria has often been described as an internal psychological process; however, researchers have begun connecting the experience of gender dysphoria to external minority stressors, oppressive systems, and social contexts (Goldbach & Knutson, 2023). Rather than viewing gender dysphoria as a singular internal conflict and construct, it might be better understood as a complex interplay between external interpersonal experiences and internal gender dissonance (Cooper et al., 2020). Further, gender dysphoria is often conceptualized within a binary framework of gender (Galupo et al., 2021), and, as such, nonbinary people's experiences of dysphoria are not always fully understood, recognized, or integrated into the literature. Although not all nonbinary people experience gender dysphoria, for those who do, it can cause significant distress (Austin, Holzworth, & Papciak, 2022) and is associated with a host of negative mental health outcomes such as depression and suicide (see Dhejne et al., 2016).

Gender euphoria, on the other hand, is often conceptualized as the joy, satisfaction, or contentment someone feels when their body or appearance feels in congruence with their gender (Beischel et al., 2021). Gender euphoria emerged from within the TNB community to combat the pathologizing and negative narratives perpetuated by a focus on gender dysphoria (Beischel et al., 2021). Gender euphoria can be experienced as a physical, psychological, or social ease with one's gender just feeling "right" (Austin, Papciak, & Lovins, 2022). Research on gender euphoria is scant, but existing qualitative studies highlight the positive mental health impacts (Austin, Papciak, & Lovins, 2022; Jacobsen & Devor, 2022).

To alleviate dysphoria or increase gender euphoria, nonbinary people may seek to affirm their gender identity via social or medical transition steps. Social transition steps can include using a different name, changing pronouns, wearing clothes and accessories that feel affirming, as well as changing one's hairstyle, appearance of facial or body hair, or use of makeup to accentuate various features. Some nonbinary people may regularly present in feminine, masculine, or androgynous ways, while others may shift their gender presentation daily to match their inner sense of self. Many nonbinary people also seek gender-affirming medical interventions (e.g., hormone therapy, gender-affirming surgeries), while some do not. Importantly, there is no one way to be nonbinary, as each nonbinary person will have their own unique experience of gender euphoria and dysphoria, and will have their own desires for social or medical transition steps. A large, robust literature exists the positive effects of social and medical transition in decreasing gender dysphoria and negative mental health outcomes, as well as increasing life satisfaction and well-being (Dhejne et al., 2016; King & Gamarel, 2021).

RESILIENCE AMONG NONBINARY COMMUNITIES

Scholars have called for more focus on resilience among TNB communities given the historical emphasis on TNB mental health risks and ongoing pathologization of TNB experiences (Matsuno & Israel, 2018; Singh & McKleroy, 2011). The minority stress model was expanded to include more resilience factors specific to TNB communities within the transgender resilience intervention model (TRIM; Matsuno & Israel, 2018), which separates group and individual resilience factors to emphasize the fact that resilience does not solely stem from an individual trait. The TRIM identified having role models, being a role model, family acceptance, community belonging, social support, and transgender activism as group resilience factors and hope, identity pride, self-definition, self-worth, and taking transition steps as individual resilience factors. TRIM also posits that group resilience factors strongly influence individual resilience factors. While nonbinary people likely have similar resilience processes as other trans communities, there may be unique factors contributing to their specific resilience.

Group Resilience Factors

Only a couple of research studies have focused on resilience among nonbinary people specifically. These studies found similar group resilience factors as previous research, including community connection and social support (Hall, 2020). Community connection was commonly reported as a source of resilience among nonbinary people, as being with other nonbinary people allowed for more authenticity and a sense of safety (Matsuno, Balsam, et al., 2021). Finding connections to other nonbinary people may be difficult, especially in rural areas. Therefore, many nonbinary people seek community connection online. Nonbinary people who do not fit the stereotypical image or dominant narrative of what it means to be nonbinary (e.g., being young, White, thin, androgynous, or masc presenting) may have more difficulty finding a sense of community belonging (Matsuno, Bricker, Collazo, Huynh, et al., 2024; Matsuno, Bricker, Collazo, Mohr, & Balsam, 2024). For this reason, making connections with others who share multiple identities may be particularly helpful and validating (Abreu et al., 2021; Stone et al., 2020).

Finding positive role models was another component of community connection that fostered resilience (Hall, 2020; Matsuno et al., in press). When role models were not available in person, nonbinary people used social media to find positive representation and mentorship (e.g., YouTube bloggers or TikTok creators). In addition, several nonbinary participants discussed giving back to nonbinary communities as enhancing their resilience. This often entailed either being a role model to other nonbinary people, providing support and advice to other nonbinary people, or engaging in activism or advocacy efforts (Hall, 2020; Matsuno et al., in press).

Individual Resilience Factors

At an individual level, nonbinary people engage in several strategies to resist oppressive systems and enhance their resilience. Having a sense of pride in one's gender appears to be strongly associated with nonbinary resilience (Matsuno, Bricker, Collazo, Huynh, et al., 2024). Matsuno et al. (in press) found that nonbinary participants described being proud of actively resisting the gender binary system. Participants engaged in intentional authenticity by going against gender norms as a way of resisting cis and binary normativity. Some participants found pride in illuminating to others the falsehoods in the notion that gender is a naturally and universally binary construct. Nonbinary participants reported that reflecting on the strength of nonbinary people throughout history and knowing that nonbinary people have always existed and had important, sacred roles in Indigenous communities enhanced participants' own self-acceptance and empowerment. These findings were particularly prominent among nonbinary POC participants. These processes align with the concept of recovering historical memory within liberation psychology (Martín-Baró, 1994) and can contribute to healing and increasing hope among minoritized communities (Mosley et al., 2020; Singh, 2020).

In addition to pride, nonbinary people describe various coping strategies that facilitate resilience. Contrary to much of the literature on coping and resilience, Hall (2020) discovered that nonbinary participants found using distraction techniques as a positive tool to help alleviate mental health distress. Distractions such as media, sleep, or work helped participants take breaks from the ongoing stressors in their lives. Hall (2020) also found participants engaged in several other coping strategies such as meditation or engaging in creative outlets helped participants overcome hardships. Matsuno et al. (in press) found that participants described actively seeking out affirming people and environments and setting boundaries with and distancing themselves from nonaffirming people as a strategy to protect their well-being.

STRENGTHS AND POSITIVE ASPECTS OF BEING NONBINARY

Considering all of the minority stressors and barriers nonbinary clients face, it is also important to honor and highlight the many strengths that nonbinary people have. Similar to prior research on the positive aspects of being trans (Riggle et al., 2011), nonbinary people report increased empathy and enhanced interpersonal relationships as a result of their experiences as a nonbinary person (Matsuno et al., 2022). Additionally, identifying as nonbinary gave many participants a sense of freedom from the gender binary which had a significantly positive impact on their lives. Nonbinary people have unique perspectives by living outside of and resisting gender binary systems. Nonbinary people report experiencing personal growth, increased self-understanding, authenticity, and resilience because they are nonbinary (Matsuno et al., 2022).

It is important that MHPs take a strengths-based approach with nonbinary clients and resist the narrative that being nonbinary only has a negative impact on one's life (Matsuno, 2019). MHPs can support clients in developing a positive relationship with their nonbinary identity by helping them find community connections, gain more self-awareness and authenticity, and reflect on the positive aspects of being nonbinary. Preliminary research shows promising outcomes of interventions that expose TNB people to positive TNB narratives through media or support groups or group therapy (Clements et al., 2021). Therefore, connecting nonbinary clients to these positive narratives through positive media, role models, or communities can help increase their positive identity development.

CASE EXAMPLE–LUCAS

Lucas (they/them) is a 33-year-old, nonbinary, trans masculine, second-generation Mexican American.[1] Lucas lives in a small college town whose population is predominantly White. They come to therapy after the end of a 5-year relationship. They report experiences of grief, sadness, and fears about their future. They

---

[1] The case of Lucas represents a composite of multiple clients and has been modified to disguise each client's identity and protect their confidentiality.

report feeling "stuck" and blame themselves for the breakup. Their ex-partner, a White cisgender man, disagreed with Lucas's decision to start hormones and often tried to convince Lucas not to take testosterone by saying things such as "If you really loved me, you wouldn't do this." He questioned whether Lucas wanted to "transition to being a man" several times and did not seem to understand Lucas's nonbinary identity. Three months after Lucas began taking testosterone, their partner ended the relationship abruptly, by moving out when Lucas was away for the weekend at their cousin's wedding. Lucas works at a university campus as a librarian but has missed several shifts since the breakup. Lucas feels hopeless and states, "I don't know if anyone will date me as a nonbinary person."

Working With Lucas

Lucas appears to be coming to therapy to process their grief after an abrupt breakup. Lucas also experienced gender-related rejection and frequent invalidation from their ex-partner, which may have contributed to internalizing the message that nonbinary people are not desirable. Lucas's current distress has been impacting their ability to go to work and may be impacting other areas of their life. There are many approaches and therapeutic interventions that could support Lucas. However, for this example, we demonstrate how a MHP can take a strength-based approach and utilize resilience factors to support Lucas.

Assess for Resilience Factors

One of the first steps in working with Lucas in addition to listening to them and validating their emotions, is to assess for resilience factors currently present in their life as well as the ways they typically cope with stress. When prompted to describe their social relationships, Lucas reported that they had strong ties to their family. They described being close with their two younger sisters and three cousins who all live in the same neighborhood. Lucas reported that *familismo* is a strong value to them and that they often have gatherings with their parents, aunts, uncles, and cousins. Lucas shares that they use a different name and pronouns around their family, but that they do not mind doing so. Lucas stated, "Keeping things this way is okay with me because it keeps the peace." Lucas said they feel that their family, especially their siblings, understand and accept their gender although it is not discussed explicitly. Although Lucas states that their parents would not understand "what nonbinary means," they report looking up to and respecting them because they know "how much they sacrificed when immigrating to the U.S."

A MHP may view Lucas' decision to not disclose their gender to their family as an indicator that their family is unsupportive and may be hesitant in recommending that Lucas spend time with them. However, Lucas states that not disclosing their gender does not bother them and does not report experiencing increased gender dysphoria from using a different name and pronouns with their family. Indeed, situational disclosure or code-switching is quite common among nonbinary people (Flynn & Smith, 2021) and may be a helpful way to maintain harmony in the family. Additionally, research demonstrates that tacit or nonverbal forms of disclosure of sexual orientation or gender are common among Latinx communities (Villicana et al., 2016) and are a way that LGBTQ+ Latinx people can facilitate both authenticity and harmony among the family. It is important for the MHP to respect and honor Lucas's cultural values and recognize the ways Lucas benefits from their family support.

Increase Community Connectedness
It would also be worthwhile for the MHP to explore Lucas's connection to other TNB people. Lucas reported that they participate in online social media groups for nonbinary people, but do not know any other nonbinary people "in real life." Lucas describes a deep desire to make friends with other TNB people. They state that they feel like they missed out on developing a sense of community because they did not come to realize their identity until they were 30 years old. Lucas noted having anxiety about going to local LGBTQ+ events or support groups because they feared "being older than everyone" and "that it would only be White people."

Lucas's MHP could help increase their community connectedness by first validating the role of online community connection. Finding community online has been shown to support resilience among TNB people (Cipolletta et al., 2017) and may be particularly helpful in connecting Lucas with other Latinx TNB people within their age cohort. Additionally, it is important to take Lucas's concerns about attending local in-person community events seriously. For example, it would not be helpful to make statements such as, "I'm sure you won't be the oldest person there" or "I know that POCs go to those events" as it would be impossible to know what Lucas will experience. Instead, it would be more helpful to collaboratively investigate local community events to try to identify spaces where Lucas may feel more welcomed and comfortable. If Lucas did identify a community event they would like to engage in, it could be helpful to explore Lucas's hopes and fears about attending and establish a plan for how Lucas will handle potential stressors or challenges that may occur.

Increase Pride and Hope
Lastly, in addition to helping Lucas engage in community and social support, it may be beneficial to address individual resilience factors in therapy such as pride and hope. Lucas showed signs of having internalized negative beliefs

about their nonbinary identity and reported feeling hopeless about finding a partner in the future. Over the course of therapy, it may be useful to identify Lucas's internalized beliefs about being nonbinary. Once these beliefs are brought to Lucas's awareness, the MHP can help the client externalize these beliefs by identifying where the messages come from. Lucas may be able to make connections between their experiences of invalidation from their partner and their internalized belief about their desirability. Lucas may also be able to reflect on how societal gender norms have influenced their perceptions of themselves as a nonbinary person. Once these systems of normative oppression are brought to consciousness, it may be easier for Lucas to resist these messages rather than internalize them. Lucas' MHP can also help Lucas identify positive media representations of nonbinary communities to cultivate pride and hope.

CHAPTER SUMMARY

Across this chapter, we provided an in-depth overview of nonbinary people's experiences, specifically as it relates to MHP considerations for working with nonbinary clients. The chapter described the importance of language and pronoun use with nonbinary clients, the historical and colonial context of the gender binary, and the role of distal and proximal minority stressors for nonbinary people. The common misconceptions about nonbinary people's identities and experiences provide MHPs with a roadmap for understanding the unique and specific microaggressions that nonbinary people may be experiencing, and the research about why these misconceptions are false and strength-based approaches are crucial. By attending to minority stressors and internalized negative messages, MHPs can support clients to challenge these messages while also exploring and bolstering resilience factors. Fostering a connection to community, identity pride, and exploring the positive aspects of being nonbinary are powerful interventions in this regard. The chapter offers several options that MHPs can use to support clients to heal from, cope with, and resist oppressive binary conceptualizations of gender while also living in their full authenticity with pride, hope, and joy.

REFERENCES

Abreu, R. L., Gonzalez, K. A., Capielo Rosario, C., Lockett, G. M., Lindley, L., & Lane, S. (2021). "We are our own community": Immigrant Latinx transgender people community experiences. *Journal of Counseling Psychology, 68*(4), 390–403. https://doi.org/10.1037/cou0000546

Akpome, A. (2021). Discourses of corruption in Africa: Between the colonial past and the decolonizing present. *Africa Today, 67*(4), 10–28. https://doi.org/10.2979/africatoday.67.4.02

American Psychological Association. (2015). Guidelines for psychological practice with transgender and gender nonconforming people. *American Psychologist, 70*(9), 832–864. https://doi.org/10.1037/a0039906

American Psychological Association. (2020). *Publication manual of the American Psychological Association* (7th ed.). https://doi.org/10.1037/0000165-000

Aparicio-García, M. E., Díaz-Ramiro, E. M., Rubio-Valdehita, S., López-Núñez, M. I., & García-Nieto, I. (2018). Health and well-being of cisgender, transgender and non-binary young people. *International Journal of Environmental Research and Public Health, 15*(10), 2133. https://doi.org/10.3390/ijerph15102133

Ashley, F. (2021). The misuse of gender dysphoria: Toward greater conceptual clarity in transgender health. *Perspectives on Psychological Science, 16*(6), 1159–1164. https://doi.org/10.1177/1745691619872987

Ashley, F. (2022). "Trans" is my gender modality. In L. Erickson-Schroth (Ed.), *Trans bodies, trans selves: A resource by and for trans communities* (2nd ed., p. 22). Oxford University Press.

Ashley, F., Brightly-Brown, S., & Rider, G. N. (2024). Beyond the trans/cis binary: Introducing new terms will enrich gender research. *Nature, 630*(8016), 293–295. https://doi.org/10.1038/d41586-024-01719-9

Austin, A., Holzworth, J., & Papciak, R. (2022). Beyond diagnosis: "Gender dysphoria feels like a living hell, a nightmare one cannot ever wake up from." *Psychology of Sexual Orientation and Gender Diversity, 9*(1), 12–20. https://doi.org/10.1037/sgd0000460

Austin, A., Papciak, R., & Lovins, L. (2022). Gender euphoria: A grounded theory exploration of experiencing gender affirmation. *Psychology and Sexuality, 13*(5), 1406–1426. https://doi.org/10.1080/19419899.2022.2049632

Beemyn, G. (2022). *The changing nature of gender in the 21st century: How trans and nonbinary students applying to college today self-identify*. Campus Pride. https://www.campuspride.org/wp-content/uploads/CampusPride_ChangingNatureofGender21stCentury.pdf

Beischel, W. J., Gauvin, S. E. M., & van Anders, S. M. (2021). "A little shiny gender breakthrough": Community understandings of gender euphoria. *International Journal of Transgender Health, 23*(3), 274–294. https://doi.org/10.1080/26895269.2021.1915223

Bettergarcia, J. N., & Israel, T. (2018). Therapist reactions to transgender identity exploration: Effects on the therapeutic relationship in an analogue study. *Psychology of Sexual Orientation and Gender Diversity, 5*(4), 423–431. https://doi.org/10.1037/sgd0000288

Binaohan, B. (2014). *Decolonizing trans/gender 101*. Biyuti Publishing. https://transreads.org/wp-content/uploads/2019/03/2019-03-22_5c9532ee72975_DecolonizingTransgender101binaohan.pdf

Boag, P. (2011). *Re-dressing America's frontier past*. University of California Press. https://doi.org/10.1525/9780520949959

Bradford, N. J., & Syed, M. (2019). Transnormativity and transgender identity development: A master narrative approach. *Sex Roles, 81*(5–6), 306–325. https://doi.org/10.1007/s11199-018-0992-7

The Brown Boi Project. (2012). *Toward health and whole: Rethinking gender and transformation for bois of color*. Brown Boi Project.
Cipolletta, S., Votadoro, R., & Faccio, E. (2017). Online support for transgender people: An analysis of forums and social networks. *Health & Social Care in the Community, 25*(5), 1542–1551. https://doi.org/10.1111/hsc.12448
Clements, Z. A., Rostosky, S. S., McCurry, S., & Riggle, E. D. B. (2021). Piloting a brief intervention to increase positive identity and well-being in transgender and nonbinary individuals. *Professional Psychology: Research and Practice, 52*(4), 328–332. https://doi.org/10.1037/pro0000390
Conover, K. J., Matsuno, E., & Bettergarcia, J. (2021). *Pronoun fact sheet*. American Psychological Association, Division 44: The Society for the Psychology of Sexual Orientation and Gender Diversity. https://www.apadivisions.org/division-44/resources/pronouns-fact-sheet.pdf
Cooper, K., Russell, A., Mandy, W., & Butler, C. (2020). The phenomenology of gender dysphoria in adults: A systematic review and meta-synthesis. *Clinical Psychology Review, 80*, 101875. https://doi.org/10.1016/j.cpr.2020.101875
Croteau, T. A., & Morrison, T. G. (2022). Development of the nonbinary gender microaggressions (NBGM) scale. *International Journal of Transgender Health, 24*(4), 417–435. Advance online publication. https://doi.org/10.1080/26895269.2022.2039339
Cusack, C. E., & Galupo, M. P. (2021). Body checking behaviors and eating disorder pathology among nonbinary individuals with androgynous appearance ideals. *Eating and Weight Disorders, 26*(6), 1915–1925. https://doi.org/10.1007/s40519-020-01040-0
Darwin, H. (2020). Challenging the cisgender/transgender binary: Nonbinary people and the transgender label. *Gender & Society, 34*(3), 357–380. https://doi.org/10.1177/0891243220912256
Davidson, S. (2016). Gender inequality: Nonbinary transgender people in the workplace. *Cogent Social Sciences, 2*(1), 1236511. Advance online publication. https://doi.org/10.1080/23311886.2016.1236511
Dhejne, C., Van Vlerken, R., Heylens, G., & Arcelus, J. (2016). Mental health and gender dysphoria: A review of the literature. *International Review of Psychiatry, 28*(1), 44–57. https://doi.org/10.3109/09540261.2015.1115753
Dolan, C. V., & Matsuno, E. (2023). Safety strategies and the impact of misgendering among nonbinary college students: A minority stress perspective. *Journal of Diversity in Higher Education*. Advance online publication. https://doi.org/10.1037/dhe0000544
Domínguez, S., & Budge, S. (2021). Gender nonconformity. In A. E. Goldberg & G. Beemyn (Eds.), *The SAGE encyclopedia of trans studies* (Vol. 2, pp. 320–323). SAGE Publications. https://doi.org/10.4135/9781544393858.n110
Estrada, G. (2011). Two spirits, nádleeh, and LGBTQ2 Navajo gaze. *American Indian Culture and Research Journal, 35*(4), 167–190. https://doi.org/10.17953/aicr.35.4.x500172017344j30
Flynn, S., & Smith, N. G. (2021). Interactions between blending and identity concealment: Effects on non-binary people's distress and experiences of victimization. *PLOS One, 16*(3), e0248970. https://doi.org/10.1371/journal.pone.0248970
Galupo, M. P., Pulice-Farrow, L., & Pehl, E. (2021). "There is nothing to do about it": Nonbinary individuals' experience of gender dysphoria. *Transgender Health, 6*(2), 101–110. https://doi.org/10.1089/trgh.2020.0041

Gender Census 2023: Worldwide Report. (2023, June 6). https://www.gendercensus.com/results/2023-worldwide/

Goldbach, C., & Knutson, D. (2023). Gender-related minority stress and gender dysphoria: Development and initial validation of the Gender Dysphoria Triggers Scale (GDTS). *Psychology of Sexual Orientation and Gender Diversity, 10*(3), 383–396. https://doi.org/10.1037/sgd0000548

Goldberg, A. E., Kuvalanka, K. A., Budge, S. L., Benz, M. B., & Smith, J. Z. (2019). Health care experiences of transgender binary and nonbinary university students. *The Counseling Psychologist, 47*(1), 59–97. https://doi.org/10.1177/0011000019827568

Hall, C. J., III. (2020). *A phenomenological study of nonbinary resilience and mental health* [Doctoral dissertation, Virginia Commonwealth University]. VCU Scholars Compass. https://doi.org/10.25772/1CM8-JP12

Hendricks, M. L., & Testa, R. J. (2012). A conceptual framework for clinical work with transgender and gender nonconforming clients: An adaptation of the Minority Stress Model. *Professional Psychology: Research and Practice, 43*(5), 460–467. https://doi.org/10.1037/a0029597

Herbitter, C., & Levitt, H. M. (2016). Butch-femme. In A. E. Goldberg (Ed.), *The SAGE encyclopedia of LGBTQ studies* (Vol. 3). SAGE Publications. https://doi.org/10.4135/9781483371283.n64

Hu, T., Jin, F., & Deng, H. (2024). Association between gender nonconformity and victimization: A meta-analysis. *Current Psychology, 43*(1), 281–299. https://doi.org/10.1007/s12144-023-04269-x

Ibrahim, F. M. (2019, February 27). *This Indonesian community has five genders—One of them is under threat of dying out*. ABC News. https://www.abc.net.au/news/2019-02-27/indonesia-fifth-gender-might-soon-disappear/10846570

Jacobsen, K., & Devor, A. (2022). Moving from gender dysphoria to gender euphoria: Trans experiences of positive gender-related emotions. *Bulletin of Applied Transgender Studies, 1*(1-2), 119–143. https://doi.org/10.57814/ggfg-4j14

James, S., Herman, J., Rankin, S., Keisling, M., Mottet, L., & Anafi, M. (2016). *The report of the 2015 U.S. Transgender Survey*. National Center for Transgender Equality.

Johnson, K. C., LeBlanc, A. J., Deardorff, J., & Bockting, W. O. (2020). Invalidation experiences among non-binary adolescents. *Journal of Sex Research, 57*(2), 222–233. Advance online publication. https://doi.org/10.1080/00224499.2019.1608422

Kassel, G. (2022, March 21). What does 'enby' mean? https://www.healthline.com/health/enby

Kattari, S. K., & Begun, S. (2017). On the margins of marginalized: Transgender homelessness and survival sex. *Affilia, 32*(1), 92–103. https://doi.org/10.1177/0886109916651904

Kennis, M., Duecker, F., T'Sjoen, G., Sack, A. T., & Dewitte, M. (2022). Gender affirming medical treatment desire and treatment motives in binary and non-binary transgender individuals. *The Journal of Sexual Medicine, 19*(7), 1173–1184. https://doi.org/10.1016/j.jsxm.2022.03.603

King, W. M., & Gamarel, K. E. (2021). A scoping review examining social and legal gender affirmation and health among transgender populations. *Transgender Health, 6*(1), 5–22. https://doi.org/10.1089/trgh.2020.0025

Lefevor, G. T., Boyd-Rogers, C. C., Sprague, B. M., & Janis, R. A. (2019). Health disparities between genderqueer, transgender, and cisgender individuals: An extension of minority stress theory. *Journal of Counseling Psychology, 66*(4), 385–395. https://doi.org/10.1037/cou0000339

Lykens, J. E., LeBlanc, A. J., & Bockting, W. O. (2018). Healthcare experiences among young adults who identify as genderqueer or nonbinary. *LGBT Health, 5*(3), 191–196. https://doi.org/10.1089/lgbt.2017.0215

Martín-Baró, I. (1994). *Writings for a liberation psychology*. Harvard University Press.

Matsuno, E. (2019). Nonbinary-affirming psychological interventions. *Cognitive and Behavioral Practice, 26*(4), 617–628. https://doi.org/10.1016/j.cbpra.2018.09.003

Matsuno, E., Balsam, K. F., Bricker, N. L., Savarese, E. (2021, August 12–14). The Enby Project: Understanding minority stress and resilience among non-binary people. In K. F. Balsam (Chair), *Gender out of the box—New directions in research with nonbinary populations* [Symposium]. Annual Convention of the American Psychological Association. https://irp.cdn-website.com/b491598e/files/uploaded/APA21-Program.pdf

Matsuno, E., Bricker, N. L., Collazo, E. N., Huynh, K., Mohr, R., Jr., Colson, A. E., & Balsam, K. F. (2024). Development and validation of the nonbinary distal minority stressors, proximal minority stressors, and resilience scales. *Psychology of Sexual Orientation and Gender Diversity*. Advance online publication. https://doi.org/10.1037/sgd0000719

Matsuno, E., Bricker, N. L., Collazo, E. N., Mohr, R., Jr., & Balsam, K. F. (2024). "The default is just going to be getting misgendered": Minority stress experiences among nonbinary adults. *Psychology of Sexual Orientation and Gender Diversity, 11*(2), 202–214. https://doi.org/10.1037/sgd0000607

Matsuno, E., & Budge, S. L. (2017). Non-binary/genderqueer identities: A critical review of the literature. *Current Sexual Health Reports, 9*(3), 116–120. https://doi.org/10.1007/s11930-017-0111-8

Matsuno, E., Collazo, E. N., Bricker, N. L., Balsam, K. F. (in press). "We've always been here": Identifying resilience factors among nonbinary adults. *Journal of Prevention and Health Promotion*.

Matsuno, E., Collazo, E. N, Bricker, N. L., Mohr, R., Colson, A. E. (2022, January 5–7). *"I love being me": A qualitative study on strengths and positive aspects of being nonbinary*. In D. Miller (Chair), *Strengths, resilience, and resistance of trans and nonbinary people* [Symposium]. National Multicultural Conference and Summit. https://www.multiculturalsummit.org/session-information

Matsuno, E., Domínguez, S., Waagen, T., Roberts, N., & Hashtpari, H. (2020). The importance of empowering nonbinary psychology trainees and guidelines on how to do so. *Behavior Therapist, 43*(4), 137–143.

Matsuno, E., & Israel, T. (2018). Psychological interventions promoting resilience among transgender individuals: Transgender resilience intervention model (TRIM). *The Counseling Psychologist, 46*(5), 632–655. https://doi.org/10.1177/0011000018787261

Matsuno, E., Webb, A., Hashtpari, H., Budge, S., Krishnan, M., & Balsam, K. F. (2021). *Nonbinary fact sheet*. American Psychological Association, Division 44: The Society for the Psychology of Sexual Orientation and Gender Diversity. https://www.apadivisions.org/division-44/resources/nonbinary-fact-sheet.pdf

Meyer-Bahlburg, H. F. (2010). From mental disorder to iatrogenic hypogonadism: Dilemmas in conceptualizing gender identity variants as psychiatric conditions. *Archives of Sexual Behavior, 39*(2), 461–476. https://doi.org/10.1007/s10508-009-9532-4

Mizock, L., & Lundquist, C. (2016). Missteps in psychotherapy with transgender clients: Promoting gender sensitivity in counseling and psychological practice. *Psychology of Sexual Orientation and Gender Diversity, 3*(2), 148–155. https://doi.org/10.1037/sgd0000177

Monro, S. (2019). Non-binary and genderqueer: An overview of the field. *International Journal of Transgenderism, 20*(2–3), 126–131. https://doi.org/10.1080/15532739.2018.1538841

Mosley, D. V., Neville, H. A., Chavez-Dueñas, N. Y., Adames, H. Y., Lewis, J. A., & French, B. H. (2020). Radical hope in revolting times: Proposing a culturally relevant psychological framework. *Social and Personality Psychology Compass, 14*(1), e12512. https://doi.org/10.1111/spc3.12512

Nonbinary Wiki. (2023, November 18). *List of nonbinary identities*. https://nonbinary.wiki/index.php?title=List_of_nonbinary_identities&oldid=38577

Price-Feeney, M., Green, A. E., & Dorison, S. H. (2021). Impact of bathroom discrimination on mental health among transgender and nonbinary youth. *The Journal of Adolescent Health, 68*(6), 1142–1147. https://doi.org/10.1016/j.jadohealth.2020.11.001

Puckett, J. A., Cleary, P., Rossman, K., Mustanski, B., & Newcomb, M. E. (2018). Barriers to gender-affirming care for transgender and gender nonconforming individuals. *Sexuality Research & Social Policy, 15*(1), 48–59. https://doi.org/10.1007/s13178-017-0295-8

Reisner, S. L., & Hughto, J. M. W. (2019). Comparing the health of non-binary and binary transgender adults in a statewide non-probability sample. *PLOS One, 14*(8), e0221583. https://doi.org/10.1371/journal.pone.0221583

Resnick, A. (2023, April 29). *What does it mean to be transfemme?* https://www.verywellmind.com/what-does-it-mean-to-be-transfemme-7368672

Riggle, E. D. B., Rostosky, S. S., McCants, L. E., & Pascale-Hague, D. (2011). The positive aspects of a transgender self-identification. *Psychology and Sexuality, 2*(2), 147–158. https://doi.org/10.1080/19419899.2010.534490

Rimes, K. A., Goodship, N., Ussher, G., Baker, D., & West, E. (2017). Non-binary and binary transgender youth: Comparison of mental health, self-harm, suicidality, substance use and victimization experiences. *International Journal of Transgenderism, 20*(2–3), 230–240. https://doi.org/10.1080/15532739.2017.1370627

Robertson, C. E. (1989). The mahu of Hawai'i. *Feminist Studies, 15*(2), 312–322. https://doi.org/10.2307/3177791

Saguy, A. C., & Williams, J. A. (2021). A little word that means a lot: A reassessment of singular they in a new era of gender politics. *Gender & Society, 36*(1), 5–31. https://doi.org/10.1177/08912432211057921

Samrock, S., Kline, K., & Randall, A. K. (2021). Buffering against depressive symptoms: Associations between self-compassion, perceived family support and age for transgender and nonbinary individuals. *International Journal of Environmental Research and Public Health, 18*(15), 7938. Advance online publication. https://doi.org/10.3390/ijerph18157938

Schuller, K. (2018). *The biopolitics of feeling: Race, sex, and science in the nineteenth century*. Duke University Press. https://doi.org/10.1215/9780822372356

Shultz, D., Wong, G. T. F., Matsuno, E. (2023, Aug 3–5). *Examining differences in minority stressors across race and gender expression among nonbinary people* [Poster presentation]. Annual Convention of the American Psychological Association, Washington, DC, United States.

Simms, D. (2020). How myths about nonbinary people impede delivering quality care. *Creative Nursing, 26*(2), 101–104. https://doi.org/10.1891/CRNR-D-19-00088

Singh, A. (2020). Building a counseling psychology of liberation: The path behind us, under us, and before us. *The Counseling Psychologist, 48*(8), 1109–1130. https://doi.org/10.1177/0011000020959007

Singh, A. A., & McKleroy, V. S. (2011). "Just getting out of bed is a revolutionary act": The resilience of transgender people of color who have survived traumatic life events. *Traumatology, 17*(2), 34–44. https://doi.org/10.1177/1534765610369261

Stone, A. L., Nimmons, E. A., Salcido, R., Jr., & Schnarrs, P. W. (2020). Multiplicity, race, and resilience: Transgender and non-binary people building community. *Sociological Inquiry, 90*(2), 226–248. https://doi.org/10.1111/soin.12341

Stryker, S. (2017). *Transgender history: The roots of today's revolution* (2nd ed.). Basic Books.

Sue, D. W. (2010). *Microaggressions in everyday life: Race, gender, and sexual orientation*. Wiley.

Thomas, G. (2007). *The sexual demon of colonial power: Pan-African embodiment and erotic schemes of empire*. Indiana University Press.

Thorne, N., Witcomb, G. L., Nieder, T., Nixon, E., Yip, A., & Arcelus, J. (2019). A comparison of mental health symptomatology and levels of social support in young treatment seeking transgender individuals who identify as binary and non-binary. *International Journal of Transgenderism, 20*(2–3), 241–250. https://doi.org/10.1080/15532739.2018.1452660

Tobia, J. (2018, November 7). *InQueery: The history of the word "genderqueer" as we know it*. https://www.them.us/story/inqueery-genderqueer

Valente, P. K., Schrimshaw, E. W., Dolezal, C., LeBlanc, A. J., Singh, A. A., & Bockting, W. O. (2020). Stigmatizaiton, resilience, and mental health among a diverse community sample of transgender and gender nonbinary individuals in the U.S. *Archives of Sexual Behavior, 49*(7), 2649–2660. https://doi.org/10.1007/s10508-020-01761-4

Villicana, A. J., Delucio, K., & Biernat, M. (2016). "Coming out" among gay Latino and gay White men: Implications of verbal disclosure for well-being. *Self and Identity, 15*(4), 468–487. https://doi.org/10.1080/15298868.2016.1156568

Vincent, B. (2019). Breaking down barriers and binaries in trans healthcare: The validation of non-binary people. *International Journal of Transgenderism, 20*(2–3), 132–137. https://doi.org/10.1080/15532739.2018.1534075

Worthen, M. G. F. (2021). Why can't you just pick one? The stigmatization of nonbinary/genderqueer people by cis and trans men and women: An empirical test of norm-centered stigma theory. *Sex Roles, 85*(5–6), 343–356. https://doi.org/10.1007/s11199-020-01216-z

8
AFFIRMATIVE PRACTICE WITH TRANS AND NONBINARY PARENTS AND CAREGIVERS

DANIEL WALINSKY, JULIE M. KOCH, AND ANNELIESE SINGH

In this chapter, we aim to uplift trans and nonbinary (TNB) families, specifically through exploring the experiences of TNB parents and caregivers. During the time we have written this chapter, there have been continuous and intentional attacks on TNB communities—from legislation limiting gender-affirming care for young people, to school boards seeking to ban books centering TNB communities of color and their history. When we look across history in the United States, we know these attacks are predictable and part of a performance by the conservative religious right to drive voter increases. We also have learned how these sociopolitical attacks influence TNB mental health and well-being, as TNB communities feel less safe and more vigilant about their everyday experiences moving through various sectors of society (Bockting et al., 2020). However, there is little attention to and information about, not only the influence these attacks have on TNB families, but also how TNB families resist these attacks and build healthy and thriving lives.

Therefore, in this chapter, we examine cisheteronormative assumptions and definitions of parenting and how mental health providers (MHPs) can challenge these inaccurate perceptions, social norms, and gender roles. We also review the unique stressors TNB parents and families experience, as well as the resilience-as-resistance strategies and mutual aid resources they create to

---

https://doi.org/10.1037/0000471-009
Affirmative Counseling and Psychological Practice With Trans and Nonbinary Clients, Second Edition, A. Singh and R. McCullough (Editors)
Copyright © 2026 by the American Psychological Association. All rights reserved.

protect and support their families. While the focus of the chapter is on TNB parents and caregivers, at times we make reference to children as well. We make this choice to highlight reciprocal and relational influence that parents or caregivers and their children have on each other. Finally, throughout the chapter, we share recommendations MHPs can use to ensure TNB parents and caregivers have affirming and liberatory experiences with their MHPs. We highlight how MHPs can address interlocking oppressions, such as racism, sexism, classism, and other intersectional oppressions.

TRANS AND NONBINARY PARENTS AND CAREGIVERS

It is difficult to estimate the number of TNB people in the United States who are parents or caregivers. In an analysis of the U.S. Transgender Population Health Survey, approximately 18.8% of respondents identified as parents, with a little over half (52.5%) being trans women (Carone et al., 2021). Despite the difficulty in identifying population estimates, TNB parents have typical concerns about parenting (e.g., child's health, mental health, development, social relationships, etc.) that cisgender parents and caregivers have, as well as unique challenges (Haines et al., 2014; Kappus et al., 2022). The current political and social climate contributes both to potential limitations on access to gender-affirming care and heightened minority stress for TNB people. *Minority stress* refers to the notion that sexual and gender minorities experience stress due to discrimination and oppression such as anti-LGBTQ+ bias (Brooks, 1981; Meyer, 2003). These layers of complexity may increase the stresses or challenges for many TNB parents. Yet, in some TNB families and communities, unique, diverse, and creative models of community care may provide additional resources for parenting that offer family opportunities not always afforded to many cisgender parents who caretake within a cisheteronormative model (Stotzer et al., 2014).

Some TNB and other LGBTQ+ parents and caregivers carefully manage decisions about disclosing their identities. Haines et al. (2014) describe the importance of viewing parenting and TNB identity through an intersectional framework. The authors suggest that although parenting can be "culturally normalizing" for TNB persons, their TNB identities will likely be "treated as their dominant, yet disadvantaged, identity" in settings such as schools or medical facilities (Haines et al., 2014, p. 240). The authors further note that TNB parents may therefore manage their visibility in parenting spaces for the safety of their child (Haines et al., 2014). TNB parents and caregivers may disclose their gender identity to a trusted teacher or school counselor, for example, but they may not disclose to the school system in general or to other parents. Some TNB parents may move their children to more supportive school systems, or may work with school administrators to create affirming environments (Kappus et al., 2022). MHPs can support TNB parents by understanding and validating choices that they make about whom they come out to and when, as well as educating themselves on the potential risks and benefits of being out in systems such as schools and health care settings (Downing, 2015; Pfeffer & Jones, 2020).

CISHETERONORMATIVE ASSUMPTIONS OF PARENTING STRUCTURE AND TRANS AND NONBINARY PARENTAL IDENTITY

Although published literature on TNB parenting has increased in the past several years, substantial gaps in the literature remain (Kelley, 2020; Veldorale-Griffin, 2014). Notably, gaps are seen through the limited use of an intersectional lens in study design that often aims to isolate gender identity without consideration of diverse life, including vast cultural and identity experiences. A preponderance of literature on TNB parents and caregivers isolates the intersection of gender identity and parenting in a way that privileges methodological parsimony over lived experiences. While such a process of investigation makes sense in many ways and lends itself well to an academic model of understanding experience, it also risks minimizing other contextual factors that may well inform perspectives both on gender identity and on parenting practices.

In addition, scholarship that isolates the study of participants' gender identities without explicitly considering the contextual and developmental impact of identities such as race, ethnicity, socioeconomic status, sexual orientation, religion, or ability status risks overlooking the influence of systems of white supremacy, ableism, racism, heterosexism, and classism—as examples of systems that help to shape the development of people in the United States. In another example, existing scholarship in the larger parenting and caregiving literature tends to focus on parents who form binary gender dyads (C. Brown & Rogers, 2020) while there is less information published on experiences of nonbinary parents. Such a gap suggests that further studies of work with nonbinary parents would be of substantial value.

Scholarship that focuses on the parenting and caregiving experiences of polyamorous and ethically nonmonogamous (P&ENM) parents is also rare. However, data from a national sample study suggests that roughly one in five U.S. adults have engaged in some form of P&ENM relationship during their lifetime (Haupert et al., 2017). While such family constellations may be unfamiliar to some MHPs, those family connections may be a critical part of a P&ENM

parent's support and community network. Increasingly, resources are available to help MHPs understand P&ENM experiences. For those socialized within a monogamy-focused relationship model, it may be necessary to explore assumptions about relationships and parenting to support TNB parents who are part of P&ENM relationship constellations.

Defining Parenting or Caregiving

The *APA Dictionary of Psychology* defines parenting as "all actions related to the raising of offspring" (American Psychological Association, n.d.). In this definition, there is no requisite identity of parents or caregivers implied, and the definition is not explicitly situated within a gendered or dyadic paradigm. Yet, many of the experiences of TNB parents and caregivers that are documented in the psychology literature occur in context of larger, socially normalized narratives about parents and families. Still, the gendered systems in which these narratives are situated present unique barriers and, perhaps, opportunities for TNB parents. For example, in interviews with 54 trans women about parenting experiences, Siegel (2023) found narratives about joy and community support. Considering TNB parenting and caregiving experiences, there is a need to consider both a political climate that may induce fear for many people and some of the real challenges that some TNB people face within families and communities. However, such challenges should never overwhelm or exclude the potential for joy, relationships, connection, and community that many TNB people experience in raising children. Often MHPs have the challenging task of both validating the real fears and the culture of violence directed toward TNB people in general—and disparate risks faced by TNB people of color and any accompanying traumas—while also holding space for narratives of joy, connection, and other positive experiences.

Cisheteronormative Assumptions Interact With Trans and Nonbinary Parenting Processes

A cisheteronormative understanding of families assumes that families are structured around two-adult, male–female dyads who care for children, who are commonly thought to be either biologically related to parents or adopted by parents. Yet, while diverse family constellations that fall outside of the cisheteronormative model (e.g., single parents, families with adopted or fostered children, same-sex parents) are common, TNB parents face unique choices and experiences based on cisheteronormative models of families. Some of the specific issues that may come up in different ways for TNB parents relate to cisheteronormative assumptions about gender, gender roles, and the respective division of parenting responsibilities starting from conception. For example, the process of conception and carrying a child, adoption and fostering-related issues, parenting pre- and post-transition, and intersections of gender identity with caregiving or parenting roles may all present challenges and choices to TNB caregivers and parents that might not emerge in cisgender parenting dyads of a woman and a man. Assumptions about parenting norms may be imposed from external sources, such as family members, medical and behavioral health communities, schools, religious organizations, etc., but may also be internalized by TNB people.

Additionally, the ways in which any parent understands their gender identity may influence their parenting. For some TNB parents, an understanding of how gender identity develops may influence their approach to parenting. This is particularly noteworthy as Riskind and Tornello (2022) found that TNB parents of very young (e.g., toddler) children were less likely to label the child's gender identity than TNB parents of older (e.g., elementary school) children. Such results suggest that very young children of TNB parents may experience less gender-role socialization from infancy within their family than might happen within a cisgender heteronormative model of parenting. Given the extensive literature on the early age at which children begin to recognize and internalize gender roles (e.g., Martin & Little, 1990; Trautner et al., 2005; Weisman et al., 2015), such actions may have significant implications.

Assumptions about family composition and parenting roles are deeply embedded in larger social contexts that may differ based on any number of variables. For example, cultural and ethnic norms play significant roles in creating assumptions around parenting and caretaking of children, with diverse roles of grandparents, aunts, uncles, and close family friends. Legal and political realities within the United States also shape pathways, barriers, and practices related to parenting and often work to maintain or mimic cisheteronormative parenting practices. As the political climate in the United States evolves, increasing regulations in some states and municipalities interrupt access to TNB-affirming care, including prenatal care. For example, recent Supreme Court rulings have had a significant impact on childbearing (e.g., *Dobbs v. Jackson Women's Health Organization*, 2022) and open the door to discriminatory denial of services to TNB people for ideological reasons (e.g., *303 Creative LLC vs. Elenis*, 2022). As MHPs work with TNB parents, it is critical to be aware of the roles and impacts of law and regulation on the lives of TNB clients, along with the detrimental impact of such legislation on TNB mental health such as increased suicide risk (The Trevor Project, 2024).

Considering regulations and laws being passed are reflective of the current cultural context and vary state-by-state, the United States is not unique in developing legislation that regulates TNB identities. For example, Swedish laws for accessing transition-related medical services previously required an individual to go through sterilization (Payne & Erbenius, 2018). The impact of such legislation on parenting practice is clear. Although such a practice did not preclude parenting via adoption and fostering, such requirements inherently shaped the process for TNB parents as they worked toward building families.

In an example of how a sample of Canadian TNB parents creatively worked to adapt cisheteronormative structures within parenting dyads, Petit, Julien, and Chamberland (2017) studied the ways in which TNB parents name themselves, as well as the processes that contribute to such naming. For example, they note the flexible use of gendered language of a participant who describes their parenting role as *la paternelle*, a feminine conjugation of the word *paternal*. Other examples of creative renaming in queer communities include the use of the term *guncle* to refer to a gay uncle or a gay friend of a child's parent or use of the drag-inspired and gender-neutral term of endearment *hunty* as opposed to *aunty*, and intentionally using gender-flexible terms such as *sibling*, rather than brother or sister. MHPs can use examples such as these as models of ways in which TNB people have adapted limited and exclusive language and grammar to name themselves in an effort to authentically exist and resist cisheteronormative standards and assumptions. Of course, it is important to note that these acts of naming are organic and emerge from communities—not from the academics who have studied and documented those community experiences. In the following case study, consider ways in which assumptions about parenting, along with opportunities, challenges, and resources emerge.

Case Study: Richie and Sheila
Richie and Sheila are partners. Richie is a white, 31-year-old trans man, and Sheila is a 35-year-old South Asian nonbinary person.[1] The two partners are coparenting a 5-year-old child with the support of their polycule. A polycule is a grouping of partners that comprise a polyamorous constellation of relationships (Cardoso & Klesse, 2022). Richie and Sheila have taken a vacation: their first long weekend away from their child since they were born. The child is being cared for by another member of the polycule, Renee, a 28-year-old nonbinary person, who has known the child for the past 2 years. On Friday afternoon, Renee went to pick the child up from school but was greeted with suspicion, even though they were listed on the child's paperwork as someone okay to pick up from school. It wasn't until Renee was able to reach Richie on the phone that the school gave permission for Renee to bring the child home.

---

[1]This case is a fictional sketch composite of multiple clients.

Once home, Renee was joined with their partner Jack. Renee and Jack spent a wonderful weekend with the child, enjoying some of the amusing remarks that seem so typical of a child of that age. Throughout the weekend, Renee and Jack commented on their good fortune in playing a role in the child's life. Returning home from vacation, Richie and Sheila also shared their appreciation for a community that was able to offer support and care for their child. While their weekend away was a welcomed getaway, as an interracial TNB couple, they still felt concern related to safety as they traveled.

Sheila is very close with their parents who do not know that Richie is trans. Sheila's parents live in a neighboring state that has recently proposed several anti-TNB laws. Sheila's parents have asked Sheila and Richie to come and visit with their grandchild for several weeks during the summer. Both Sheila and Richie feel mixed—but different—feelings about accepting the invitation. The discussion about the visit has brought up unprocessed feelings for both Richie and Sheila, and they feel that couples therapy would be helpful. However, as they look at in-network therapists, they are struggling to find someone who is aware of some of the issues facing TNB people of color and P&ENM people. An extensive search for a provider and suggestions from friends led to them finding a telehealth MHP in another state who was able to see them at a reasonable sliding scale cost. Sheila and Richie were relieved to find a therapist and found themselves both grateful for the community support in seeking a therapist, and also frustrated at the amount of time and energy that went into finding someone who felt both safe and knowledgeable.

Sheila and Richie were appreciative of a provider who was familiar with issues and concerns that can be present for TNB parents, and specifically for interracial TNB couples navigating structures of white supremacy. Further, the MHP's understanding of P&ENM relationships helped Sheila and Richie feel that they would not be judged and that their parenting would not be questioned because they approach child raising in a nonmonogamous community.

PARENT DISCLOSURE OF IDENTITY

Disclosure of TNB identity is not unique to TNB parents, and many TNB people manage decisions about identity disclosure throughout their lifespan. For TNB people who share their medical or social transition with others, there can be a *cotransition*, a term used to refer to the process that family members may experience related to the TNB identity disclosure of a family member (e.g., N. R. Brown, 2009; Haines et al., 2014). In a qualitative study of adult children of TNB parents, Veldorale-Griffin (2014) observed cotransition-related stressors surrounding identity disclosure for both TNB parents as well as adult children.

While adult parents feared family rejection, job discrimination, and loss of friends or community, adult children recalled feeling fear of bullying from peers and stress related to how they viewed their parent. Veldorale-Griffin (2014) also noted that the age of the child at the time of disclosure and stage in the family life cycle may impact the family's experience of TNB identity disclosure. To further illustrate such differences, Kelley suggested that children born into a family with a TNB parent will have a different experience than a child with a parent currently transitioning (Kelley, 2020). For example, some research indicates that younger children may have an easier time with their parents' transition than adolescents (Kelley, 2020). Hines (2006) found that children were more affected by parental divorce and separation after disclosure than by the actual disclosure or transition itself.

Likewise, Dierckx et al. (2017) found that children did not experience their parents' gender transition as a loss because of four key family protective factors. These protective family factors that were supportive to the family included continuity, communication, acceptance by significant others, and attributing meaning. Continuity referred to things like maintaining family activities or some responsibilities (e.g., the parent who always took out the trash still took out the trash; the gender transition did not interfere with roles or responsibilities parents held). Continuity also included things like the transitioning parent still having the same sense of humor or interest in sports that they previously did prior to disclosing their gender identity or transition. Another protective factor was communication, specifically open and honest communication and both parents answering children's questions consistently. The third protective factor was acceptance from significant others, where children would look to parents, family members, and peers for acceptance and validation.

For example, if a child worried about their nontransitioning parent and that parent modeled using a new name and pronouns, the child felt reassured. The last protective factor was attributing meaning, or the time and space for children to reflect, imagine, and navigate or negotiate meanings for themselves about what the transition meant to them and their family (Dierckx et al., 2017). The authors found that although the transition posed a challenge to these families and the children involved, the children also viewed the transition experience as a means for the family and individuals to become more resilient (Dierckx et al., 2017). The children described opportunities for better communication, learning to be more open about gender, and developing skills such as focusing on the positive outcomes. The authors concluded that gender transition of a parent should not be "problematized," rather what is important is how people react and work through the situation (Dierckx et al., 2017, p. 409). It may be helpful for TNB parents to understand findings (e.g., Dierckx et al., 2017; Kelley, 2020) that explicate potential impacts of gender transition on children.

As MHPs work with TNB parents and families during periods of identity disclosure or transition, it is useful to remember that enhancing internal protective factors can be beneficial to the well-being of their clients. Participants in Veldorale-Griffen's (2014) study also highlighted the role of resilience as a protective factor during these times, along with other beneficial strategies such as finding support groups or therapy, and receiving affirming support from friends, family members, and children.

FAMILY PLANNING AND PREGNANCY

Although there are external issues that may challenge TNB people in the process of family planning, Dietz (2021) argued that TNB parenting is "unexceptional"; in other words, TNB people who parent "encounter a cavalcade of barriers that, while more likely to accrue them, are by no means specific to them" (p. 191). Dietz stated that TNB people do not pose extraordinary challenges to health systems, but rather that health systems assume TNB pregnancy will be "exceptional," or difficult and unfamiliar (Dietz, 2021). Dietz's position which highlights unfamiliarity that some providers may have with TNB pregnancies may be bolstered by recent changes in regulations passed by some U.S. state legislatures that privilege the belief system of the health care provider over the health and well-being of a TNB parent.

For example, South Carolina's General Assembly has codified the right of a health care provider to deny care to a patient based on the "the practitioner's or entity's conscience" (Medical Ethics and Diversity Act, 2022), and defines *conscience* as "the religious, moral, or ethical beliefs or principles held by any medical practitioners, health care institutions, and health care payers." Therefore, health care access for TNB parents or prospective parents in South Carolina is codified as being potentially secondary to the beliefs and principles of certain medical providers, hospitals and institutions, or third-party payors whose beliefs or principles delegitimize TNB people. The Supreme Court decision that stated that a business cannot be compelled into speech that is counter to its belief system—even if that means discriminating against a customer—opens numerous and yet unknown pathways to discrimination against TNB people (303 Creative LLC v. Elenis, 2023). For a provider lacking familiarity with TNB people, parents, and families, such a provision may allow the unknowns associated with TNB pregnancies and family planning efforts to be sufficient reasons for denying services.

Although there are many similarities between TNB and cisgender people approaching family planning and pregnancy, some experiences may be unique to some TNB people. Tornello et al. (2019) found that a vast majority (95%) of their sample of 300 TNB parents reported taking a biological pathway toward conceiving a child. Some participants took a cobiological approach with a partner, some participants took a biological approach without a partner, and for some, the child was biologically related to their partner but not to them. Only 5% of this sample reported being adoptive parents or fostering a child. Several studies have found that conceiving and delivering a child through biological processes is significantly less costly than adoption or fostering a child (dickey et al., 2016; Tornello & Bos, 2017; Tornello et al., 2019).

There are important considerations that MHPs should be aware of as they work with TNB people who take a biological approach to conception. For example, scholars (e.g., dickey et al., 2016; Ellis et al., 2015) note the medical, social, and emotional impact of pregnancy on some TNB parents. People attempting to conceive a child through vaginal intercourse may need to pause HRT, leading to a potential shift in both emotion and physical appearance. Such a process has the potential to trigger gender dysphoria. Additionally, Ellis et al. (2015) highlight the loneliness that transmasculine study participants reported while carrying a child. These unique considerations require MHPs to be aware of the ways in which a client's medical and mental health needs may shift and evolve as a client adjusts to changing HRT and physiological changes in the body during pregnancy.

TRANS AND NONBINARY PARENT-CHILD RELATIONSHIPS

A TNB parent's transition can impact their relationships with children. While parental transition can present stressors in the family system, they are also opportunities for increased empathy between parents and children. MHPs can support TNB parents and their children by viewing the transition as a family process.

Empathy and Support

A transitioning parent may have a positive impact on families. Most evident, a parent or caretaker's transition may improve that parent's self-concept. Other benefits may be less evident. For example, Kelley (2020) interviewed 20 adolescents and young adults about their experiences while one of their parents transitioned. They found that participants saw themselves as becoming more compassionate and empathic toward the trans community as well as to their parents through the process (Kelley, 2020). Participants' self-reported ability to navigate and negotiate changes varied depending on whether they still lived in the home with their parents (Kelley, 2020). All the participants reported wanting to support their parents, including offering love and acceptance to their parent (Kelley, 2020). Participants discussed observing shifts in both of their parents' identities and changing definitions of their parents' relationships (Kelley, 2020). Other studies have demonstrated similarly positive relational outcomes between children and parents. For example, Imrie et al.'s (2020) findings suggest that children of the TNB parents in the study were psychologically well-adjusted and that the children and parents had positive relationships.

Stressors

In addition to positive outcomes of parent transition, such as increased empathy and support, TNB parents and their children may also experience transition-related stressors. TNB parents who experience nonaffirmation have higher parenting stress (Imrie et al., 2020). In a study of TNB parents and their adult children, Veldorale-Griffin (2014) found that adult children of TNB parents and the parents themselves experienced similar levels of stress related to parental gender transition, but the types of stress were different. Parents reported experiences or fears of familial rejection and workplace discrimination (Veldorale-Griffin, 2014). The most common stressors for children were bullying at school and having to shift the way they viewed their parent, which included worries about what to call their parent and use of different pronouns (Veldorale-Griffin, 2014). Parents reported that support groups, therapy, and social support were helpful sources of strength (Veldorale-Griffin, 2014).

Adult children indicated that they benefited from therapy and psychoeducation (Veldorale-Griffin, 2014). Parents shared that they wished they had better quality and more information available, and adult children said they wished they had someone else who could relate to their situation (Veldorale-Griffin, 2014). In addition, parents and their adult children reported mixed reactions within their families to the initial disclosure (Veldorale-Griffin, 2014). However, parents and their adult children indicated no change or positive change in the parent–child relationship after transition, which is supported by other literature (Charter et al., 2022; Imrie et al., 2020; Veldorale-Griffin, 2014).

Scholars recommend that, based on the number of parents and adult children who report familial-based stress, MHPs should focus on assisting the family and viewing the transition as a family process or *family emergence* rather than an individual process, (e.g., assessing readiness of the individual for transition) and recommend MHPs advocate for better information and advocacy on TNB parenting to combat transprejudice (Veldorale-Griffin, 2014; Pfeffer & Jones, 2020). When discussing transition with TNB parents, it is important for practitioners and clinicians to be able to talk to clients about scholarly findings that highlight both stressors and positive relational outcomes of transition between TNB parents and children.

QUEER TIME

Models of lifespan development have framed developmental tasks in an ordered fashion, often assuming that satisfactory completion of one task is required in order to complete subsequent tasks (e.g., Erikson, 1950). Similarly, models of sexual identity development follow a structured path in which individuals navigate phases or stages to achieve a hypothesized outcome related to identity. Yet, critics of these models highlight the potential for identity foreclosure and associate assumptions underlying these models as being based heavily on outdated systems of class and gender (Aronson, 2008; Langdridge, 2008). Despite its longstanding influence, Odets (2019) noted that Erikson viewed gaps in his model related to absent developmental experiences of LGBTQ+ people. Through the lens of some developmental theorists, one can view choices such as parenting and partnering as being structured, in part, by similar class and gender assumptions.

Such assumptions may not hold the same validity within TNB and queer families, even when desires to parent and build relationships are innately held by TNB people. Yet, the lives of many TNB and queer people often follow unique and diverse pathways, resulting in a unique relationship to time. Scholars such as Halberstram (2005) highlight ways in which queer and trans people's development may occur in opposition to social and temporal (e.g., cis-heteronormative) expectations, or *queer time*. Understanding TNB family relationships, parenting and caretaking choices, and family-unit structure through the lens of queer time may help some to contextualize the influence of cisheteronormative assumptions that are so commonly internalized both in clients and providers alike. For example, a queer time lens may help to disrupt assumptions about the number of primary caregivers, the structure of the relationships among parental figures (e.g., monogamous vs. polyamorous), approaches to conception, and even the definition of who comprises a family.

TRANS- AND NONBINARY-AFFIRMING CARE WITH PARENTS AND CAREGIVERS

Affirming care covers address not just ensuring TNB parent and caregiver's health and well-being but also helping them address legal issues, connect to mutual aid networks, and navigating public spaces.

Physical and Mental Health

Carone et al. (2021) compared TNB and cisgender parents and nonparents on health outcomes including psychological distress, life satisfaction, social well-being, happiness, quality of life, substance use, and physical health. Although TNB people overall reported more distress, less satisfaction, and poorer quality of life than did cisgender people, the researchers found no differences based on gender identity among parents. In other words, neither TNB nor cisgender parents scored better or worse on any of the factors they examined when controlling for demographic factors such as age, education, and relationship status (Carone et al, 2021). They concluded that the stressors and joys of parenting may not be dependent upon gender identity and that, in fact, for TNB people, having children may be a fulfilling and valuable life event that increases well-being and counteracts some effects of stigmatization (Carone et al., 2021). In another study, Charter et al. (2022) found that TNB parents experienced fear and anxiety prior to coming out to coparents and children but balanced this with their desire to transition and pursue gender affirmation. Participants reported a sense of joy, relief, improved mental health, and improved relationships with coparents and children upon coming out and pursuing gender affirmation (Charter et al., 2022).

Legal Issues

During the past decades, TNB people have increasingly been a subject of national discourse in the United States. Recognizing and understanding the impact of specific changes in federal, state, and local policies on TNB lives is crucial, as is understanding the impact of efforts to legislate and invisibilize one's gender identity. Legal and structural issues that emerge in times of heightened politicization of TNB identities, along with accompanying threats to safety, can be seen as profound stressors impacting TNB people, including TNB parents and caregivers. A recent study published by The Williams Institute estimated that recent state bans and policies left over 156,300 TNB youth at risk of losing access to gender-affirming care (Redfield et al., 2023). Of course, the impact of such a loss has been devastating and the range of intersecting family-related issues is vast. Tebbe et al (2022), for example, found that compared with TNB people who were not aware of anti-TNB legislation in their state, TNB people with knowledge of anti-TNB legislation experienced a heightened potential for hopelessness and less of a sense of belonging. And Abreu and colleagues (2022) found that parents of TNB children observed their children experiencing increased anxiety, depression, suicidal ideation, gender dysphoria in relation to anti-TNB legislation. Further, if a state prohibits TNB children from receiving Medicaid-covered care, the impact would disproportionately affect lower income families. Beyond legislative changes, executive interpretation of federal statutes related to gender identity may create additional barriers to accessing identity affirming care through federally funded agencies. For example, TNB veterans may be less able to access TNB-affirming medical services related to family planning.

The increased access to interstate telehealth practice (e.g., PSYPACT, Counseling Compact, Social Work Licensure Compact) offers significantly expanded opportunities for MHPs to see clients outside of their local jurisdiction and states and may offer some TNB people access to a larger pool of TNB-affirming and knowledgeable clinicians. Yet, expanded opportunity for interjurisdictional practice requires that MHPs understand the disparate range of laws and state regulations. Practically, an MHP being located and licensed in a state that does not have anti-TNB regulations does not allow that same MHP to ignore anti-TNB regulations when working with a client who is physically located in a state where anti-TNB regulations are on the books. This situation may both frustrate and confuse both MHPs and TNB clients. And while there is a unique opportunity for MHPs who practice in TNB-affirming ways to nationally coordinate with colleagues to brainstorm and address barriers to TNB-affirming care, clients should be made aware of the MHP's legal responsibilities and limitations during an informed consent process.

Connecting With Mutual Aid Networks

Although there are numerous challenges TNB caregivers, parents, children, and family members face in family building and other domains of their lives, it is notable that these communities have created mutual aid networks that support them in navigating these complexities. *Mutual aid* has been defined as collaborative and voluntary efforts where people self-organize communities to increase resource sharing and other forms of assistance where needed (Norman, 1977; Spade, 2020). Although research about these networks remains sparse, MHPs can learn about these mutual aid networks created by TNB families that can expand and deepen, especially during crises, societal backlashes, and attacks on TNB families.

For instance, the recent attacks on gender-affirming care for young TNB people under 18 years old across multiple states (Trans Track Legislation, n.d.) have had devastating impacts on TNB families, forcing them to move to states with more supportive legislatures (Alfonseca, 2023). These families have relied on mutual aid networks forming on social media and on the ground in these states to help them access TNB-affirming resources, while also documenting their journeys and creating resources as they face barriers and leverage support (Parks, 2023). Mutual aid networks have roots in Black communities, as they were considered a crucial strategy to survive human trafficking, enslavement, and many levels of anti-Black racism (Norman, 1977). Through the Black history of mutual aid organizations and evolving TNB mutual aid networks, MHPs can learn how to support social connections, increase family resilience, and fill gaps that exist in services for TNB families and caregivers (e.g., legal resources, health care access, religious and spiritual supports).

There are three key areas of mutual aid that MHPs can focus their learning in with TNB communities of color that can enhance mental health care for all TNB families and caregivers: (a) supporting TNB empowerment, (b) TNB community-building, and (c) addressing TNB social inequities (Singh et al., 2023). In supporting TNB empowerment, MHPs can help TNB families and caregivers build collective power and solidarity with one another. For example, identifying existing mutual aid networks and uplifting stories of success while negotiating challenges can help enhance empowerment and self-efficacy in the face of what can feel like daunting odds. In doing so, networks of *chosen family* and *thick trust networks*, or networks built on deep levels of interpersonal connection, can be built as enduring sources of support (Hwahng et al., 2021).

MHPs can also support mutual aid networks through community-building with other local, regional, and national networks of MHPs and other providers who are TNB-affirming to strengthen resource-sharing and access to care. This community-building can include fundraising campaigns using platforms such as GoFundMe and Cash App. MHPs might consider creating their own resource list for TNB parents and caregivers, particularly those in rural areas who might be unfamiliar with safe providers, agencies, and even affirming retail locations. MHPs can address TNB societal inequities by including an assessment of societal barriers TNB families and caregivers face in intake and future sessions, while also providing tangible TNB resources that can assist them along their journey. These resources can include a multitude of general and emergency supports and should include access to emergency funds as well (National Center for Transgender Equality, n.d.), which exist across a multitude of states (e.g., Iowa Trans Mutual Aid Fund). Ultimately, TNB mutual aid networks are a vital source of support in the face of a persistent lack of social safety nets (Vaden, 2022). In fact, mutual aid networks can be an especially important support system given some of the challenges that may occur for some TNB people in the public spaces described in the next section.

Navigating Issues Outside the Home

Some parenting and caregiving occurs at home in private spaces and within a family (biological and chosen; dyadic or polyamorous), but MHPs should remember that parenting and caregiving also occurs very publicly in contexts like school systems; doctor's offices; places of worship; public libraries; community centers; youth sports; and activities like dance, band, and scouts (Edwards et al., 2019; Luster & Okagaki, 2005; Ryan & Martin, 2000). It occurs with extended family and community systems, concurrently with neighbors, and is facilitated by any number of workplace interactions. School-age children spend a large proportion of time in schools, and schools expect parental involvement (Ryan & Martin, 2000). This means parents will interact with teachers, school staff, and administrators as well as other parents and children through events such as volunteering in classrooms, school or activity fundraisers, track and field events, plays, basketball games, holiday events such as veteran's day appreciation, and more (Ryan & Martin, 2000). Parenting also happens in workspaces, as coworkers may ask about children, through the need to take time off for doctor appointments or navigating working from home alongside childcare (Edwards et al., 2019; Luster & Okagaki, 2005).

As MHPs, helping TNB parents and caregivers to navigate the varied systems in which parenting occurs, it is necessary to support a range of parenting decisions and experiences. As much as parents make efforts to provide specific contexts and environments for raising their children, children's interactions outside of the home also influence their development and it may be impossible for parents to shield their children from messages outside of the home. Parents who make efforts to avoid socializing a child into a specific gender identity, rather than assuming a gender identity based on the child's sex assigned at birth, may be able to control how gender-related messages in the home avoid binarism or assumptions about the child's gender identity, messages that come from outside of the home may be unavoidable. MHPs can provide support to parents by helping to bridge gaps between gender messages from outside of the home and the messages that come from within the family.

Reflection: Consider the Following Case Examples

In the following section, we offer several situations as brief examples that could emerge for TNB parents and caregivers. As a mental health professional, how would you assist your client(s) in navigating these issues? What other cultural or contextual information would you need? How might your own family system or beliefs about families and parenting play a role in your approach? How might current state or other legislation affect your work?

Gendered School Events
Stef (they/them) is a nonbinary person; their partner Jules (they/them) is also nonbinary. Their daughter Helene (3rd grade) comes home from school with a flier for an event, "Doughnuts with Dads." Helene is excited about doughnuts! Stef is angry and wants to address this sexist event with the principal; Jules disagrees and doesn't want to draw any negative attention to Helene. They also disagree about whether Helene should be able to attend and, if so, with whom.

In approaching this situation, it would be important to understand past experiences that Stef and Jules have had as parents, the extent to which Jules and Stef are out as nonbinary parents in the school, and whether Helene has had negative attention as Jules and Stef's child. MHPs can affirm and validate Stef's anger as well as Jules's efforts to avoid negative attention on Helene. If Helene attends the event, a MHP can also help Stef and Jules to find opportunities to advocate withing the school system to reduce sexism and biases in school functions.

Family Building
Logan (they/them) is a 35-year-old, nonbinary, single, and asexual person. They live near their immediate and extended family and close childhood friends. They experience much love and support. They love spending time with their young nieces and nephews and their friends' children. Logan longs for a child of their own, though they aren't sure their family would approve and are not sure they could adopt in the state where they live. They tend to be private and are not sure they want the invasive questioning and monitoring required by the state agency that facilitates fostering and adoption.

MHPs can help Logan in several ways. They can emphasize the value of family connection, and work with Logan to explore ways to talk to at least some of their family members about their desire to have a child. A MHP can also support Logan by learning more about what potential foster or adoptive parents can expect during the adoption process in the state. If Logan decides to pursue the process, a MHP could help them to prepare for the questions and oversight that they could expect as they move through the fostering or adoption process.

A Child Is Concerned About a Parent's Gender Identity
Amy (she/her) and Carlos (he/him) met in college, when they both identified as lesbian women. They had two children through a sperm donor. When the children were babies, Carlos went through a social gender transition and currently identifies as a man. Amy and Carlos appear, to acquaintances, as a straight couple; they are not out to anyone except close family and friends. Now, their son, Alfie, is in high school and is active in Boy Scouts. Alfie has been invited to

a scouts and dads camping trip and doesn't want Carlos to attend with him; he is worried someone will "find out" about Carlos on the trip because they will be in a remote area where there won't be bathroom facilities.

An MHP who is working with Alfie, Carlos, and Amy would want to learn more about the nature of Alfie's concerns, and the extent to which Carlos and Amy have participated in other scouting activities. MHPs can help Alfie to navigate his feelings about others potentially learning about his father's gender identity. It would also be important to understand the extent to which Carlos shares this concern. This situation offers an opportunity to enhance empathy and understanding between Alife and his parents.

CHAPTER SUMMARY

In this chapter, we reviewed data focused on TNB parents and caregivers, while also discussing multiple contexts in which TNB parenting is situated. Awareness and understanding of both resources and challenges experienced by TNB parents is crucial for MHPs. Awareness of biases and beliefs related to gender identity, parenting norms, socialization within a cisheteronormative structure, and quickly shifting political and legal realities can help MHPs to support TNB parents and caregivers as they make decisions about parenting in relation to gender identity.

REFERENCES

Abreu, R. L., Sostre, J. P., Gonzalez, K. A., Lockett, G. M., Matsuno, E., & Mosley, D. V. (2022). Impact of gender-affirming care bans on transgender and gender diverse youth: Parental figures' perspective. *Journal of Family Psychology, 36*(5), 643–652. https://doi.org/10.1037/fam0000987

Alfonseca, K. (2023, June 11). *'Genocidal: Transgender people begin to flee states with anti-LGBTQ laws.* https://abcnews.go.com/US/genocidal-transgender-people-begin-flee-states-anti-lgbtq/story?id=99909913

American Psychological Association. (n.d.) . Parenting. In *APA dictionary of psychology.* https://www.dictionary.apa.org/parenting

Aronson, P. (2008). The markers and meanings of growing up: Contemporary young women's transition from adolescence to adulthood. *Gender & Society, 22*(1), 56–82. https://doi.org/10.1177/0891243207311420

Bockting, W., Barucco, R., LeBlanc, A., Singh, A., Mellman, W., Dolezal, C., & Ehrhardt, A. (2020). Sociopolitical change and transgender people's perceptions of vulnerability and resilience. *Sexuality Research & Social Policy, 17*(1), 162–174. https://doi.org/10.1007/s13178-019-00381-5

Brooks, V. R. (1981). *Minority stress and lesbian women*. Free Press.
Brown, C., & Rogers, M. (2020). Removing gender barriers: Promoting inclusion for trans and non-binary carers in fostering and adoption. *Child & Family Social Work, 25*(3), 594–601. https://doi.org/10.1111/cfs.12731
Brown, N. R. (2009). "I'm in transition too": Sexual identity renegotiation in sexual-minority women's relationships with transsexual men. *International Journal of Sexual Health, 21*(1), 61–77. https://doi.org/10.1080/19317610902720766
Cardoso, D., & Klesse, C. (2022). Living outside the BOX: Consensual non-monogamies, intimacies, and communities notes on research and terminology. In M. D. Vaughan & T. R. Burnes (Eds.), *The handbook of consensual non-monogamy affirming mental health practice* (pp. 15–49). Rowman & Littlefield.
Carone, N., Rothblum, E. D., Bos, H. M. W., Gartrell, N. K., & Herman, J. L. (2021). Demographics and health outcomes in a U.S. probability sample of transgender parents. *Journal of Family Psychology, 35*(1), 57–68. https://doi.org/10.1037/fam0000776
Charter, R., Ussher, J. M., Perz, J., & Robinson, K. H. (2022). Transgender parents: Negotiating "coming out" and gender affirmation with children and co-parents. *Journal of Homosexuality, 70*(7), 1287–1309. https://doi.org/10.1080/00918369.2021.2020542
dickey, l. m., Ducheny, K. M., & Ehrbar, R. D. (2016). Family creation options for transgender and gender nonconforming people. *Psychology of Sexual Orientation and Gender Diversity, 3*(2), 173–179. https://doi.org/10.1037/sgd0000178
Dierckx, M., Mortelmans, D., Motmans, J., & T'Sjoen, D. (2017). Resilience in families in transition: What happens when a parent is transgender? *Family Relations, 66*, 399–411. https://doi.org/10.1111/fare.12282
Dietz, E. (2021). Normal parents: Trans pregnancy and the production of reproducers. *International Journal of Transgender Health, 22*(1–2), 191–202. https://doi.org/10.1080/26895269.2020.1834483
Dobbs v. Jackson Women's Health Organization, 597 U.S. (2022). https://supreme.justia.com/cases/federal/us/597/19-1392/
Downing, J. B. (2013). Transgender-parent families. In A. E. Goldberg & K. R. Allen (Eds.), *LGBT-parent families: Innovations in research and implications for practice* (pp. 105–115). Springer Science + Business Media. https://doi.org/10.1007/978-1-4614-4556-2_7
Edwards, L., Goodwin, A., & Neumann, M. (2019). An ecological framework for transgender inclusive family therapy. *Contemporary Family Therapy, 41*(3), 258–274. https://doi.org/10.1007/s10591-018-9480-z
Ellis, S. A., Wojnar, D. M., & Pettinato, M. (2015). Conception, pregnancy, and birth experiences of male and gender variant gestational parents: It's how we could have a family. *Journal of Midwifery & Women's Health, 60*(1), 62–69. https://doi.org/10.1111/jmwh.12213
Erikson, E. (1950). *Childhood and Society*. Norton & Company.
Haines, B. A., Ajayi, A. A., & Boyd, H. (2014). Making trans parents visible: Intersectionality of trans and parenting identities. *Feminism & Psychology, 24*(2), 238–247. https://doi.org/10.1177/0959353514526219
Halberstam, J. (2005). *In a queer time and place: Transgender bodies, subcultural lives*. New York University Press.

Haupert, M. L., Gesselman, A. N., Moors, A. C., Fisher, H. E., Garcia, J. R. (2017). Prevalence of experiences with consensual nonmonogamous relationships: Findings from two national samples of single Americans. *Sex Marital Therapy, 43*(5), 424–440. http://doi.org/10.1080/0092623X.2016.1178675

Hines, S. (2006). Intimate transitions: Transgender practices of partnering and parenting. *Sociology, 40*(2), 353–371. https://doi.org/10.1177/0038038506062037

Hwahng, S. J., Allen, B., Zadoretzky, C., Barber Doucet, H., McKnight, C., & Des Jarlais, D. (2021). Thick trust, thin trust, social capital, and health outcomes among trans women of color in New York City. *International Journal of Transgender Health, 23*(1–2), 214–231. https://doi.org/10.1080/26895269.2021.1889427

Imrie, S., Zadeh, S., Wylie, K., & Golombok, S. (2020). Children with trans parents: Parent–child relationship quality and psychological well-being. *Parenting: Science and Practice, 21*(3), 185–215. https://doi.org/10.1080/15295192.2020.1792194

Kappus, B. D., Lucero, L., Cascalheira, C. J., & Ijebor, E. E. (2022). Invisible stories: A phenomenological study of bi and trans parent experiences within elementary schools in the southwestern United States. *Journal of Homosexuality, 69*(12), 2084–2103. https://doi.org/10.1080/00918369.2021.1987746

Kelley, A. D. (2020). Cisnormative empathy: A critical examination of love, support, and compassion for transgender people by their loved ones. *Sociological Inquiry, 91*(3), 625–646. https://doi.org/10.1111/soin.12390

Langdridge, D. (2008). Are you angry or are you heterosexual? A queer critique of lesbian and gay models of identity development. In L. Moon (Ed.), *Feeling queer or queer feelings? Radical approaches to counselling sex, sexualities and genders* (pp. 23–35). Taylor & Francis Group.

Luster, T., & Okagaki, L. (Eds.). (2005). *Parenting: An ecological perspective* (2nd ed.). Lawrence Erlbaum Associates Publishers.

Martin, C. L., & Little, J. K. (1990). The relation of gender understanding to children's sex-typed preferences and gender stereotypes. *Child Development, 61*(5), 1427–1439. https://doi.org/10.2307/1130753

Medical Ethics and Diversity Act, S.C. Stat. § 44-139 (2022). https://www.scstatehouse.gov/sess124_2021-2022/bills/4776.htm

Meyer, I. H. (2003). Prejudice, social stress, and mental health in lesbian, gay, and bisexual populations: Conceptual issues and research evidence. *Psychological Bulletin, 129*(5), 674–697. https://doi.org/10.1037/0033-2909.129.5.674

National Center for Transgender Equality. (n.d.). *Mutual aid and emergency funds*. https://transequality.org/covid19/mutual-aid-and-emergency-funds

Norman, A. J. (1977). Mutual aid: A key to survival for Black Americans. *The Black Scholar, 9*(4), 44–49. https://doi.org/10.1080/00064246.1977.11413974

Odets, W. (2019). *Out of the shadows: Reimagining gay men's lives*. Farrar, Straus, and Giroux.

Parks, C. (2023, July 28). *After Mississippi banned his hormone shots, an 8-hour journey*. https://www.washingtonpost.com/dc-md-va/interactive/2023/mississippi-youth-transgender-care-ban-aftermath/

Payne, J. G., & Erbenius, T. (2018). Conceptions of transgender parenthood in fertility care and family planning in Sweden: From reproductive rights to concrete practices. *Anthropology & Medicine, 25*(3), 329–343. https://doi.org/10.1080/13648470.2018.1507485

Petit, M., Julien, D., & Chamberland, L. (2017). Negotiating parental designations among trans parents' families: An ecological model of parental identity. *Psychology of Sexual Orientation and Gender Diversity, 4*(3), 282–295. https://doi.org/10.1037/sgd0000231

Pfeffer, C. A., & Jones, K. B. (2020). Transgender-parent families. In A. E. Goldberg & K. R. Allen (Eds.), *LGBTQ-parent families: Innovations in research and implications for practice* (2nd ed., pp. 199–214). Springer.

Redfield, E., Conron, K. J., Tentindo, W., & Browning, E. (2023). *Prohibiting gender-affirming medical care for youth*. The Williams Institute.

Riskind, R. G., & Tornello, S. L. (2022). "I think it's too early to know": Gender identity labels and gender expression of young children with nonbinary or binary transgender parents. *Frontiers in Psychology, 13,* 916088. https://doi.org/10.3389/fpsyg.2022.916088

Ryan, D., & Martin, A. (2000). Lesbian, gay, bisexual, and transgender parents in the school systems. *School Psychology Review, 29*(2), 207–216. https://doi.org/10.1080/02796015.2000.12086009

Siegel, D. (2023). Trans women and reproductive (in)justice—How race, class, and gender shape experiences of family formation and parenthood. *Data and Datasets, 167.* https://doi.org/10.7275/98VH-2K15

Singh, A. A., Awachie, T., Estevez, R., & Breaux, H. (2023, August). *BIPOC trans and nonbinary liberation: Advocacy and healing strategies* [CEU Workshop]. Annual Convention of the American Psychological Association, Washington, DC, United States.

Spade, D. (2020). *Mutual aid: building solidarity during this crisis (and the next)*. Verso.

Stotzer, R. L., Herman, J. L., & Hasenbush, A. (2014). *Transgender parenting: A review of existing research*. The Williams Institute.

Tebbe, E. A., Simone, M., Wilson, E., & Hunsicker, M. (2022). A dangerous visibility: Moderating effects of antitrans legislative efforts on trans and gender-diverse mental health. *Psychology of Sexual Orientation and Gender Diversity, 9*(3), 259–271. https://doi.org/10.1037/sgd0000481

303 Creative LLC v. Elenis, 600 U.S. 570 (2023). https://www.supremecourt.gov/opinions/22pdf/21-476_c185.pdf

Tornello, S. L., & Bos, H. (2017). Parenting intentions among transgender individuals. *LGBT Health, 4*(2), 115–120. https://doi.org/10.1089/lgbt.2016.0153

Tornello, S. L., Riskind, R. G., & Babic, A. (2019). Transgender and gender non-binary parents' pathways to parenthood. *Psychology of Sexual Orientation and Gender Diversity, 6*(2), 232–241. https://doi.org/10.1037/sgd0000323

Trans Track Legislation. (n.d.). *2023 Anti-trans legislation*. Retrieved from https://www.tracktranslegislation.com/

Trautner, H. M., Ruble, D. N., Cyphers, L., Kirsten, B., Behrendt, R., Hartmann, P. (2005). Rigidity and flexibility of gender stereotypes in children: Developmental or differential? *Infant and Child Development, 14*(4), 365–381. http://doi.org/10.1002/icd.399

The Trevor Project. (2024). *State-level anti-transgender laws increase past-year suicide attempts among transgender and non-binary young people in the USA*. https://www.thetrevorproject.org/research-briefs/state-level-anti-transgender-laws-increase-past-year-suicide-attempts-among-transgender-and-non-binary-young-people-in-the-usa/

Vaden, M. (2022, September 6). *Without social safety nets, mutual aid is a lifeline for Black trans communities*. Prism. https://prismreports.org/2022/09/06/mutual-aid-lifeline-black-trans-communities/

Veldorale-Griffin, A. (2014). Transgender parents and their adult children's experiences of disclosure and transition. *Journal of GLBT Family Studies, 10*(5), 475–501. https://doi.org/10.1080/1550428X.2013.866063

Weisman, K., Johnson, M. V., Shutts, K. (2015). Young children's automatic encoding of social categories. *Developmental Science, 18*(6), 1036–1043. http://doi.org/10.1111/desc.12269

9 AFFIRMATIVE COUNSELING WITH TRANS AND NONBINARY CHILDREN

AIDAN KEY AND RAFE McCULLOUGH

Affirmative mental health care for trans and nonbinary (TNB) children is an exciting and developing field. As children's developmental stages are quite different than those of adults, or even adolescents, gender-affirming mental health care needs to be tailored to individual children with these developmental stages in mind. Gender-affirming care can be lifesaving and can significantly improve the quality of life for children (Durwood et al., 2017; Horton, 2023; Turban, 2017). Though there is much more research to be done, mental health providers (MHPs) should be aware there is important, empirically-based guidance for how to best support TNB youth—which is a critically important endeavor given the attacks on gender-affirming care for TNB youth. Although we would like to know more, particularly about longer term outcomes data of currently supported gender-affirming treatments for children, taking the approach of not intervening until we know more is not a neutral option and can inhibit emotional and psychological wellness (Rosenthal, 2021). This chapter will focus on ways to promote the health and well-being of TNB children.

In order to identify the needs of TNB children, it is necessary to understand their mental health needs. Though there is a dearth of studies on TNB children, historically, studies of prepubescent children with gender dysphoria suggest higher rates of mental health issues, especially internalizing manifestations

---

https://doi.org/10.1037/0000471-010
Affirmative Counseling and Psychological Practice With Trans and Nonbinary Clients, Second Edition, A. Singh and R. McCullough (Editors)
Copyright © 2026 by the American Psychological Association. All rights reserved.

such as anxiety and depression (Olson et al., 2016), and self-harm and suicidality particularly in the second half of childhood (Aitken et al., 2016). It may be that parents underreport internalizing mental health symptoms because they are unaware of their children's internal experiences, and because children are often less able to also express these experiences (Durwood et al., 2017). TNB identities tend to be inherently pathologized, but for TNB children, poor mental health outcomes often stem from higher levels of social rejection, including rejection from families and peers in the form of bullying and harassment (Pariseau et al., 2019; Tordoff et al., 2022). We are also at a time in our country when purposeful efforts to reduce constitutional rights of TNB people—especially TNB children and youth—are escalating. This has been particularly impactful to TNB people of color and their families, as targeted attempts to block voting rights have also been enacted across multiple states and municipalities. In 2023, 87 bills removing rights of TNB people were signed into law across all states. In 2024, 50 of these bills passed out of the 674 proposed across the country (Trans Legislation Tracker, 2025), including bills that forcibly out TNB youth and block TNB kids and teachers from being visible in schools. Moreover, in 2025, 482 bills blocking rights of TNB people are active at the time of writing; many of these intend to impede access to health care and gender-affirming care for TNB children.

The good news is that family, school, community, and public policy support seem to increase the likelihood of resilience and better mental health outcomes for TNB youth (Durwood et al., 2021; Gower et al., 2018; L. V. Grossman et al., 2019; Lefevor et al., 2018; Pariseau et al., 2019). This is particularly true for TNB children (Olson et al., 2016). Additionally, lower odds for lifetime suicidal ideation have been shown for TNB youth who wanted and received access to pubertal suppression versus those who wanted pubertal suppression and did not receive it (Turban et al., 2020). Moreover, emerging literature suggests that enabling young children to socially transition and live as their affirmed gender, or to support a child's shift in identified gender, can lower their anxiety and depression metrics to similar rates as non-TNB (cisgender) youth (Durwood et al., 2017; Horton, 2023; Turban, 2017). Even though it is not always the case, research suggests that TNB children who are assertive about their gender identity, including children who socially transition before puberty, are more likely to persist in their gender identity over time (Coleman et al., 2022; Olson et al., 2016). In addition, much of the research conducted with TNB young people has predominantly included samples of White children and families who have social and financial resources to access gender-affirming care (Moradi et al., 2016). The underrepresentation of solid data and the perspectives of TNB children of color and their experiences continues to be an issue and needs to be prioritized.

This chapter provides an overview of some helpful knowledge and skills to support MHPs' successful navigation of the remarkable worlds of TNB children and their families. Through research and the narratives of TNB youth and their loved ones, we are becoming more informed about what mental health practices and collaborations are most affirming and supportive to TNB youth as they grow up to be healthy, strong, and empowered adults. We include personal anecdotes alongside empirically supported information to describe how MHPs can best serve TNB children and their families so TNB children feel connected and supported during the therapeutic process.

STIGMA AND MINORITY STRESS

Researchers have posited that stress related to the stigma of holding gender minority status—including discrimination, victimization, and rejection stemming from underlying oppressive structures—is more closely related to poor TNB mental health outcomes rather than a person's own anxieties about their TNB identity (Hendricks & Testa, 2012; Meyer, 2003; Toomey, 2021). There is evidence to suggest that TNB children may experience higher levels of minority stress compared to TNB adults due to their limited ability to access protective resources, such as supportive peer groups and MHPs, leading to feelings of isolation and disenfranchisement (Chavanduka et al., 2020). Further, TNB children may not be able to exercise the same level of control over minority stressors in their school and family contexts due to their lack of autonomy and bodily freedoms (Toomey, 2021). We have clear evidence that TNB children who are well supported by their families have similar levels of anxiety and depression as their non-TNB siblings and peers (Durwood at al., 2021; Olson et al., 2016). Even when TNB youth are certain of their gender identity (Olson et al., 2016), adults often question the validity of TNB children's asserted gender identity because of their developmental stage, especially if TNB youth are in early or middle childhood (Toomey, 2021; Yong, 2019).

This worry has been exploited by politicians in efforts to undermine gender-affirming care for youth and restrict access to books about TNB young people and other topics across the United States. Further complicating matters, deliberate misinformation is rampant, making it difficult for parents to discern reputable information sources from fear-stoking ones. Medical personnel and MHPs understand the importance of providing accurate information and a supportive environment for TNB children to determine which gender-affirming steps may be most helpful and the optimal timelines for social and medical interventions. Caregivers can play a significant role in fostering resistance and resilience in their TNB child. MHPs can provide caregivers with resources that help highlight these needs so they can increase their understanding of their child's experience.

ASSESSMENT AND THERAPEUTIC CONCERNS

According to the World Professional Association for Transgender Health's *Standards of Care, Version 8* (Coleman et al., 2022), for prepubescent children, it is assumed that gender diversity is expected and nonpathological. Further, diverse gender expressions are not necessarily an assumption of a child's TNB identity. Research in this area is nascent and there are currently no reliable, culturally competent, psychometrically sound assessments that can fully evaluate a TNB child's understanding of their gender identity and gender support needs (Bloom et al., 2021). Thus, it is important for MHPs to have a flexible, collaborative, and individualized approach to gender-affirming care (Coleman et al., 2022).

A full psychosocial assessment may not be needed for all gender-expansive children but may be helpful in determining and garnering the best support for TNB youth. If other mental health concerns are present, it is important for MHPs to ascertain whether those concerns exacerbate the child's gender dysphoria or discomfort and should be addressed, or whether they may be a result of the gender dysphoria or discomfort (Keo-Meier & Ehrensaft, 2018). Any assessment should take into consideration important aspects of the child's and caregiver's racial, ethnic, religious, socioeconomic, and other cultural identities and lived experiences, including beliefs, attitudes, and worldviews (Telfer et al., 2018). MHPs should further assess the child's and caregivers' experiences of minority stress, discrimination, hostility, and rejection. The developmentally appropriate assessment process should identify child, parent, and community strengths, as well as family concerns and potential risks to the child, including the family's ability to support a TNB child and the potential for conflict (Coleman et al., 2022).

Further, it is important to explore a child's gender history, whether a child experiences feelings of dysphoria, level of support in multiple contexts, such as school and extended family, and aspects of family stress and mental health. TNB children should be evaluated for coinciding medical or mental health concerns. The type of support that a gender-expansive child needs will be different from the gender-affirming care needs of a child who is struggling with gender identity concerns (Keo-Meier & Ehrensaft, 2018). Therapy should focus not only on the child, but it should involve key family members and other support adults as necessary.

SUPPORTING FAMILIES

It can be challenging for MHPs to ascertain the best ways to support the gender identity pathways of TNB children, which is quite different than for adults. A TNB adult who seeks out an MHP has likely spent extensive time considering their gender identity before enlisting outside help. MHPs who work with adults will likely find themselves in a collaborative process with their client, including providing a safe sounding board for concerns regarding disclosure to others, discussion of which medical interventions are desired (if any), timing of transition-related actions, and implications of social or medical transition steps on the client's personal relationships with spouse, children, friends, extended family, coworkers, and others (Pepping et al., 2025). In short, the MHP role in these cases is not to make a determination about the gender identity of their adult client, but rather provide emotional support and assistance for improvement.

On the other hand, the therapeutic relationship with a child or young teen needs a different approach (Pariseau et al., 2019). For one, TNB children must be connected to families and caregivers who are responsible for their well-being and safety, and thus, make decisions for their child (Ehrensaft et al., 2018; Keo-Meier & Ehrensaft, 2018). MHPs will need to work in concert with the families of TNB youth to understand and interpret the gender messages their children are expressing. The straightforwardness of a TNB child's statement such as, "I am a girl, not a boy" or "I am both a boy and a girl" or even "I don't have a gender, I'm just me" is sometimes met with skepticism from the adults in their lives. Parents and caregivers may experience worry, distress, or confusion about their child's assertions about their gender (Buckloh et al., 2022). These concerns can include wondering if their child's TNB identity is a temporary phase, worrying that their child is being influenced by peers or social media, or considering whether the child could be confused, perhaps conflating their personal interests—such as a young boy playing with dolls—with actual gender identity differences. The MHP's role then is to support the gender-expansive child while providing support to the adults in the child's life (Buckloh et al., 2022).

The caregiving adults will need to be partners in the decision-making for their child and, with very few exceptions, they will not have the benefit of being able to personally relate to the gender experience of their child (Nealy, 2017). It is important that MHPs encourage parents and caregivers not to be the "gender decider," but to facilitate supportive environments for gender exploration. Parents may experience a loss of social support from their networks when others find out about their TNB child's gender identity (Schlehofer & Cortez-Regan, 2022). When adults feel distressed about their child's gender journey, it can impair their ability to fully support their TNB child. A provider equipped with a deeper understanding of these factors and how to appropriately address them can optimize the entire family's journey to support their TNB child's well-being (Costa et al., 2015; A. H. Grossman et al., 2011; Pariseau et al., 2019).

Establishing a Relationship With Parents and Caregivers

When a child discloses their gender identity to a parent, their first reaction is often shock and disbelief. For some caregivers, there may have been signs. For others, they feel as if there were none. Often parents attempt to rationalize the child's behavior and expressions by stating, "My child never mentioned this until they started hanging out with *that* group of kids and watching *TikTok*," or "My son can't be a girl. He loves football and sports," or "A neighbor molested my child when they were younger. That's why she is saying this. Maybe she's just depressed," or "There is no way someone so young can know this about themselves." Providing a foundational understanding of gender to caregivers minimizes the conflation of issues and decreases confusion. For instance, help caregivers to understand that TNB children who have benefited from similar levels of social acceptance can know and understand their gender identity as clearly as their developmentally equivalent cisgender peers (Olson et al., 2015; Rafferty et al., 2018). Optimizing a therapeutic relationship with a TNB child must include clear and true information in order to establish a trusting relationship with the child's caregiver(s).

The support provided to children by parents is crucial for their well-being, and it is essential that MHPs understand some of parents' obstacles that can delay or prevent proactive care for their child (Durwood et al., 2021; Olson et al., 2016). Some of these obstacles include conflicting values such as religious beliefs, political leanings, cultural norms, and other personal biases or viewpoints regarding gender identity, expression, or sexual orientation. These can also encompass conflicts with, or differing perspectives from, a spouse, partner, or a caregiver. Other barriers may include feelings of isolation, confusion, grief, anger, fear, hesitancy, and apprehension—or lack of access to clear, true, and empirically based information and resources. Parents may express these conflicts in various ways. As the magnitude of what their child has shared begins to sink in, so do many other thoughts: "God doesn't make mistakes. My child is not transgender," or "My in-laws are Southern Baptist. They will blame me and my husband!" or "What will my parents and friends say about this? Will they question my parenting?"

In addition to some of the previously mentioned barriers, families, and caregivers of TNB children of color face additional challenges, such as the synergistic impacts at the intersection of racism and anti-TNB prejudice (Singh, 2013; Vance et al., 2021). For Black and Latino TNB youth and their families, past negative encounters and fear of future intolerance in medical systems have been cited as major reasons for postponing seeking care (Panchal et al., 2022; Zhou et al., 2023). Additionally, TNB youth of color and their families often face the potential for cultural estrangement from their racial and ethnic communities due to the forces of transprejudice. TNB youth of color may also simultaneously experience alienation from queer and trans communities who are predominantly White and may not fully understand or affirm their racial and cultural experiences (Zhou et al., 2023).

Further complicating counseling experiences for TNB children of color, many MHPs who serve trans youth often hold damaging beliefs about families of color not being as supportive of their TNB children. Marx and colleagues (2023) and Connell (2016) discussed the assumption of many that White people are more supportive than people of color. Examples of statements such as, "How do you talk about gender with Latine families who are so religious?" or "What about Asian parents, who don't understand all this gender stuff?" (Marx et al., 2023, p. 4) underscore these racialized discourses of anti-TNB prejudice. It is important for MHPs to keep this in mind; question their assumptions, biases, and practices regarding young TNB people of color and their and families; seek consultation and supervision; and be open to proactively addressing issues of power and privilege in the context of counseling (see Chapter 6, this volume, for further information on working with TNB communities of color).

Seeking Certainty

With an increasing number of children feeling more comfortable with gender expansiveness, many parents sometimes feel uncomfortable when thinking about whether a child is ready to make important decisions regarding their gender identity, given their developmental stage (Alegría, 2018; Ehrensaft et al., 2018). There can be a strong inclination amongst parents to desire unequivocal assurance that a gender-expansive child will grow up to identify with the gender they are asserting presently (Buckloh et al., 2022; Coolhart & Shipman, 2017). In the past, the prevailing wisdom was to wait and see (called *watchful waiting*) if a child's gender identification could be solidly categorized by examining three different markers: insistence, consistency, and persistence over time (Ehrensaft et al., 2018). This outdated criterion was subjective and ill-defined, resulting in parents and MHPs waiting an indefinite period of time—sometimes until the child reached legal age of consent—before considering the possibility of gender-affirming steps, resulting in increased distress from the TNB child.

This approach also assumes that notions of gender identity are fixed at a particular age or developmental period (Rafferty et al., 2018). Differentiating from children who consistently identify as a gender different from the one they were assigned versus children who simply do not conform to traditional expectations of gender expression or behavior, sometimes known as *gender expansive*, is not always clear. For many families, the fear of making an "irreversible mistake" still prevails today. Presenting gender-related options for TNB children as a single, binary decision—either the "right" or "wrong" choice—can be limiting. A more helpful approach is to guide families in understanding the distinction between gender identity and gender expression while encouraging caregivers to support their child in exploring a range of gender expressions (Buckloh et al., 2022). Suppressing gender expression may lead TNB children to question their own self-awareness or feel compelled to conceal their authentic gender (Ehrensaft et al., 2018).

Helping Caregivers to Create Gender-Supportive Environments

MHPs can help caregivers foster the creation of gender-supportive environments at home, where TNB children can feel safe to explore and express their gender fluidly without shame. It can be difficult for parents to navigate gender fluidity when this clashes with commonly held assumptions about gender identity. Seeking certainty from a child before they have a clearer understanding of their own needs may prematurely pressure them to name and define their experience (Nealy, 2019). Engaging in gender-supportive practices helps a TNB child feel seen, heard, and validated. If a child can safely explore their gender with support, and find the path of greatest personal resonance, the adults in their lives then can feel relieved of the notion that a terrifying mistake will occur.

Additionally, not rushing to the conclusion that a child needs to either socially transition or wait until they turn 18 leaves room open for the possibility that a child may instead identify as queer or grow up to be a cisgender straight man who loves sewing and floral arranging. The child, of course, may also identify as trans or nonbinary. In any case, providing affirming support serves to boost the TNB child's confidence, resiliency, and self-esteem. It is crucial that MHPs provide caregivers pathways to nonpathologizing approaches for gender-affirming care. This results in a family that is more informed, less fearful, and better equipped to embrace all the steps that may be part of a child's gender journey. As Keo-Meier and Ehrensaft (2018) suggested, "If you want to know a child's gender, ask in multiple ways, from multiple perspectives, over multiple time frames" (p. 101).

Meeting Parents and Caregivers Where They Are

When an unknown situation occurs in relation to one's child, it can elevate distressing feelings. Parents are sometimes surprised when they first learn of their child's TNB identity. Parenting a TNB child can be an isolating experience, and families can feel like they are suddenly thrust into circumstances unfamiliar to themselves and their friends, coworkers, and even their pediatrician or child's MHP. Therefore, caregivers are often flooded with emotions, feeling there is nowhere to turn to for information or support. It can be common for parents to experience a sense of dissonance when confronted with the reality of their child's expressed gender identity. Consider the following example and how MHPs can support caregivers and TNB children.

Regina and Ben are parents of a TNB child named Nadia, who disclosed at age 9 that she was not a boy but a girl.[1] Regina and Ben struggled to understand how their child could be trans. They felt stunned as they thought there were no prior indicators, although Regina described her child as "sullen, anxious, and reserved much of the time." Regina said, "I truly don't see how he can say he's a girl. He's a Boy Scout, and he plays soccer." Ben's resistance came more in the form of anger and disbelief, "He is just being defiant. It's probably just the attention-deficit and hyperactivity disorder. We just need to set stricter boundaries." As a result of participating in an online support group for parents of TNB youth, Regina gained greater clarity as she witnessed her daughter's positive transformation. Nadia made friends easily and became more outgoing. Her child's visible gender-related changes helped Regina more clearly recognize that her child was a girl. Ben took longer to get to a supportive place. He eventually felt like he was risking losing his relationship with his child if he did not try harder to understand and accept her, so he decided to spend more time with her, listening more deeply to her. Though the process had been difficult, as Ben saw that Nadia seemed so much more at ease and comfortable with herself, he became an unwavering advocate for her during a period when things got tough at school.

If an MHP understands the context under which a parent enters their office, it will then be much easier to recognize the emotional stages a parent is experiencing. Before the family experiences acceptance and celebration, it is common for parents to experience loss, uncertainty, and helplessness (Alegría, 2018; Gregor et al., 2015). Often it can be helpful to meet privately with the caregivers of a TNB child and allow them to process their feelings of grief or uncertainty. In a sense, the caregivers often need to be able to grieve the loss of the child they thought they had in order to receive and embrace the child in

---

[1] The case examples in this chapter have been modified to disguise the clients' identities and protect their confidentiality.

front of them. A struggle for many caregivers is reconciling the desire to love and support their child with the fear that their child may experience hardship, ostracism, discrimination, and danger. This may be especially true for parents of TNB children of color, who already experience the daily dangers of racism. A family may also feel more intense uncertainty around an autistic or neurodivergent child who proclaims a TNB identity due to the impact of societal ableist notions that suggest an autistic child may be less able to understand what it means to identify as TNB.

It is tempting for MHPs to feel protective of and side with the TNB child and be critical of the parents. This may look like trying to coax a parent to a place of support by citing the high-risk statistics for gender-expansive youth who are in *unsupportive* environments. The challenge with using this as an approach is that these caregivers do not see themselves or their actions as unsupportive, so it is essential that MHPs manage their own emotions that can manifest as anger, frustration, or impatience directed at caregivers. In meeting caregivers where they are, offering emotional support and guidance will often facilitate a parent's eventual arrival to a place of support (Nealy, 2017). Additional strategies may include asking parents directly about their concerns, encouraging them to tell their story while listening and validating, and supporting the usage of a child's old name and pronouns in parent-only sessions to facilitate trust and help them speak with greater ease about their child (Buckloh et al., 2022). MHPs can also try to help caregivers avoid making premature, definitive statements about a child's gender identity and ask permission to give parents resources and respectful language to talk about gender identity when they are ready (Nealy, 2019; Ryan & Diaz, 2011).

Addressing Expectations

Caregivers may have expectations that are unrealistic and seek the support of an MHP in achieving those. One expectation is that an MHP can change the gender identification of a child and "make it go away." Another expectation parents have is to assume that a child is no longer struggling with people interacting negatively with their TNB identity if their gender history is undisclosed at school. TNB children experience gender minority stress whether their status is known or private. Another expectation from some parents is that once certain transition-related steps are taken, the child will be *done*, and life will get back to *normal*. One parent of a teen trans boy said, "I can't wait until my child is 18 and has all this transgender stuff behind him!" The reality is that her child will always be TNB and will most likely have to negotiate factors related to his TNB identity in areas that include medical care, privacy considerations, and intimate or other social relationships. MHPs can help parents to come to terms with reality and accept that there may always be difficulties, but that their child can be equipped to successfully navigate those challenges as many TNB adults have.

CLINICAL CONCERNS

MHPs should support interventions that are specific to each individual TNB child and their family and that foster resilience in the event of potential peer or adult negative responses to a child's gender identity or expression (Malpas et al., 2018; Spencer et al., 2021). Interventions should bolster environmental and personal supports for TNB youth and their families (e.g., access to true information, fostering of relationships based in warmth and connection, the ability to define and explain their own identities), which allow for opportunities for TNB children to develop a better understanding of their internal sense of felt gender (Ehrensaft et al., 2018; Malpas et al., 2018; Singh, 2013). MHPs should pay special attention to understanding the differences between a child who is exploring gender expression and one who is asserting a gender that is different than the one they were assigned. MHPs who are collaborative in their approach to learning a TNB child client's understanding of themselves are able to distinguish between when caregivers are cautious and concerned or if they are perhaps insistent about changes before a child is ready (Leibowitz et al., 2020). In the following sections, gender-affirming interventions and considerations for aiding in social and medical transitions will be discussed. This chapter focuses more on social transition than medical aspects of transition because, for TNB children before they reach Tanner Stage 2 of puberty (approximately 9–11 years), social transition is the only aspect of transition that is indicated as part of gender-affirming care.

Social Transition

A *social transition* refers to a time where a child begins to live part or full time in the gender that resonates most with them. Social transition, which often precedes medical steps (Nealy, 2019), can involve crucial steps taken to validate a child's gender identity, allowing the child to "try it on" and gain perspective to discover whether these changes resonate. These steps, such as new clothing, name, pronouns, or hair changes, are all reversible and don't require identity certainty or diagnosis. These supportive steps may feel daunting for families at first, when they feel uncertain about the permanency of their child's TNB identity. When a TNB child is supported in their social transition, they have time and space for self-discovery while receiving encouragement and affirmation, which can decrease pressure to definitively name a gender identity before they are ready (Ehrensaft et al., 2018; Coleman et al., 2022). Social transition can also provide more time and space for parents, siblings, extended family, and others to adjust to these changes.

For those concerned and cautious about allowing TNB youth to socially transition because of their belief that children could change their minds and not continue to identify as TNB beyond childhood, it is important to keep in mind that it is not possible to truly measure the number of children who no longer identify as TNB as adults because we do not even have an accurate and valid way to measure gender identity in children (Ehrensaft et al., 2018). Also, inherent in the fear of children "desisting" is the assumption that changing one's mind about gender identity and expression is negative, which is not necessarily the case. It is possible for TNB children to explore their gender identity more deeply with these methods, in part because they have the option to socially transition and use puberty blockers at the onset of puberty, both of which are fully reversible. In essence, when TNB youth reach 16 years of age, having socially transitioned and used puberty blockers, they might have 10 years of experience already living as their affirmed gender. There is little scientific data on "retransition" or "detransition" (Olson et al., 2022), and data on rates of discontinuing gender-affirming care is mixed, largely due to inconsistencies in how "detransition" is defined and misunderstandings about individuals' reasons for discontinuation (Feigerlova, 2025). It is also difficult to accurately determine desistance rates without valid measures of gender identity in children, which are difficult to measure (Ehrensaft et al., 2018); however, studies generally suggest that once individuals begin social or medical transition, most continue (Davies et al., 2019; James et al., 2016; Olson et al., 2022; Turban, 2018).

One study indicated that 5 years after beginning their social transition, an overwhelming 94% of TNB youth are living as the same gender to which they socially transitioned (Olson et al., 2022). More specifically, of the 7.3% of TNB youth who "retransitioned," 1.3% were reported transitioning to nonbinary then back to "binary" trans, 3.5% were reported living as nonbinary, and 2.5% reported using gender pronouns associated with their assigned sex. According to another study, while some adolescents detransitioned, they reported that they did not regret the decision to initiate gender-affirming care because it helped them better understand their gender-related needs (Turban, 2018). As it is possible for young TNB adolescents to change their minds, it is important for MHPs to present a full range of options for them to consider (Coleman et al., 2022). Though regret rate for gender-affirming medical care is thought to be relatively low (Davies et al., 2019; James et al., 2016; Olson et al., 2022; Turban, 2018), it is important to note that even though other fields of medicine report some rates of regret for medical procedures, they do not have their treatment efficacy challenged in the face of some patient regret, highlighting a double-standard for lifesaving gender-affirming care.

The reasons why TNB youth discontinue socially transitioning mirror the reasons why adults detransition. In a national study of over 27,000 trans adults, 8% reported that they detransitioned temporarily or permanently at some point (James et al., 2016). Of the many reasons these participants cited, pressure to detransition from family, friends, clergy, employers, partners, MHPs, or others were noted. Of the 8% of TNB folks stating that they detransitioned, only 5% said that it was because they realized that gender transition was "not for them." Additionally, 4% of the 8% stated that the "initial transition did not reflect the complexity of their gender identity" (James et al., 2016, p. 111). Others stated that their reasons were about medical and financial issues and discrimination. Overall, MHPs should give caregivers accurate information about the likelihood that their TNB child may change their minds at any time, but treatment pathways become clearer as TNB children demonstrate more consistent gender identities and expressions over time. In the event that a 16-year-old TNB adolescent asserts a need for gender-affirming hormone therapy after coming out as trans at age 7, it might be helpful for parents to think that their now 16-year-old has 9 years of experience as a transitioned TNB person and they have gained much wisdom and insight about their needs.

Name Changes
A request for a name change is often one of the first social transition steps articulated by a young person. That said, assigning a name is traditionally the role of the child's parent, who may have considered many factors: legacy names (such as the name of a grandparent), culturally specific names, certain name spellings, those related to religious figures, etc. A TNB child may be more inclined to consider character names found in books, movies, cartoons, current popular names, other contemporary figures, or even a beloved pet (Key, 2023). The request for a gender-related name change can inspire significant consternation for caregivers. Some parents will experience sadness and grief at letting go of the name they gave their child at birth. They may disagree or be frustrated at their child's new chosen name. Providers can support the family and child to find a name that honors both of their preferences, especially as a way to support and strengthen the bonds between parent and child. In some cases, TNB children are happy to be given a new name by their parent(s). Often this may be a name the parents already considered before their child was born. Sometimes

siblings or extended family can be involved, providing collective love, connection, and support for a TNB child.

Name changes can be completed within a family, school, youth program, or with peers at any time. MHPs should be aware that no diagnosis is needed, nor does a legal name change order need to occur. Due to new legislation that seeks to reduce rights for TNB youth, some states are requiring that school personnel report students' requests to be called a name other than what is on their birth certificates. For example, Tennessee passed a senate bill in May 2024 that states:

> If a student enrolled in a Local Educational Agency (LEA) or public charter school requests an accommodation from an employee of the LEA or public charter school that is intended to affirm the student's gender identity, including a request that the student be addressed using a name that differs from the name assigned to the student on the student's school registration forms or in the student's educational record . . . then the employee of the LEA or public charter school shall report the student's request to a school administrator, and the school administrator shall report the student's request to the student's parent. (Tennessee Senate Bill 1810, p. 1)

Legislation like this can create intense stress and safety issues for TNB children whose caregivers are not supportive. It is important for MHPs to understand these laws and how they may impact the roles of educators. Many youths go by names other than their legal name at school (e.g., a middle name, nickname, or initials like P.J.) and are scarcely noticed. Some TNB youth will refer to their former name as their "dead name," which can be both distressing to their parents and a testimony to the importance of the new name and how it relates to their affirmed identity. Regardless of how a new name is selected, there is almost always a time of adjustment for families, peers, and teachers. Often that adjustment is more prolonged than the child would prefer. MHPs can help families understand the significance and meaning of a new name for their TNB child and support them to adapt as early as possible, as well as to advocate for their child when other family, friends, peers, and teachers use their incorrect name.

Pronouns

Until more recently, it was rare for anyone to have to accommodate a person's pronoun change request. There were so few visible TNB adults and next to no visible TNB youth. For many, making the mental shift to a new pronoun is difficult, unfamiliar terrain. For MHPs, it is crucial to understand the impact of correct pronoun usage for a child and to help families also understand. For TNB children, using a correct pronoun delivers a clear message that they are heard, believed, and that their gender identity is validated. MHPs should use the requested pronoun and name when engaging with the child in session. This act builds and strengthens the trust between child and provider. Additionally, MHPs can request that caregivers also use the new pronoun and name at the child's request. For parents who struggle with this, MHPs can support them by asking parents to practice often and regularly picture the child in their mind then say the name and pronoun aloud. The internal visualization coupled with the vocal and auditory reinforcement is a good way to increase consistency (Key, 2023).

Sometimes parents struggle and may dismiss their child's request to use their identified pronouns as being whimsical or unnecessary. In these cases, MHPs can encourage parents and family members to take the child's requests seriously (Key, 2023). It may be helpful for caregivers to know that it takes courage for their child to ask for a new pronoun, because regardless of their age, TNB youth are often aware of the resistance they are likely to encounter and anticipate it. MHPs should have compassion for parents who struggle and validate the fact that pronoun changes are hard for most people and that the initial learning curve is steep. MHPs can provide space in sessions with parents to practice using the child's name and pronouns and process their feelings around the experience of using these new terms. Additionally, it is important to allow people to make honest mistakes. When a mistake happens, MHPs can encourage parents to offer a quick apology and correction, then get on with the conversation. Over-apologizing, explaining, and justifying the error can result in greater distress than the initial slip itself. It is reasonable to check in with a parent and ask if they want help or reminders about pronoun usage. Encourage the caregiver to enlist additional help from their own friends and family.

It may be necessary for a provider to use the child's name and pronoun given at birth for a period of time when engaging with the parent. If an MHP determines that this could be a helpful step that serves to decrease tension (and build trust with the parent), it is recommended to discuss this with the child. An explanation for the child can go like this:

> Sometimes parents need more time than we think to change to a different pronoun, but it doesn't mean that they don't love you. It just means they might need more time to adjust. I don't need that time so I will use your correct name or pronoun. However, let's talk about how it might be helpful for me to use your old name or pronoun with your parents at first. Would that be ok with you? Know that I will be working hard to help them get to a place where they can start using your correct name and pronouns as soon as they can.

Many TNB youth are using they/them as a singular pronoun. The use of "he" or "she" may feel limiting or inaccurate to best reflect their experience. Some TNB children will use they/them as an interim pronoun while continuing to explore their identity, and some TNB youth and adults will ultimately choose they/them as their definitive pronoun. It is important for MHPs to help parents understand that their child may change a pronoun or name a few times before they ultimately decide what fits best for them.

Assessing Readiness
Is it important for MHPs, together with caregivers, to assess a child's readiness to begin social transition. Gender-expansive children need to be supported in exploring the wide range of gender expressions possible so they do not feel as though they need to foreclose on a particular way of expressing their gender that is based on ideas about stereotypical behavior (Buckloh et al., 2022; Nealy, 2017). MHPs need to assess whether they are currently clear about their affirmed gender identity, and it can be helpful to determine if their gender identity and expression has been fairly consistent for some time (Nealy, 2019). If gender-expansive children have been asserting the need to become more public, go to school and live part or full time in a particular gender identity and expression, it is important to assess whether they have all the information they need and are prepared to take the steps to socially transition.

TNB children must also be prepared to disclose to siblings, friends, teachers, and peers and be ready to handle intrusive questions or unplanned disclosure by a peer who knew them before socially transitioning and demands for information about their gender history (Nealy, 2019). In these situations, MHPs can role-play with TNB youth how to respond and what to do to ask for help when needed, while modeling for caregivers how to use role-playing techniques if further issues arise. Many TNB children fear the possibility of inadvertent disclosure. In a simulated activity, one parent role-played different situations with her child who was less than thrilled with the activity. One day at school, however, her child put that work into action when another student approached her and said, "Didn't you used to have a boy's name?" She very quickly responded with an eyeroll and said, "Yeah, do you believe my parents did that to me!" In another instance, a TNB child responded candidly to a child's request to know whether they were a girl or a boy with, "Actually, I'm neither."

Sometimes, TNB youth are undisclosed about their gender history to their peers but are later interested in sharing their history with a close friend. The MHP can help the child strategize an approach and enlist the help of their parent to achieve the best outcome. That approach could include reaching out in advance to the close friend's parent to discuss how to best share the information. The child's friend may have questions that could be addressed by their own parent and their parent can help them understand that their friend is sharing something important, but private.

Weighing Risks and Benefits
As part of the preparation, MHPs should discuss—in developmentally appropriate ways—the risks and benefits of socially transitioning with the family and child (Ehrensaft et al., 2018). The benefits are that, according to current data, children who desire social transition feel more affirmed in their gender identity and have better mental health outcomes (Durwood et al., 2017; Ehrensaft et al., 2018; Olson et al., 2016). In short, children are happier and healthier when they are living more authentic lives in their identified gender. The risks of socially transitioning are that children may experience more bullying and discrimination by peers and school staff. This is especially true for nonbinary children who tend to experience other children and adults around them reacting in a more negative or uncomfortable way to their blended gender expressions and potential use of they/them pronouns (Ehrensaft et al., 2018).

Parents and caregivers of TNB children who live in states where TNB youth are restricted in their access to trans-affirming medical care can also experience negative mental health outcomes such as anxiety, depression, fear, and feelings of hypervigilance when being questioned about their child's gender identity (Abreu, Sostre, Gonzalez, Lockett, & Matsuno, 2022; Abreu, Sostre, Gonzalez, Lockett, Matsuno, & Mosley, 2022; Bull & D'Arrigo-Patrick, 2018). These should be addressed with families in counseling. Some of these supports may include validating their concerns, processing their grief and rejection, and externalizing strategies that allow TNB families and caregivers to understand that the problem of rejection is situated outside of themselves and inside other individuals and systems. There are risks involved in social transitioning, like navigating bullying or harassment, or social ostracism for families (Ehrensaft et al., 2018); however, when a TNB child and their supportive caregivers work together, they can combat the impacts of minority stress and the effects of navigating unsupportive environments, all the while strengthening their connection to each other and cultivating new, more supportive communities.

Considerations for Trans and Nonbinary Families of Color
For any TNB child of color, having a TNB identity can compound marginalization and increase feelings of isolation, making social transition more difficult. Further, TNB children of color can experience transprejudice within their own racial and ethnic communities and racism in predominantly White spaces at school that are supposed to be affirming (Zhou et al., 2023) for all TNB youth, such as gender and sexuality alliance groups. Black and Latino TNB youth may have a higher chance of experiencing race-based harassment compared to cisgender peers because they are seen as different from their peers due to both their race and gender, meaning they may face more harassment in general (Vance et

al., 2021). If TNB children of color have additional identities that are marginalized, the impact to their mental health and well-being can be even greater. A provider with a strong understanding of intersectionality will be better prepared to more holistically support a young TNB person of color and their family through the gender exploration process. Consider the following case study.

Pedro is a 10-year-old Dominican trans boy who has cerebral palsy and uses a walker. He attends a mostly White school. Pedro socially transitioned last year at school. At first, his mom was nervous because Pedro told her that kids stare at him a lot. Pedro's mom is not sure if the other kids stare because he looks different from them because of his race or disability, or because they are uncomfortable with his identifying as a boy now. Pedro's mom has also expressed concerns to Pedro's therapist because teachers have begun to call home more often this year to report behavior issues. She is worried that he will have more negative encounters with the school system now that he's seen as a Black male.

It is helpful for Pedro's mother and counselor to be able to discuss all aspects of Pedro's lived intersectional experiences as a young, Black, Dominican trans boy with a disability. As Pedro is seen and experienced by others as a boy, he can decide whether he wants to disclose his gender history, but his fears about unplanned, forced disclosure of his TNB identity by others can increase the impacts of gender minority stress (Hendricks & Testa, 2012). His identities as a Black and disabled person can never be invisible to others, which can lead to ongoing racial and disability microaggressions, stigma, and discrimination. It would be important for an MHP to help validate Pedro's mother's concerns about Pedro being treated differently now because of our society's pathologizing behaviors of Black males. Also, it would be beneficial to validate her lack of clarity about where the discrimination is originating, addressing the nature of microaggressions with her and how this makes Pedro's social transition more difficult.

An approach for MHPs initiating intersectional identity discussions is called *broaching* (Day-Vines et al, 2021). Broaching is when MHPs identify aspects of clients' race, class, culture, disability, and other important identities that impact clients' presenting concerns and directly initiate conversations around those experiences. White and nondisabled MHPs may experience discomfort around these conversations because many have learned that discussions of race, culture, and disability are strongly discouraged in professional spaces—but in not broaching important aspects of clients' identities, clients' lived experiences and realities are rendered invisible in a space that is supposed to be therapeutic. Broaching increases trust, more in-depth self-disclosures by clients, satisfaction with the therapy process, and the likelihood that clients will return for more sessions (Day-Vines, 2021).

School Safety Concerns

Some families have felt that the only way to keep their child safe was to relocate to a new community to start fresh, and some have the social and financial means to change their physical location. It is important for MHPs to understand that a harmful school environment is not a problem for the child to solve, and it can foster feelings of internalized oppression to focus on the situation being the child's responsibility by only providing tools for coping with bullying without also addressing the hostile environment (Coolhart, 2018; Nealy, 2019). Some schools are in the early stages of gender inclusivity. Especially for families for whom relocation is not an option, MHPs can be instrumental in offering guidance and advocacy for the child by assisting school staff with gaining a deeper understanding and acceptance of TNB children. However, some situations are so harmful that they could have deleterious and lifelong impact on the child's physical and mental health. MHPs can serve families in these situations by presenting possible alternatives (i.e., online schooling or homeschooling), providing resources, and connecting families with advocates within the school systems, such as a supportive school counselor or family liaison.

Medical Interventions for Trans and Nonbinary Children

Although this chapter focuses more on social transitions, MHPs should be prepared to have discussions about medical transition processes and options, as TNB children may bring these topics up themselves and their caregivers often have important questions and concerns to discuss about their child's potential trajectories as they enter adolescence. MHPs can also help dispel myths that anti-TNB legislation restricting gender-affirming care have promoted (e.g., fear-based claims about TNB children "transitioning" by having their anatomies permanently altered). Preventing youth from accessing gender-affirming care has caused significant stress for TNB young people in multiple states (Dhanani & Totton, 2023). In a statement written on behalf of World Professional Association for Transgender Health, providers and facilitators of gender-affirming care for youth from around the country stated, "Withdrawing care for all transgender and gender-expansive young people or adults or threatening to criminalize conscientious healthcare providers who work with transgender patients or clients using evidence-based care is a clear abuse of administrative and legislative power" (Leibowitz et al., 2020, p. 4). Please see Chapter 10 exploring TNB adolescents for a more comprehensive discussion about gender-affirming hormone therapy, which can follow pubertal suppression for many TNB youth.

CHAPTER SUMMARY

Given the ongoing sociopolitical attacks on gender-affirming care where the rights of TNB children and adolescents are severely at risk, it is now more important than ever for MHPs to understand how to provide the best gender-affirming care for TNB children. Part of providing care that reduces mental health risks for TNB children is learning to work collaboratively with the parents, caregivers, and families. Supportive caregivers and families provide lifesaving protection and bolster resilience that help TNB children grow up to be confident adults who feel affirmed in who they are (Durwood at al., 2021; Olson et al., 2016; Pariseau et al., 2019), yet these factors do not eliminate hardships that can have a painful impact. MHPs play a crucial role in supporting caregivers during challenging periods characterized by feelings of overwhelm, emotional turmoil, and the acquisition of essential knowledge related to raising their TNB child. It is imperative for MHPs to demonstrate empathy, possess comprehensive understanding, and exhibit proficiency in the care they provide. This ensures that TNB children and adolescents are equipped with a clear understanding of available options and receive explanations tailored to their developmental stage, supporting their journey toward living authentically.

REFERENCES

Abreu, R. L., Sostre, J. P., Gonzalez, K. A., Lockett, G. M., & Matsuno, E. (2022). "I am afraid for those kids who might find death preferable": Parental figures' reactions and coping strategies to bans on gender affirming care for transgender and gender diverse youth. *Psychology of Sexual Orientation and Gender Diversity, 9*(4), 500–510. https://doi.org/10.1037/sgd0000495

Abreu, R. L., Sostre, J. P., Gonzalez, K. A., Lockett, G. M., Matsuno, E., & Mosley, D. V. (2022). Impact of gender-affirming care bans on transgender and gender diverse youth: Parental figures' perspective. *Journal of Family Psychology, 36*(5), 643–652. https://doi.org/10.1037/fam0000987

Aitken, M., VanderLaan, D. P., Wasserman, L., Stojanovski, S., & Zucker, K. J. (2016). Self-harm and suicidality in children referred for gender dysphoria. *Journal of the American Academy of Child & Adolescent Psychiatry, 55*(6), 513–520. https://doi.org/10.1016/j.jaac.2016.04.001

Aramburu Alegría, C. (2018). Supporting families of transgender children/youth: Parents speak on their experiences, identity, and views. *International Journal of Transgenderism, 19*(2), 132–143. https://doi.org/10.1080/15532739.2018.1450798

Bloom, T. M., Nguyen, T. P., Lami, F., Pace, C. C., Poulakis, Z., Telfer, M., Taylor, A., Pang, K. C., & Tollit, M. A. (2021). Measurement tools for gender identity, gender expression, and gender dysphoria in transgender and gender-diverse children and adolescents: A systematic review. *The Lancet Child & Adolescent Health, 5*(8), 582–

588. Advance online publication. https://doi.org/10.1016/S2352-4642(21)00098-5

Buckloh, L. M., Poquiz, J. L., Alioto, A., Moyer, D. N., & Axelrad, M. E. (2022). Best practices in working with parents and caregivers of transgender and gender diverse youth. *Clinical Practice in Pediatric Psychology, 10*(3), 325–335. https://doi.org/10.1037/cpp0000442

Bull, B., & D'Arrigo-Patrick, J. (2018). Parent experiences of a child's social transition: Moving beyond the loss narrative. *Journal of Feminist Family Therapy, 30*(3), 170–190. https://doi.org/10.1080/08952833.2018.1448965

Chavanduka, T. M. D., Gamarel, K. E., Todd, K. P., & Stephenson, R. (2020). Responses to the gender minority stress and resilience scales among transgender and nonbinary youth. *Journal of LGBT Youth, 18*, 135–154. https://doi.org/10.1080/19361653.2020.1719257

Coleman, E., Radix, A. E., Bouman, W. P., Brown, G. R., de Vries, A. L. C., Deutsch, M. B., Ettner, R., Fraser, L., Goodman, M., Green, J., Hancock, A. B., Johnson, T. W., Karasic, D. H., Knudson, G. A., Leibowitz, S. F., Meyer-Bahlburg, H. F. L., Monstrey, S. J., Motmans, J., Nahata, L., . . . Arcelus, J. (2022). Standards of care for the health of transgender and gender diverse people, Version 8. *International Journal of Transgender Health, 23*(Suppl. 1), S1–S259. https://doi.org/10.1080/26895269.2022.2100644

Connell, C. (2016). Contesting racialized discourses of homophobia. *Sociological Forum, 31*(3), 599–618. https://doi.org/10.1111/socf.12265

Coolhart, D. (2018). Helping families move from distress to attunement. In C. Keo-Meier & D. Ehrensaft (Eds.), *The gender affirmative model: An interdisciplinary approach to supporting transgender and gender expansive children* (pp. 125–140). American Psychological Association. https://doi.org/10.1037/0000095-008

Coolhart, D., & Shipman, D. L. (2017). Working toward family attunement: Family therapy with transgender and gender-nonconforming children and adolescents. *The Psychiatric Clinics of North America, 40*(1), 113–125. https://doi.org/10.1016/j.psc.2016.10.002

Costa, R., Dunsford, M., Skagerberg, E., Holt, V., Carmichael, P., & Colizzi, M. (2015). Psychological support, puberty suppression, and psychosocial functioning in adolescents with gender dysphoria. *The Journal of Sexual Medicine, 12*(11), 2206–2214. https://doi.org/10.1111/jsm.13034

Davies, S., McIntyre, S., & Rypma, C. (2019, April 11). Detransition rates in a national UK gender identity clinic [Abstract]. In *3rd biennal EPATH Conference Inside Matters. On Law, Ethics and Religion* (p. 118). https://epath.eu/wp-content/uploads/2019/04/Boof-of-abstracts-EPATH2019.pdf

Day-Vines, N. L., Cluxton-Keller, F., Agorsor, C., & Gubara, S. (2021). Strategies for broaching the subjects of race, ethnicity, and culture. *Journal of Counseling and Development, 99*(3), 348–357. https://doi.org/10.1002/jcad.12380

Dhanani, L. Y., & Totton, R. R. (2023). Have you heard the news? The effects of exposure to news about recent transgender legislation on transgender youth and young adults. *Sexuality Research & Social Policy, 20*(4), 1345–1359. https://doi.org/10.1007/s13178-023-00810-6

Durwood, L., Eisner, L., Fladeboe, K., Ji, C. G., Barney, S., McLaughlin, K. A., & Olson, K. R. (2021). Social support and internalizing psychopathology in transgender youth. *Journal of Youth and Adolescence, 50*(5), 841–854. https://doi.org/10.1007/s10964-020-01391-y

Durwood, L., McLaughlin, K. A., & Olson, K. R. (2017). Mental health and self-worth in socially transitioned transgender youth. *Journal of the American Academy of Child & Adolescent Psychiatry, 56*(2), 116–123.e2. https://doi.org/10.1016/j.jaac.2016.10.016

Ehrensaft, D., Giammattei, S. V., Storck, K., Tishelman, A. C., & St. Amand, C. (2018). Prepubertal social gender transitions: What we know; what we can learn—A view from a gender affirmative lens. *International Journal of Transgenderism, 19*(2), 251–268. https://doi.org/10.1080/15532739.2017.1414649

Feigerlova, E. (2025). Prevalence of detransition in persons seeking gender-affirming hormonal treatments: A systematic review. *The Journal of Sexual Medicine, 22*(2), 356–368. https://doi.org/10.1093/jsxmed/qdae186

Gower, A. L., Rider, G. N., Brown, C., McMorris, B. J., Coleman, E., Taliaferro, L. A., & Eisenberg, M. E. (2018). Supporting transgender and gender diverse youth: Protection against emotional distress and substance use. *American Journal of Preventive Medicine, 55*(6), 787–794. https://doi.org/10.1016/j.amepre.2018.06.030

Gregor, C., Hingley-Jones, H., & Davidson, S. (2015). Understanding the experience of parents of pre-pubescent children with gender identity issues. *Child & Adolescent Social Work Journal, 32*(3), 237–246. https://doi.org/10.1007/s10560-014-0359-z

Grossman, A. H., D'Augelli, A. R., & Frank, J. A. (2011). Aspects of psychological resilience among transgender youth. *Journal of LGBT Youth, 8*(2), 103–115. https://doi.org/10.1080/19361653.2011.541347

Grossman, L. V., Masterson Creber, R. M., Benda, N. C., Wright, D., Vawdrey, D. K., & Ancker, J. S. (2019). Interventions to increase patient portal use in vulnerable populations: A systematic review. *Journal of the American Medical Informatics Association, 26*(8–9), 855–870. https://doi.org/10.1093/jamia/ocz023

Hendricks, M. L., & Testa, R. J. (2012). A conceptual framework or clinical work with transgender and gender nonconforming clients: An adaptation of the minority stress model. *Professional Psychology: Research and Practice, 43*(5), 460–467. https://doi.org/10.1037/a0029597

Horton, C. (2023). "Euphoria": Trans children and experiences of prepubertal social transition. *Family Relations, 72*(4), 1890–1907. https://doi.org/10.1111/fare.12764

James, S. E., Herman, J. L., Rankin, S., Keisling, M., Mottet, L., & Anafi, M. (2016). *The report of the 2015 U.S. Transgender Survey*. National Center for Transgender Equality.

Keo-Meier, C., & Ehrensaft, D. (2018). Introduction to the gender affirmative model. In C. Keo-Meier & D. Ehrensaft (Eds.), *The gender affirmative model: An interdisciplinary approach to supporting transgender and gender expansive children* (pp. 3–19). American Psychological Association. https://doi.org/10.1037/0000095-001

Key, A. (2023). *Trans children in today's schools*. Oxford University Press. https://doi.org/10.1093/oso/9780190886547.001.0001

Lefevor, G. T., Sprague, B. M., Boyd-Rogers, C. C., & Smack, A. C. P. (2018). How well do various types of support buffer psychological distress among transgender and gender nonconforming students? *International Journal of Transgenderism, 20*(1), 39–48. https://doi.org/10.1080/15532739.2018.1452172

Leibowitz, S., Green, J., Massey, R., Boleware, A. M., Ehrensaft, D., Francis, W., Keo-Meier, C., Olson-Kennedy, A., Pardo, S., Rider, G. N., Schelling, E., Segovia, A., Tangpricha, V., Anderson, E., T'Sjoen, G., & the WPATH, USPATH, and EPATH Executive Committee and Board of Directors. (2020). Statement in response to calls for banning evidence-based supportive health interventions for transgender and gender diverse youth. *International Journal of Transgender Health, 21*(1), 111–112. https://doi.org/10.1080/15532739.2020.1703652

Malpas, J., Glaeser, E., & Giammattei, S. V. (2018). Building resilience in transgender and gender expansive children, families, and communities: A multidimensional family approach. In C. Keo-Meier & D. Ehrensaft (Eds.), *The gender affirmative model: An interdisciplinary approach to supporting transgender and gender expansive children* (pp. 141–156). American Psychological Association. https://doi.org/10.1037/0000095-009

Marx, R. A., Peña, F. J., McCurdy, A. L., & Maier, A. (2024). "They won't push me away": Transgender and gender-expansive youth of color's perceptions of parental gender-identity-specific support. *Family Relations, 73*(2), 993–1013. https://doi.org/10.1111/fare.12923

Meyer, I. H. (2003). Prejudice, social stress, and mental health in lesbian, gay, and bisexual populations: Conceptual issues and research evidence. *Psychological Bulletin, 129*(5), 674–697. https://doi.org/10.1037/0033-2909.129.5.674

Moradi, B., Tebbe, E. A., Brewster, M. E., Budge, S. L., Lenzen, A., Ege, E., Schuch, E., Arango, S., Angelone, N., Mender, E., Hiner, D. L., Huscher, K., Painter, J., & Flores, M. J. (2016). A content analysis of literature on trans people and issues: 2002-2012. *The Counseling Psychologist, 44*(7), 960–995. https://doi.org/10.1177/0011000015609044

Nealy, E. C. (2017). *Transgender children and youth: Cultivating pride and joy with families in transition*. W. W. Norton.

Nealy, E. C. (2019). *Trans kids and teens: Pride, joy, and families in transition*. W. W. Norton.

Olson, K. R., Durwood, L., DeMeules, M., & McLaughlin, K. A. (2016). Mental health of transgender children who are supported in their identities. *Pediatrics, 137*(3), e20153223. https://doi.org/10.1542/peds.2015-3223

Olson, K. R., Durwood, L., Horton, R., Gallagher, N. M., Devor, A. (2022). Gender identity 5 years after social transition. *Pediatrics, 150*(2), e2021056082. http://doi.org/10.1542/peds.2021-056082

Olson, K. R., Key, A. C., & Eaton, N. R. (2015). Gender cognition in transgender children. *Psychological Science, 26*(4), 467–474. https://doi.org/10.1177/0956797614568156

Panchal, Z., Piper, C., Whitmore, C., & Davies, R. D. (2022). Providing supportive transgender mental health care: A systemized narrative review of patient experiences, preferences, and outcomes. *Journal of Gay & Lesbian Mental Health, 26*(3), 228–264. https://doi.org/10.1080/19359705.2021.1899094

Pariseau, E. M., Chevalier, L., Long, K. A., Clapham, R., Edwards-Leeper, L., & Tishelman, A. C. (2019). The relationship between family acceptance-rejection and transgender youth psychosocial functioning. *Clinical Practice in Pediatric Psychology, 7*(3), 267–277. https://doi.org/10.1037/cpp0000291

Pepping, C. A., Cronin, T. J., & Davis, A. W. (2025). Mental health care for transgender and non-binary adults: An investigation of affirmative practice, therapy experiences and outcomes, and reasons for treatment termination. *Sexuality Research & Social Policy*. Advanced online publication. https://doi.org/10.1007/s13178-024-01065-5

Rafferty, J., AAP Committee on Psychosocial Aspects of Child and Family Health, AAP Committee on Adolescence, & AAP Section on Lesbian, Gay, Bisexual, and Transgender Health and Wellness. (2018). Ensuring comprehensive care and support for transgender and gender-diverse children and adolescents. *Pediatrics, 142*(4), e20182162. https://doi.org/10.1542/peds.2018-2162

Rosenthal, S. M. (2021). Challenges in the care of transgender and gender-diverse youth: An endocrinologist's view. *Nature Reviews: Endocrinology, 17*(10), 581–591. https://doi.org/10.1038/s41574-021-00535-9

Ryan, C., & Diaz, R. (2011). *Family Acceptance Project: Intervention guidelines and strategies*. Family Acceptance Project.

Schlehofer, M. M., & Cortez-Regan, L. (2022). Early reactions of parents to their trans and gender non-conforming children. *LGBTQ+ Family: An Interdisciplinary Journal, 18*(1), 81–99. https://doi.org/10.1080/27703371.2021.2023374

Singh, A. (2013). Transgender youth of color and resilience: Negotiating oppression and finding support. *Sex Roles, 68*(11–12), 690–702. https://doi.org/10.1007/s11199-012-0149-z

Spencer, K. G., Berg, D. R., Bradford, N. J., Vencill, J. A., Tellawi, G., & Rider, G. N. (2021). The gender-affirmative life span approach: A developmental model for clinical work with transgender and gender-diverse children, adolescents, and adults. *Psychotherapy, 58*(1), 37–49. https://doi.org/10.1037/pst0000363

Telfer, M. M., Tollit, M. A., Pace, C. C., & Pang, K. C. (2018). Australian standards of care and treatment guidelines for transgender and gender diverse children and adolescents. *The Medical Journal of Australia, 209*(3), 132–136. https://doi.org/10.5694/mja17.01044

Tennessee Senate Bill 1810, 113th General Assembly, Title 49 (2024). https://wapp.capitol.tn.gov/apps/BillInfo/Default.aspx?BillNumber=SB1810&ga=112

Toomey, R. B. (2021). Advancing research on minority stress and resilience in trans children and adolescents in the 21st century. *Child Development Perspectives, 15*(2), 96–102. https://doi.org/10.1111/cdep.12405

Tordoff, D. M., Wanta, J. W., Collin, A., Stepney, C., Inwards-Breland, D. J., & Ahrens, K. (2022). Mental health outcomes in transgender and nonbinary youths receiving gender-affirming care. *JAMA Network Open, 5*(2), e220978–e220978. https://doi.org/10.1001/jamanetworkopen.2022.0978

Trans Legislative Tracker. (2025). *2025 anti-trans bills tracker* [Unpublished raw data]. https://translegislation.com

Turban, J. L. (2017). Transgender youth: The building evidence base for early social transition. *Journal of the American Academy of Child & Adolescent Psychiatry, 56*(2), 101–102. https://doi.org/10.1016/j.jaac.2016.11.008

Turban, J. L., Carswell, J., & Keuroghlian, A. S. (2018). Understanding pediatric patients who discontinue gender-affirming hormonal interventions. *JAMA Pediatrics, 172*(10), 903–904. https://doi.org/10.1001/jamapediatrics.2018.1817

Turban, J. L., & Ehrensaft, D. (2018). Research review: Gender identity in youth: Treatment paradigms and controversies. *Journal of Child Psychology and Psychiatry, and Allied Disciplines, 59*(12), 1228–1243. https://doi.org/10.1111/jcpp.12833

Turban, J. L., King, D., Carswell, J. M., & Keuroghlian, A. S. (2020). Pubertal suppression for transgender youth and risk of suicidal ideation. *Pediatrics, 145*(2), e20191725. https://doi.org/10.1542/peds.2019-1725

Vance, S. R., Jr., Boyer, C. B., Glidden, D. V., & Sevelius, J. (2021). Mental health and psychosocial risk and protective factors among Black and Latinx transgender youth compared with peers. *JAMA Network Open, 4*(3), e213256–e213256. https://doi.org/10.1001/jamanetworkopen.2021.3256

Yong, E. (2019, January 19). Young trans children know who they are. *The Atlantic*. https://www.theatlantic.com/science/archive/2019/01/young-trans-children-know-who-they-are/580366/

Zhou, A. N., Huang, K. J., & Howard, T. L. (2023). Beyond race, sex, and gender: Mental health considerations of transgender youth of color, intersex youth, and nonbinary youth. *Child and Adolescent Psychiatric Clinics of North America, 32*(4), 683–705. Advance online publication. https://doi.org/10.1016/j.chc.2023.04.002

10

GENDER-AFFIRMING CARE WITH TRANS AND NONBINARY ADOLESCENTS

LISA GRIFFIN

M, a 12-year-old child who was assigned male at birth, was referred to me for evaluation for gender identity concerns.[1] M's South American parents shared that M had always preferred clothing, toys, and activities more common for girls and that these preferences had been present since toddlerhood. The parents reported that M loved to read and write, and had written stories for years whose main characters were all girls. M said to me in the first visit, "This [sweeping arms down body] is not this [pointing to heart]." Regarding genitals, M said, "That's the oddest part; if I feel more feminine, why is this here?"

Adolescence can be a time of excitement, angst, and dramatic changes for everyone, but especially for trans and nonbinary (TNB) youth who come to realize that their sex assigned at birth does not align with their internal experience of their gender (Wilson & Cariola, 2020), as in the case of M, who we will revisit at the end of this chapter. Challenges facing TNB youth, such as elevated risks for bullying, self-harm, and suicidality, are well known (Tankersley et al., 2021); less appreciated are the unique joys and sometimes surprising benefits the TNB experience can bring a young person. To help youth and their families navigate difficulties while also fostering optimism, the affirming mental

---

[1]The case of M has been modified to disguise the client's identity and protect their confidentiality.

https://doi.org/10.1037/0000471-011
Affirmative Counseling and Psychological Practice With Trans and Nonbinary Clients, Second Edition, A. Singh and R. McCullough (Editors)
Copyright © 2026 by the American Psychological Association. All rights reserved.

health provider (MHP) working with TNB adolescents must come to the table equipped with proficiency in an array of knowledge areas and how they intersect with one another, as well as a strengths-based philosophy.

The MHP ideally functions as an ally and teammate to both the youth and the family, offering support, tools, and vision of a positive future. The stakes are perhaps higher than at any other developmental stage, since decisions made during puberty will have lifelong concrete, bodily consequences. Appropriate support and medical care during adolescence can not only halt or prevent irreversible development of secondary sex characteristics inconsistent with youths' internal identities, but also can literally save lives through amelioration of suicidal feelings and behaviors (Turban et al., 2020). Clearly, the current disruption of gender-affirming care for youth driven by political forces in the United States is thus life-threatening. Adding to the sense of urgency is the recognition that the timeframe for making these medical decisions may be short, since many young people do not understand the reasons for their discomfort—or may not even have discomfort—until the pubertal process has begun to change their bodies. Thus, specialized expertise and a comprehensive assessment process are crucial, along with steadfast commitment to evidence-based care, regardless of the winds of politics.

This chapter provides MHPs with an overview of the complex landscape of affirmative care for TNB preteens and teens, with a broad view of adolescent development and how gender incongruence can affect its trajectory, and an exploration of environmental characteristics and intersections influencing TNB youth and their families. I discuss the assessment and therapeutic process, options for how MHPs can act as agents of change more broadly, and common therapeutic themes in affirming TNB youth and their families. Surveying this landscape will hopefully inspire readers to embrace this exciting, rewarding, and critical area of care.

FOUNDATIONAL KNOWLEDGE FOR GENDER-AFFIRMING PRACTICE WITH TRANS AND NONBINARY ADOLESCENTS

To understand TNB youth, it is necessary to understand adolescents as a group, as this phase of development is marked by unique, exciting, and frequently tumultuous changes. These include an increase in the ability to think abstractly and with more concern about the world at large, a growing reliance upon peer relationships, a push toward independence from parents, and exploration of romantic feelings and sexuality (Newman & Newman, 2021). At the same time, adolescents are experiencing bodily and emotional changes brought about by puberty that influence brain maturation and perceptions of social interactions (Pfeifer & Allen, 2021). The transformations of adolescence form the bridge from childhood to adulthood, ideally carrying the young person to a solid sense of identity, healthy relationships with peers, and a renegotiated respectful relationship with parents.

Of course, adolescence is not without its challenges, which include emotional turbulence, painful self-consciousness, social awkwardness, and the tendency of young people with stigmatized traits (e.g., perceived unattractiveness or lack of athleticism) to be punished by peers, which can lead to increased adjustment difficulties (e.g., Leggett-James et al., 2023). Associations have also been found between bodily changes in early puberty and increases in depressive symptoms for those assigned female at birth (e.g., McGuire et al., 2019).

Gender Minority Stress and Trans and Nonbinary Adolescents

With all the changes going on in the process of identity formation during the transition from childhood to adulthood, it is difficult to overstate the impact on this process of an individual having a bodily gender phenotype that, as puberty progresses, is increasingly incongruent with their internal gender identity. Studies have found TNB adolescents to have elevated levels of anxiety, depression, suicidality, self-harm behavior, substance use, and disordered eating (Geilhufe et al., 2021; Price-Feeney et al., 2020; Taliaferro et al., 2019; Tankersley et al., 2021; Toomey et al., 2018). However, much of the hardship experienced by these youth has been attributed to minority stress; that is, stress uniquely faced by members of marginalized groups. Gender minority stress factors that may affect TNB youth include anti-trans cultural elements, political rhetoric and anti-trans legislation, some religious views, and direct bullying and harassment (Chodzen et al., 2019; Delozier et al., 2020; Dhanani & Totton, 2023; Johns et al., 2021). Unlike many other minoritized group members, TNB youth are usually living in families made of up members that are not TNB, which can be isolating. Their status prior to coming out is invisible to others, and many must endure being disbelieved or unsupported by their parents, at least initially. In such a climate, it is no wonder that TNB young people can feel unloved, misunderstood, and even hopeless.

Gender incongruence itself can also directly negatively impact a young person's quality of life. It is possible that the effects of increasing levels of (incorrect) sex hormones during puberty can cause discomfort directly, even before anatomical changes are evident, but this discomfort is likely to increase as the young person's body transforms with the development of secondary sex characteristics that are dissonant with their inner identity. In fact, evidence points to an association between earlier access to gender-affirming medical care and more positive psychological functioning (Chen et al., 2023; Sorbara et al. 2020), whereas greater depression (Holt et al., 2016) and body dissatisfaction (de Vries et al., 2014) have been found in adolescents who start treatment at later ages when more physical pubertal changes have occurred.

The foregoing suggests that both decreased environmental transprejudice (and thus reduction in minority stress) and early interventions leading to better alignment between mind and body could improve the quality of TNB youths' lives. Indeed, evidence to date supports both of these predictions. In the realm of minority stress reduction, one study found that community validation, such as using TNB youths' chosen names in school, was associated with more positive mental health outcomes compared to those of TNB youths whose chosen names were not used (Pollitt et al., 2019). Studies have demonstrated positive outcomes when TNB youth have access to medical interventions aimed at bringing their bodies more into alignment with their identities (Chen et al., 2023; de Vries et al., 2014; Kuper et al., 2020; Turban et al, 2020).

For example, one study identified an increase in positive affect and life satisfaction, and a decrease in depression and anxiety, for TNB youth after two years of gender-affirming hormone therapy (GAHT; Chen et al., 2023). Another study found lower rates of self-reported lifetime suicidality among adults whose innate pubertal development had been suppressed medically with puberty blockers (described in a later section) compared with those who had wanted such treatment but were unable to get it (Turban et al., 2020). Though psychotherapeutic interventions have for the most part not been studied separately from medical interventions, some evidence suggests that psychological support is associated with improved psychosocial functioning (Costa et al., 2015). In contrast, evidence abounds that protocols aimed at changing a person's gender identity to align with birth-assigned sex, sometimes called reparative therapies, do not work and are moreover harmful (Fish & Russell, 2020).

Finally, it is important to note that being TNB does not entail only distress (and hopefully its alleviation); it can also confer benefits. The term *gender euphoria* has been used to describe positive sensations associated with gender-affirmative experiences (Beischel et al., 2021). Many TNB youth feel pride in their identities and find joyful, rewarding communities with other LGBTQ+ youth and older role models. The process of exploring one's own gender experience can hone an adolescent's burgeoning insightfulness and self-awareness. Additionally, gaining the courage to share their identities with others, even when reactions are not unanimously supportive, can grow the young person's self-confidence and comfort with authenticity—qualities that can benefit them throughout their lives.

Moderating Effects of Demographics and Other Characteristics

As is true for any aspect of identity formation and affirmation, gender incongruence may manifest and be impacted differently in the presence of a variety of personal, family, background, and other contextual factors, as well as in response to various treatment modalities. The age and developmental stage at which a youth begins transition (Chen et al., 2021), the sex to which a young person was assigned at birth (Verbeek et al, 2020), the degree to which a youth's identity adheres to the traditional gender binary (Poquiz et al., 2021), a youth's racial or ethnic identities (Park et al., 2022), the degree to which a youth is neurodiverse or neurotypical (Strang et al., 2023), and the level of parental and community support a youth receives (Dhanani & Totton, 2023), all have particular influence on adolescents' experiences, so these factors will be explored next. Factors, such as one's cultural, religious, and socioeconomic context, and the state or national policy and political climate, are addressed in detail elsewhere in this volume so will only be touched on here as they impact youth in specific ways, but a central theme is that youth who are unable to access care because of financial, geographic, legal, or other barriers will suffer most.

Age and Developmental Stage at Transition

A young person's experience of the gender transition process is greatly affected by the age and developmental stage during which it occurs. A child may enter adolescence already having lived in their asserted and affirmed gender for years, or come to understand their actual gender is incongruent to the one assigned to them at birth as their sex hormones surge and their body starts changing with puberty, or they may realize well into puberty that their uncomfortable feelings are a result of being TNB. Parents of a child in the first category may already have established a plan for medical intervention long before puberty blockers are needed, whereas in the latter two categories, youth and parents alike may feel daunted by the many considerations and decisions facing them. Often, the young person is in a very different stage of processing their gender difference than their parent(s), and sometimes a gulf exists between parents who have different ideas about what is best for their child. The MHP is a crucial element in the successful navigation of these dynamics, mediating conflicts and helping each member of the family system understand and gain empathy for other members' concerns, even when full agreement is elusive (techniques for establishing and maintaining alliances with families in conflict are offered in a later section).

The pubertal stage at which a youth receives medical intervention for gender incongruence has a profound impact not only on their emotional well-being during adolescence but also their lived experience as an adult. Youth who, shortly after pubertal onset, undergo medical pubertal blockade followed by GAHT do not develop the secondary sex characteristics of their birth-assigned sex, and thus avoid associated dysphoria (and potentially some corrective surgeries years down the road) for the duration of adolescence and into adulthood. This cohort is similar to cisgender counterparts in terms of overall psychological functioning and well-being (de Vries et al., 2014), which is unsurprising given the finding that the more congruent TNB youths' body contours are with youths' identity, the fewer symptoms of anxiety and depression and the greater levels of positive affect and life satisfaction (Chen et al., 2023). Youth who begin medical treatment for dysphoria during the middle to late stages of adolescence manifest relatively higher levels of distress (Chen et al., 2021; Sorbara et al., 2021). These findings suggest that best practice for many TNB youth is to treat gender dysphoria as soon as possible after its presence is confirmed via appropriate assessment.

Sex Assigned at Birth
While TNB teenagers encounter common experiences, both environmental and biological factors can make the transition process different for those assigned female versus male at birth. In the environmental domain, traditional sex roles and expectations can set a stage in which children raised as boys may be judged, ridiculed, or otherwise punished for exhibiting traditionally feminine characteristics (e.g., sensitivity and nurturance), whereas children raised as girls may receive praise and admiration for having what are perceived as masculine traits (confidence and athleticism). A boy playing with dolls may be a target for bullying and a girl playing football may not. This could be a social conditioning setup in which those assigned male at birth may be identified as TNB early in life and perhaps supported in their interests and identities, or they may learn to hide and even feel ashamed of their authentic selves, overcompensating via hypermasculine behavior. Those assigned female at birth may be rewarded for traditionally masculine behaviors and thus may fly under the TNB radar and avoid negative social shaping. They may live as tomboys until their bodies start to change, illuminating a newly felt incongruence with identity. Of course, in many families and communities adhering to more traditional gender norms, birth-assigned females can be as rigidly regulated in their expression as birth-assigned males, and the previously described patterns may not apply.

Some TNB youth have a more complicated gender journey because their gender expression or sexual orientation aligns with cultural expectations for their assigned sex. For example, a trans boy can be feminine in presentation or attracted to males, which may confound those around him or even himself.

For these youth and their families, it can be illuminating to encourage them to think of examples of cisgender individuals who do not conform to traditional gender norms. Some cisgender men enjoy wearing makeup, skirts, and nail polish, and some of them are gay. Some cisgender women never wear makeup, skirts, or nail polish, and some of them are lesbians.

In addition to social factors, physiological factors, including bodily configuration and the timing of pubertal onset, may explain differences in the experience of dysphoria. Often, a significant source of dysphoria for trans women is genitals, whereas for trans men, it is their chest. Some female-assigned children recognize that they are TNB only after the onset of puberty, since breasts do not develop until the pubertal period. On the other hand, birth-assigned females begin puberty, on average, about a year sooner than do birth-assigned males and thus may experience hormonally mediated dysphoria at earlier ages than their birth-assigned male peers. It is hoped that future investigations will elucidate the influences of these differences on differential experiences of gender incongruence between birth-assigned males and females, supporting more customized treatment strategies.

An additional category of assigned sex differences arises from medical treatment and its impact. Birth-assigned males and females who begin GAHT during latter stages of puberty will have quite distinct experiences of "second puberty." Transmasculine teens may experience more social dysphoria early in transition than their transfeminine counterparts, simply because it is harder for these teens to project maleness via clothing and hairstyles alone. This is true in part because, for many decades, it has been more acceptable for females than males to adopt gender nonconforming styles. Also, the contour of breasts can cause others to automatically gender a person as female. However, later in transition, the tables turn; transfeminine young people may have a more difficult time projecting an accurate gender to others than their transmasculine counterparts, because feminizing GAHT does not correct secondary sex characteristics as readily as does masculinizing GAHT. Whereas adequate time on masculinizing GAHT will confer the facial hair and deep voice that facilitate an individual being seen as male, feminizing GAHT does not reverse some of the effects of an original puberty, such as skeletal features and vocal pitch, which may trigger misgendering. Indeed, Verbeek and colleagues (2020) found that trans women experienced stronger social stigma than trans men.

Identity on the Gender Spectrum
Increasingly, youth are asserting genders outside or beyond the binary, reflecting the actual complexity of the brain and consequent experiential phenomena we call gender or gender identity. Scholars have found both similarities and

differences in the experiences of binary trans (transmasculine and transfeminine) as compared to nonbinary youth. For example, Poquiz et al. (2021) found that among adolescents and young adults, transmasculine and transfeminine individuals experienced more discrimination compared to nonbinary individuals, possibly related to greater visibility of their gender minority status.

Trans and Nonbinary Youth in Communities of Color
Youth in communities of color are subjected to the chronic social stressors of prejudice and racism, and a number of investigations have found that the added dimension of being TNB imposes further challenges (Park et al., 2022; see also Chapter 6 in this volume). Vance and colleagues (2021) found that Black and Latinx TNB youth had levels of mental health symptoms similar to those of White TNB youth, but higher than those of cisgender Black and Latinx youth. Moreover, for TNB Black and Latinx youth, victimization and harassment increased their risk of symptoms, but school connectedness and caring adult relationships were not protective in the same way they were for cisgender Black and Latinx youth. Also, TNB Black and Latinx youth experienced more race-based harassment than their cisgender Black and Latinx peers, revealing a complex interplay of stigmatization factors and variations in how these youth perceived harassment in relation to their identities. These results highlight the need for specifically targeted school- and community-based antibullying efforts as well as future research understanding the experiences among specific communities of color.

The intersection of racism and gender also impacts health care. For example, Johns et al. (2023) found that among gender, race, and ethnicity identity cohorts, Black and Hispanic young TNB women were least likely to be insured, have a current health care provider (and be out to their provider), and they were most likely to predict they would have problems with their care because of their gender. Some TNB youth become caught up in the particularly tragic phenomenon in which they are ejected or run away from unsupportive family environments, only to land in environments that increase their risk for incarceration. This is particularly true for youth in communities of color, who can be ensnared in what Mountz (2020) terms a revolving-door dynamic. Mountz describes how LGBTQ+ youth of color, having decreased access to a social safety net, are more likely to utilize survival strategies that lead to systems involvement, which in turn leads to more marginalization. Despite evidence that TNB youth of color may hesitate to be out, experience more distress, and receive less support than their White counterparts, at least one large, longitudinal, multisite study reported some contrasting findings. TNB youth of color in this study were found to have less depression and more positive affect at baseline than non-Latinx or non-Latine White youth (Chen et al., 2023), and a later publication examining the same cohort found lower lifetime suicidality rates among TNB youth of color compared to White TNB youth (Vance et al., 2023). The authors offered several possible explanations for these findings, including the fact that youth in the sample were supported by caregivers who were willing to bring them to gender-affirmative clinics, the possibility that distress may only emerge when youth enter young adulthood and no longer have access to familial supports, and potential reporting bias due to culture-based stigma surrounding suicide. Future research should illuminate more resilience factors for TNB youth of color, providing MHPs with valuable tools for bolstering these strengths. Importantly, rather than burdening TNB youth of color with the responsibility of building resilience, the improvement of health care access and quality for TNB people of color should be included in the mission of health care settings (Goldenberg et al., 2021).

Neurodiversity Spectrum
As mentioned earlier, associations have been found between gender dysphoria and several medical and mental health conditions, some of which may differentially impact a youth's experience with gender diversity. Glidden and colleagues (2016) found that TNB individuals are more likely than their cisgender counterparts to have autism spectrum diagnoses; however, given the few studies published about this topic, the connection between autism spectrum diagnoses and TNB people is not yet conclusive. It is relevant to note that, relative to neurotypical TNB youth, higher levels of internalizing symptoms have been found in neurodivergent TNB youth, and among the latter, those with poorer executive function and more autism-related social symptoms fared worse in terms of mental health (Strang et al., 2023). However, neurodiversity can be a protective factor for those youth who are less drawn into adolescent clique systems than are their neurotypical peers. MHPs should strive to explore how a TNB adolescent's unique personhood can provide unexpected sources of resilience.

Level of Parental, School, Community, and Policy-Level Support
Environmental support has been strongly associated with positive mental and emotional health for TNB youth. Pariseau et al. (2019) found that lower levels of past acceptance in primary caretakers were associated with higher levels of anxiety and other internalizing symptoms, and indifference from caretakers was associated with higher rates of depressive symptoms; lower sibling acceptance was also associated with higher levels of suicidal ideation. Pollitt et al. (2019) found that adolescents whose chosen name was routinely used in home, school, and work environments fared better in terms of mental health.

On the policy level, there is preliminary evidence to suggest that anti-TNB legislation negatively affects not only youth directly impacted by bans on care, but also TNB youth more broadly. Specifically, Dhanani and Totton (2023) found that mere exposure to the existence of such legislation, as well as the perception that socially relevant others supported it were associated with a range of negative health consequences, increased fears of disclosing and health care avoidance. Sadly, the implication is that *all* TNB youth are potentially at greater risk for harm because of policy actions in the United States.

Other Diversity Characteristics of Trans and Nonbinary Youth
Ultimately, TNB adolescents are a diverse group of young people whose gender identities are refracted through a variety of lenses, some of which interact with one another to create even more diversity of experiences. The foregoing is only a sample of the many dimensions that can affect a given youth's trajectory. These and others, such as faith tradition (a topic covered in Chapter 14 of this volume), national origin, parental educational background, and disability status (see Chapter 9 in this volume for a brief discussion of disability status among TNB children), are important factors to consider when caring for TNB youth.

ASSESSMENT AND THERAPEUTIC PROCESS

Gender-affirming mental health care for youth encompasses wide-ranging knowledge domains and may include various assessments; individual, family, or group counseling; social transition education and support; sexual and reproductive health education; medical puberty blockade; gender-affirming hormone treatment; auxiliary services (such as permanent hair removal and voice training); and surgical intervention. Legal services may also be indicated for name and gender marker changes, or for sealing a youth's records following such changes—a protective step available in some states. It is important that MHPs keep in mind that every youth has a unique path toward a life in which they are comfortable in their skin and their world. MHPs should be ready to support TNB adolescents and family members with intentional care and guidance, regardless of where they are in the process, and to incorporate the following components in some form.

Assessment

Formal assessment may not be indicated in adult TNB care unless desired by the client, but for youth, a thorough biopsychosocial assessment is generally recommended (Coleman et al., 2022). Assessment can help to confirm that feelings of gender incongruity are not caused by conditions other than gender dysphoria (thus necessitating different treatments or approaches), identify coexisting mental health and medical conditions that may affect treatment recommendations, elucidate cultural influences that may inform decisions, uncover family dynamics that may guide the MHP's approach, and uncover personality, cognitive, and other individual factors that may be important in helping youth and their parents make good choices. A thoughtful assessment can help alleviate anxieties faced by both youth and their parents resulting from an awareness that the wrong decisions either way—pursuing medical treatment when it is *not* the right path or not pursuing medical treatment when it *is* the right path—can result in unwanted consequences. Assessment is most likely to be effective and feel affirming to all involved if the MHP frames it from within a systems perspective. Each party understands that they provide unique and important data to the complete picture. The parents provide background and developmental observations, the MHP provides tools and expertise in the area of gender diversity, and most importantly, the youth provides the raw data regarding how they feel. Emphasizing that no one else on the treatment team has this most direct piece of information centers the youth and elevates the importance of their contributions.

Assessment often begins with a parents-only session in which the MHP orients the parents or caregivers to the assessment process and gathers general family, medical, and developmental history, as well as parents' descriptions of their child's gender experience. ("Parent" session is understood to include whatever adults provide primary care to the youth.) The parent session can provide the MHP with valuable insights about parents' values and attitudes about gender diversity, particularly as it relates to their child. A parents-only session prior to the MHP meeting with the youth additionally affords an opportunity, if appropriate, to educate parents about the wide variety of possible trajectories, a process that often reassures parents that the MHP is not simply putting their child on a "sex-change conveyer belt." The parent session also ideally establishes a positive alliance between parents and MHPs, a necessary component of successful assessment and therapy (if indicated).

Having such an alliance proves especially critical when youth and parents are not on the same page regarding the youth's path forward, or when parents are in disagreement with one another, and it becomes a role of the MHP to facilitate a meeting of minds. Of course, many families enter the MHP's office well into the process, having successfully negotiated early stages of transition together. In such cases, families may only be consulting the MHP because they have been informed that this is required for some further phase of care, such as medical intervention. A final goal of the parent session is establishing boundaries. Most parents understand that their child must be able to trust that the MHP will keep their confidences and will agree to the MHP's policy of only sharing details with parents to which the child has consented, except of course when it comes to mandated reporting content.

Following the parent session, the MHP will want to meet with the adolescent alone, once, twice, or several times, depending on complexity and time allowed per session. The limits of confidentiality should be discussed at the beginning, so the young person understands exactly what will and will not be shared with parents. The MHP should then describe what will happen during the session, emphasizing that even though there will be a focus on the MHP learning as much as possible about the youth's gender experience, they are aware that the youth is a whole person with a lot of other things going on in their life. As always, the simplest language possible should be used until the MHP has a good feel for the youth's cognitive and linguistic maturity. As is true with child assessment, the MHP may need to assess the degree to which the adolescent understands the concept of gender and how they distinguish that from sex and gender expression.

During the session, and while using exclusively nonleading language, the MHP should ask about the youth's current understanding of their gender and about the process that led them to this understanding. It helps for the MHP to reassure the young person that they realize these feelings and internal experiences can be very difficult to describe, even if someone is trying. For some, this may be the first time they have been asked to describe their feelings in detail. The MHP may then go on to assess components of the young person's past and current experience that have been associated with gender incongruence, including interests, friendship preferences, preferences regarding clothing and hairstyles, etc. Prior to discussing the young person's feelings about their body, it can be helpful to give them a gentle heads-up that the next questions are about very private feelings and can make a lot of people uncomfortable, especially when they are talking to an adult they just met. For this part of the assessment, explaining why these questions are being asked can help the young person understand that you are there to support them.

It should be noted that although instruments geared toward assessing gender identity and gender dysphoria in adolescents exist, their psychometric properties are unavailable, they are based on small sample sizes, and they contain outdated content (Bloom et al., 2021). Until future research validates existing tools or more relevant and culturally appropriate tools are developed, open and structured interview techniques are likely to produce the richest, most accurate picture of a youth's gender experience. Throughout the assessment and therapeutic process, it is essential that the MHP thoughtfully consider their social positionalities relative to the youth and family and the resulting potential impacts on the therapeutic relationship. Differences in racial or ethnic background, age, education level, and other factors may affect not only the clients' stance toward the MHP, but also the MHP's approach to their clients through their own unexamined biases. Working with TNB youth also necessitates evaluation of how the MHP's own transness or cisness may affect their relationship with not only the TNB youth, but also the parents, who are likely to be cisgender. MHPs should explicitly discuss these factors as a matter of course, and especially when they appear to be affecting the therapeutic alliance.

Individual, Family, and Group Counseling

It is said that when a youth transitions, the whole family transitions. While this is a simplification, it is true that the process requires much not only of the youth, but also of their family. Often, counseling can provide valuable support and guidance to families navigating this evolution. Individual therapy can be a touchstone for a young TNB person during a time when they may feel overwhelmed. The youth can explore how their birth-designated gender category is incongruent with their experienced internal gender; whether a new name, pronouns, gender markers, and appearance will help them feel more comfortable; whether and how to talk with others about their process; and so on. They may encounter significant apprehension regarding potential reactions from peers, parents, and siblings, as well as concerns about potential rejection, which they must navigate and address. They may have absorbed vast quantities of information from internet and social media sources, both accurate and helpful, and inaccurate and harmful. The MHP can be a comforting presence during this time, sharing the heavy lifting, and reminding them of their own unique journey.

At the same time, parents may feel surprised by their child's assertion of a different gender identity, and as they learn more about gender diversity, parents may feel pressured to act before they feel ready, particularly when it comes to supporting a teen's asserted need for medical interventions. Many parents express anxieties about their child's safety in an anti-TNB world. Some believe their child's feelings are being influenced by peers, social media, or just the usual emotional storms of adolescence; they worry that their child is not actually gender dysphoric and may change their mind after irreversible treatments. Many come to the table with a belief that their child is too young to make such profound decisions, often citing their own struggles during puberty and adolescence. These are not unreasonable concerns, and the MHP's empathy and validation can help maintain an alliance with parents while they learn about gender incongruence and how to distinguish it from other conditions and processes.

Sometimes when parents fully believe and support their child in their asserted gender, they may face judgment and backlash from their own parents and other family members, neighbors, coworkers, and friends. Additionally, turning to other members of the system, siblings may face scrutiny at school, often being the target of curiosity and questions from students, causing internally conflicting feelings of resentment, defensiveness, embarrassment, and protectiveness. At the same time, they can feel forgotten as their trans sibling absorbs a lot of parental focus during the transition period. It is recommended that youth and their families seek therapeutic support from a gender specialist MHP during the transition process. Additionally, access to mentorship programs, support groups, or group therapy with others in similar situations can be affirmative, educational, and can help youth and their families feel less isolated. A resource list of books, websites, podcasts, and even social media accounts can help to fill out a family's support structure and knowledge base. For example, many youth gain insight working through *The Gender Quest Workbook* (Testa et al., 2015).

Social Transition Education and Support

As mentioned earlier, some youth will already be well along their transition path by the time they arrive at the MHP's office. However, many will be unsure what steps to take (and in what order) to live more comfortable lives. For these youth, once a determination has been made via assessment that social transition is appropriate for a youth, the MHP can aid the youth in coming out, choosing a new name (if desired), and declaring pronouns and identity descriptors. Guidance can also be offered regarding presentation concerns, including gender-specific practices such as binding (flattening the chest, for transmasculine youth) and tucking (minimizing genital bulge, for transfeminine youth), and resources covering safety guidelines for these practices can be offered. MHPs can offer youth and their parents suggestions on how to lay the groundwork for a social transition in various environments (school, work, faith community, and others) and with extended family members that is as seamless as possible.

Sexual and Reproductive Health Education

Although youth vary in the degree to which (if any) their dysphoria interferes with their interest in sexual activities, it is important for the MHP to normalize sexuality as part of healthy development. Even if the young person has significant dysphoria regarding their genitals and reproductive organs, the MHP can gently encourage them to stay open to learning about how to stay emotionally and physically safe in this arena. For TNB youth, having supportive counseling space where they can explore their thoughts and feelings about their relationship with their body (e.g., genitals, body shape) can open up not only self-acceptance, but also possibilities for fulfilling sexual relationships, with or without future surgeries. For instance, reframing genitals using new vocabulary can help, as can utilization of visualization techniques (during masturbation, for example). For youth who identify as asexual or "ase," it is possible that their current lack of sexual feelings may be temporary, and as their dysphoria eases, they may experience an awakening of sexual interest, which may warrant further exploration. If this triggers anxiety, the MHP can reassure them that they will still have full control over whether they choose to engage in sexual activities, and they can discuss management of their feelings and decisions about behaviors with the MHP if desired.

Regarding reproductive options, it is often the youth's parents who are most invested in fertility preservation. After all, most young people are not thinking about whether they want to have children, and it can be a good idea to acknowledge the strangeness of having to think about it so soon. Fertility preservation options should be reviewed; for transfeminine youth, this can involve cryopreservation of sperm, and for transmasculine youth, egg retrieval can be pursued. Still, it is important that young people understand the impacts medical treatments may have on their future ability to be biological parents, and MHPs are often in the best position among providers to explore a young person's feelings on the matter with them. This means MHPs must have accurate and current knowledge about reproductive impacts of various medical interventions at various stages of pubertal development and must also be ready to refer families to appropriate professionals for fertility preservation if desired, as discussed in the next section.

Education Regarding and Referral for Medical and Auxiliary Services

Parents and youth often feel overwhelmed by the maze of options and decisions to be made when it comes to exploring transition steps, and most know little about how to find accurate information, much less reputable professionals who can provide needed services. The MHP can be a valuable resource both in approaching decisions to be made and also in directing families to services. Some of these treatments and services are outlined here.

Puberty Blockade
For youth at the early stages of puberty, *medical puberty blockade* ("blockers") can stave off bodily changes that may be undesirable long-term, for when youth or parents are unsure about future bodily goals or when it is clear that those goals align with the development of secondary sex characteristics different from what the body would produce on its own. Blockers are gonadotropin releasing hormone agonists—agents that have been used for decades in the treatment of precocious puberty without incident, but that have more limited empirical confirmation for their use in trans youth (Lee & Rosenthal, 2023). Still, politicized efforts to label this treatment as "experimental" are dubious considering accumulated evidence to date (Murano-Kinney, 2024).

Puberty blockers are usually administered by a pediatric endocrinologist; if an implant is used, a surgeon may also be involved. Most centers require referral by an MHP, though some will administer blockers by informed consent of the child and parents. Though the medical provider is responsible for sharing details regarding risks and side effects, the MHP should help prepare the family for treatment. They should be able to educate the child and parents on the early signs of puberty so they can be on the lookout in situations where the child is already socially transitioned.

Findings indicate that blockers, followed by gender-affirming hormone treatment, are an effective protocol for treating gender dysphoria, leading to positive outcomes and low levels of regret (Chelliah et al., 2024; Chen et al., 2023; de Vries et al., 2014; Olson et al., 2024). Despite these positive findings, there is a relative paucity of available research investigating what long-term effects, if any, they may have on bone health, brain development, and growth (Lee & Rosenthal, 2023). Treatment with blockers at the earliest recommended stage of puberty, *if* followed by long-term GAHT, results in likely infertility, though possibilities for future fertility preservation innovations exist; however, blockers on their own do not cause infertility. It is important for the youth and parents to be fully informed prior to initiating puberty blockade and GAHT, and for all individuals involved to recognize that when the youth reaches young adulthood, they may come to grieve the possible loss of their ability to have their own biological children. However, the minimal negative impacts of this treatment are overshadowed by the benefits it has on the youth who find blockers and GAHT to be lifesaving; they turn out to be well-adjusted adults because of this treatment (de Vries et al., 2014).

Gender-Affirming Hormone Treatment
When youth are already in middle or late stages of puberty, GAHT can be implemented when appropriate to enable them to develop secondary sex

characteristics that are congruent with their identity. MHPs should be familiar with modes of delivery as well as the expected changes, their order, and their timing. They may need to educate the youth and parents about potential emotional impacts of hormones, which are not always as expected. For example, though testosterone is often associated in the popular mind with aggression, in transmasculine people, the strongest effects are decreases in psychological distress and depressive symptoms (Doyle et al., 2023). Transfeminine people experience similar positive mood changes when beginning hormones, but they may also notice increased emotional lability (Doyle et al., 2023); preparing youth and parents for this effect can prevent distress due to misinterpreting tearfulness or emotionality as the onset or worsening of depressive symptoms. Also, increased lability can be especially distressing for youth on the autism spectrum, who may be more prone to difficulties in emotion regulation than neurotypical peers (Beck et al., 2020).

Current research on reproduction following initiation of GAHT can be shared, and in particular, youth should receive accurate information regarding the possibility of getting pregnant or impregnating someone else, even when receiving GAHT (Light et al., 2014). In addition to or instead of GAHT, transmasculine youth who experience dysphoria secondary to menses can benefit from hormonal menstrual suppression. This treatment stops menstrual periods but does not induce masculinizing changes to the body. As with blockers, pediatric endocrinologists are often the providers of hormone therapy and menstrual suppression for youth, though many youths can receive care from their pediatricians or other primary care providers, including settings such as Planned Parenthood clinics. Many providers do not require mental health referrals but require informed consent from youth and their parents or caregivers.

Surgery
Though most types of gender confirmation surgeries are rare among teens, more common is chest masculinization, or "top surgery," for transmasculine and nonbinary teens who were assigned female at birth and were not treated with blockers. The World Professional Association for Transgender Health's *Standards of Care* (Coleman et al., 2022) acknowledge that earlier surgical intervention for chest dysphoria is often warranted, and in fact, may be the only medical intervention needed for some youth. Although many transmasculine youth wear binders to flatten the chest, these garments can restrict breathing; prevent optimized exercise and athletic performance; cause rib, back, and shoulder pain; cause gastrointestinal problems; and even cause skeletal changes (Peitzmeier et al., 2017). Thus, for many, chest masculinization surgery can be seen as a healthier alternative. Studies with youth who have undergone this surgery

resulted in good surgical outcomes, high levels of satisfaction with results, and minimal regret (Marinkovic & Newfield, 2017; Olson-Kennedy et al., 2018). MHPs should be familiar with surgical preparation, procedures, and aftercare, and should have knowledge of area surgeons to whom they can refer youth and their parents; most surgeons require a mental health referral.

Some genital gender confirmation surgeries, when appropriate, are endorsed by the World Professional Association for Transgender Health's *Standards of Care* for TNB individuals starting in late adolescence, following continuous GAHT for at least a year (Coleman et al., 2022). Exceptions can be made when GAHT is medically contraindicated or is not compatible with the individual's embodiment goals, as is true for many nonbinary individuals. Phalloplasty is not recommended prior to the age of 18 years, due to the complexity of the surgery and the higher risk for complications in comparison to other surgeries. MHPs working with youth who are seeking genital surgery must familiarize themselves with subcategories of these types of surgeries as well as pre- and postsurgical care, including lifelong aftercare practices and potential complications. Clinicians should be prepared to have frank conversations with their young clients about differences in function between natal versus reconstructed genitals and about the need for specialized aftercare routines, some of which will be required throughout the individual's lifetime. Also, adolescents must fully absorb the finality of gonadal removal, which in the absence of gamete or embryonic cryopreservation will render them infertile. These conversations can be challenging for adolescents, who may have limited capacity for long-term planning. Finally, adolescents may underestimate what is required in preparation for surgery, which may entail months of painful permanent hair removal, tissue expansion, or skin grafts. For many, reality is different from the fantasies many have of simply waking up with everything corrected.

MHPs should be familiar not only with the subcategories of surgeries, but also with suitable surgical providers, preferably in the area and in network with the family's health insurance provider. They should inform youth and families regarding the fact that different bodily characteristics may call for different surgical techniques, not all of which are performed by all surgeons. They should also keep an up-to-date list of area electrologists who can perform permanent genital hair removal (if indicated), and ideally, specialized physical therapists who can help the youth develop a strong pelvic floor in preparation for and after surgery, a service that is increasingly recommended for postsurgical healing and function (Gallagher et al., 2022).

Other surgical options that may be desired include facial feminization or masculinization procedures, liposuction and fat transfer, chest feminization surgery, and feminization laryngoplasty. All of these procedures are aimed at altering secondary sex characteristics. Again, the MHP plays an important role in ensuring that the youth has realistic goals and also are not simply acting out of impatience, as it can take several years to determine ultimate hormonal changes (although some characteristics, such as vocal pitch in transfeminine individuals, will not be impacted by GAHT). Careful exploration may help to elucidate the appropriate path forward, whether continuing to work with the client on complex and persistent dysphoria or referring for additional specialized treatment.

It should be noted that, at the time of this writing, the United States has witnessed an unprecedented escalation of legislative bans on gender-affirming care, particularly for youth. Such bans have been decried as harmful by many major national health organizations, including the American Psychological Association, the American Medical Association, the World Professional Association for Transgender Health, and the American Academy of Pediatrics. However, due to legal restrictions, many TNB youth and their families are unable to access vital and medically necessary care, which will have long-term consequences.

Other Services
MHPs should be aware that there are additional services TNB adolescents may want to access. For instance, although voice feminization surgeries are available nationally and internationally, because of the cost and risks of these surgeries, transfeminine individuals who wish to have vocal characteristics more typical of adult cisgender women most often seek vocal change through voice therapy. TNB adolescents may self-educate via apps or videos, or they can seek individual or group voice counseling, either in person or virtually. The MHP can facilitate matching the client with an appropriate resource or resources. TNB youth may also be interested in connecting with hair removal specialists when this service is needed, either in preparation for genital surgery or for youth whose facial or other body hair prevents them from living comfortably in their affirmed identities. Finally, it is useful for the MHP to keep an up-to-date list of TNB-competent legal professionals available for clients to use if they need help with a legal name change, custody dispute, discrimination experience, or other matter. Sometimes individual attorneys or firms are appropriate referrals, but in cases involving discriminatory school or workplace policies, organizations such as Lambda Legal, the National Center for Lesbian Rights, or the American Civil Liberties Union can provide valuable guidance.

Consultation, Advocacy, and Community Education
Though not directly related to individual client care, MHPs serving TNB youth often develop great passion for the communities they serve, and they seek to

better the lives of TNB persons and their families in broader ways. They may contract or volunteer to consult schools, corporations, and religious entities who wish to better support their gender diverse students, teachers, employees, clergy, and congregants. They may also engage in lobbying efforts to elevate political discourse and promote legislation founded in science versus ideologies, particularly given current regressive trends in these areas in the United States and elsewhere. Similarly, they may serve as expert witnesses or write affidavits to educate judges, attorneys, and jurors, and support case law grounded in solid scientific knowledge. They can develop and provide community trainings and workshops for a range of audiences. Finally, they can show up in solidarity with TNB people at pride rallies, Transgender Day of Remembrance and Transgender Day of Visibility commemorations, and other community events. MHPs can go beyond providing excellent care for their clients by doing their part to create a more comfortable and inclusive society for all TNB people.

COMMON THERAPEUTIC CONCERNS

While the previous section covered many of the themes encountered when supporting TNB adolescents and their families, several types of challenges are commonly seen with TNB adolescents and merit further exploration. It should be noted that research is sparse on specific psychotherapeutic techniques and their outcomes in this population, so most of the guidance found here derives from anecdotal evidence.

Gender Dysphoria

Most TNB adolescents experience *gender dysphoria*, a multifaceted phenomenon that may involve distress regarding the incongruence between their felt identities and their body conformations, how others perceive them, the gender roles they occupy, and so on. When TNB youth are misgendered by others, the MHP can assist them in making decisions about how and whether to correct the misgendering and how to enlist others to act as their allies and speak up on their behalf. MHPs can also offer suggestions for how to avoid triggers (e.g., by covering the bathroom mirror while showering) and to distract (e.g., by listening to a podcast while showering). It can be useful to have the youth create a list of such interventions they can consult when they are struggling. Finally, cognitive behavioral techniques can be utilized to explore beliefs that they will never be seen accurately or that they will always hate their body; such beliefs can be magnified in the adolescent mind, which is not fully developed in terms of long-term planning and ability to see beyond the current moment.

Self-Harm

Self-injurious behavior is also common in TNB teens and is also often related to feelings of dysphoria (Morris & Galupo, 2019). For this reason, many of the strategies that are helpful for coping with dysphoria can also be utilized for self-harm behaviors. However, unique concerns exist when TNB adolescents engage in self-harm as a result of dysphoria, for example, when youth target parts of their bodies that cause feelings of dysphoria. In combination with interventions geared toward self-harm generally, TNB adolescents struggling with bodily dysphoria may be additionally supported through strategies that enable them to reframe parts of their bodies via visualization techniques, or even apps that permit them to see their potential future body contours. Such strategies can instill a desire to care for the tissues that will ultimately make up a body that is more congruent with the young person's experienced identity. This technique aligns with the approach described previously for dysphoria reduction, in that it helps the youth imagine a future in which they are comfortable in their skin. An alternative approach is to encourage the youth to access carefully curated resources celebrating diverse bodies, such as trans-made erotica; seeing themselves reflected in bodies that are desirable and sexy can help to undo cultural training around what constitutes "acceptable" genitals.

Suicidality

Elevated levels of suicidal ideation and behavior are well documented in TNB adolescents, as discussed earlier. As with self-harm, techniques for treating suicidality in youth in general may be helpful for this population, but nuanced particularities in suicidal feelings among dysphoric youth may call for additional and different approaches. As noted earlier, youth may be unable to visualize a future in which their bodies conform with their identities. More specifically, some youth may have been unable during their development to relate to the adult role models of their own assigned sex represented in their lives and more generally in culture and media; being unable to see future selves, they may see no reason to continue. Sometimes, encouraging youth to develop alternate developmental narratives in which they imagine having been raised from birth in a manner congruent with their identities, and supported in gender mentoring consistent with cultural expectations for their identities, can enable them to see that their current lack of a future vision is an artifact of having had a lack of relatable life trajectory models. Though searching for inspiring TNB role models online can be a landmine, many youths do benefit enormously from following TNB celebrities who provide positive messaging about transness. This can lead to hopefulness and a new ability to plan for a bright, imaginable future. See Chapter 13 for a further discussion of suicidality.

Dissociation

Dissociation is generally discussed as a strategy for coping with trauma, but anecdotally, it seems to be a common experience for TNB youth, even those with no known history of trauma. For at least some young people, receiving messages inconsistent with internal identity can lead to the negation of authentic self-experience and development of a false self that enables them to meet expectations and avoid punishment. These messages are environmental reinforcement of the wrong gender, which create a microaggressive climate for the youth and constantly overwhelms them (e.g., through misgendering). The cumulative effect can be likened to gaslighting by the youth's very interface with outside reality. Even though affirming treatment can help to rectify the disconnect between identity and how the youth is treated by the world, the mechanism of dissociation can remain installed in the psyche. It can be empowering for the MHP to assist the youth in exploring how the ability to dissociate can be useful in some situations, but the youth will likely benefit from learning and employing techniques for staying present when dissociation interferes with functioning (e.g., using modalities such as dialectical behavioral therapy).

Eating Disturbances

Though TNB youth can develop eating disturbances for reasons similar to other youth, many TNB youth experiencing dysphoria alter their eating patterns in attempts to forestall pubertal changes or disguise unwanted body elements (Coelho et al., 2019). For example, transmasculine youth may restrict calories in an attempt to prevent further breast growth or to halt menses. Although MHPs may employ some of the previously described techniques in an effort to help youth envision future body changes with GAHT or surgeries, if disordered eating is entrenched or progressed, it may be necessary to refer the youth to specialized care. If so, consultation between the gender and eating specialists is strongly recommended.

Decisions About Disclosure

If GAHT treatment is part of a youth's path, once they have achieved greater congruence between body and identity, they may encounter a need to make decisions about whether they wish to disclose their status as trans or transition history to others. Having this option is sometimes called *passing privilege*, though the concept of passing can be problematic, since the person is not passing as anything: they simply are who they are. However, this privilege is real, as it enables someone who wishes to do so to be able to go about their lives without automatically being recognized as trans by others, whereas those who do not have this privilege have less choice over the matter. Those who opt to allow the assumption to be made that they are cisgender are sometimes described as living *stealth*, though this term is also problematic; again, they are simply living their lives. The issue with both terms, passing and stealth, lies in the difference between secrecy and privacy. Rather than keeping their history secret, most people who do not disclose their trans status prefer to keep this information private, just as others may not broadcast details of their own medical history. However, these terms are widely used and understood within the TNB community.

Circumstances can arise in which having one's TNB status unknown to others can create complications. If a romantic spark develops with someone, for example, the TNB teen may need to decide if or when to disclose their history, knowing that a possibility exists for physical intimacy that may reveal anatomical differences from what is expected. Alternatively, the teen may have to decide what to say to a partner if they have chosen not to be physically intimate until after surgical intervention. A transfeminine teen may also have to decide how to participate when conversations among friends turn to the topic of their periods. More nuanced situations can arise when some of a youth's friends know about their history and others do not, or when a relationship with a friend has deepened to the point that the friend can feel hurt if they eventually learn about this important aspect of the teen's life and discover it had not been previously shared. MHPs and clients can process possible scenarios before they arise to prevent young people from being caught off guard and to foster a sense of control and self-determination.

Unsupportive Parents

Dynamics in families where parents do not believe or support their child's assertion of a different gender pose one of the most difficult sets of challenges for the MHP. Lack of parental support is a major contributor to distress and maladjustment in TNB youth (Vance et al., 2023), so it is critical for the MHP to make this impasse a therapeutic priority. Once assessment has confirmed the presence of gender incongruence, the MHP must find the right balance between alliance and empathy with parents and firmness in stating recommendations for the youth—a task that requires keen therapeutic acumen.

For a strong therapeutic alliance with the parents, the MHP can listen to the parents' doubts and concerns without any preconceptions, validate and empathize with the parents' feelings of distress, and capitalize on the parents' strengths, which perhaps lie in their concern, protectiveness, and positive intentions for their child. Sometimes a seeming lack of support may stem mostly from concern that their child's coming out as trans may subject them to discrimination, bullying, or even violence. Still, this is the MHP's first opportunity to educate parents on what is known about TNB adolescents' experiences, and the MHP may wish to emphasize the strong evidence we have showing how crucial parental support is in creating positive outcomes in these youth. It can be helpful for the MHP to lay out the steps of assessment and to list the conditions and variables to be examined that can cause a young person to think they are trans when they actually are not. It should be emphasized that there are few such conditions, and that the majority of youth do not change their minds or decide to revert to living in their gender assigned at birth (Olson et al., 2022). As described earlier, parents can be offered a variety of resources for helping them move forward.

Despite their best efforts, some parents may not agree to support their child's asserted gender, either through utilizing preferred name and pronouns, or consenting to medical treatment, or advocating for their child with schools, relatives, and others. In some cases, the young person may feel unsafe even disclosing their feelings to their parents, and the MHP (e.g., a school counselor) may only be able to help the youth develop strategies for surviving until the age of majority. In either of these scenarios, the MHP can help the youth identify strengths as well as steps they can currently take to feel as comfortable as possible. It can help to engage some of the techniques described earlier for managing dysphoria, self-harm, and suicidality that permit the youth to envision a future in which they are happy, healthy, and affirmed.

Detransition and Retransition

As more youth are able to access gender-affirming medical care, it is inevitable that some will continue to shift in the way they perceive their gender over time. However, multiple investigations have found that the large majority of adolescents who undertake transition steps continue on this path. For example, van der Loos and colleagues (2022) found that most youth who began hormone treatment in adolescence continued it into adulthood, and that reversion to the original birth designation after starting GAHT was very rare (van der Loos et al., 2023). Olson and colleagues (2022) found that 5 years after social transition, 97.5% of TNB youth continued to identify as TNB. When a youth does decide to revert, it may not be because they were originally misdiagnosed or misunderstood their gender identity. For example, Turban et al. (2021) found that among adults who detransition (or retransition, as it is sometimes called), 82.5% reported at least one external driver, including family and social stigma. Durwood et al. (2022) reported a number of themes in their examination of youths' shifting identities, including transprejudice. Regardless of the forces influencing retransitions, the researchers found little merit in warnings against transition that are based in the possibility of a later distressing retransition. Among the small numbers of individuals who did retransition, the experience was met with largely neutral or even positive social responses and was unassociated with regret over the initial transition.

It is important that adolescents are made to feel comfortable in expressing any doubts or second thoughts that arise, and in fact, it can be helpful to frame the initial phase of GAHT as a diagnostic period: a time for adolescents to assess what hormone treatment feels like for them, and a time for parents and MHPs to observe any behavioral or emotional changes that can guide future decisions about continuation of treatment. When a youth expresses a desire to change course, regardless of the reason, a careful assessment will be indicated in light of their complex gender journey.

CHAPTER SUMMARY

Caring for TNB adolescents can be a richly rewarding endeavor for the MHP, who in turn can offer what is often lifesaving care to young people. The learning curve can seem steep; however, the need for quality care is great and increasing. As the current cohort of TNB youth comes of age, it is hoped that they can not only inhabit a world that embraces and celebrates gender diversity more fully, but that they themselves are at the forefront of the field of trans studies. Already, distinguished TNB researchers are shaping the dialogue about future research directions in ways unprecedented in prior decades (Veale et al., 2022), helping to build a brighter world for the diverse youth of the future.

M is currently a popular, attractive, high-performing 19-year-old college student who has continued seeing me in therapy every other week. Having undergone puberty suppression, hormone therapy, and genital surgery, she enjoys an active life that involves parties, dating, and extracurricular activities, including mountain biking and hosting a campus podcast. She has told some close friends about her gender journey, but most of her classmates are unaware of this history. She wrote the following when I asked her to provide a description of how her gender transition steps had impacted her life:

> I really cannot imagine who I would be had I not transitioned. For the most part, I feel like my life has only been improved. . . . Insecurities that I used to have about my body have been minimized, people don't question my gender, and I'm grateful to have started transitioning early enough that any pubescent changes that would have occurred were stopped. . . . I remember the little kid I used to be and how insecure and self-conscious I used to be, and I remember that kid with a lot of fondness. But also a lot of gratitude that this is who I grew up to be, and not someone whose outer body didn't match with who she was.

REFERENCES

Beck, K. B., Conner, C. M., Breitenfeldt, K. E., Northrup, J. B., White, S. W., & Mazefsky, C. A. (2020). Assessment and treatment of emotion regulation impairment in autism spectrum disorder across the life span: Current state of the science and future directions. *Child and Adolescent Psychiatric Clinics of North America, 29*(3), 527–542. https://doi.org/10.1016/j.chc.2020.02.003

Beischel, W. J., Gauvin, S. E. M., & van Anders, S. M. (2021). "A little shiny gender breakthrough": Community understandings of gender euphoria. *International Journal of Transgender Health, 23*(3), 274–294. https://doi.org/10.1080/26895269.2021.1915223

Bloom, T. M., Nguyen, T. P., Lami, F., Pace, C. C., Poulakis, Z., Telfer, M., Taylor, A., Pang, K. C., & Tollit, M. A. (2021). Measurement tools for gender identity, gender expression, and gender dysphoria in transgender and gender-diverse children and adolescents: A systematic review. *The Lancet Child & Adolescent Health, 5*(8), 582–588. https://doi.org/10.1016/S2352-4642(21)00098-5

Chelliah, P., Lau, M., & Kuper, L. E. (2024). Changes in gender dysphoria, interpersonal minority stress, and mental health among transgender youth after one year of hormone therapy. *The Journal of Adolescent Health, 74*(6), 1106–1111. https://doi.org/10.1016/j.jadohealth.2023.12.024

Chen, D., Abrams, M., Clark, L., Ehrensaft, D., Tishelman, A. C., Chan, Y. M., Garofalo, R., Olson-Kennedy, J., Rosenthal, S. M., & Hidalgo, M. A. (2021). Psychosocial characteristics of transgender youth seeking gender-affirming medical treatment: Baseline findings from the Trans Youth Care Study. *The Journal of Adolescent Health, 68*(6), 1104–1111. https://doi.org/10.1016/j.jadohealth.2020.07.033

Chen, D., Berona, J., Chan, Y. M., Ehrensaft, D., Garofalo, R., Hidalgo, M. A., Rosenthal, S. M., Tishelman, A. C., & Olson-Kennedy, J. (2023). Psychosocial functioning in transgender youth after 2 years of hormones. *The New England Journal of Medicine, 388*(3), 240–250. https://doi.org/10.1056/NEJMoa2206297

Chodzen, G., Hidalgo, M. A., Chen, D., & Garofalo, R. (2019). Minority stress factors associated with depression and anxiety among transgender and gender-nonconforming youth. *The Journal of Adolescent Health, 64*(4), 467–471. https://doi.org/10.1016/j.jadohealth.2018.07.006

Coelho, J. S., Suen, J., Clark, B. A., Marshall, S. K., Geller, J., & Lam, P. Y. (2019). Eating disorder diagnoses and symptom presentation in transgender youth: A scoping review. *Current Psychiatry Reports, 21*(11), 107. Advance online publication. https://doi.org/10.1007/s11920-019-1097-x

Coleman, E., Radix, A. E., Bouman, W. P., Brown, G. R., de Vries, A. L. C., Deutsch, M. B., Ettner, R., Fraser, L., Goodman, M., Green, J., Hancock, A. B., Johnson, T. W., Karasic, D. H., Knudson, G. A., Leibowitz, S. F., Meyer-Bahlburg, H. F. L., Monstrey, S. J., Motmans, J., Nahata, L., . . . Arcelus, J. (2022). Standards of care for the health of transgender and gender diverse people, version 8. *International Journal of Transgender Health, 23*(Suppl. 1), S1–S259. https://doi.org/10.1080/26895269.2022.2100644

Costa, R., Dunsford, M., Skagerberg, E., Holt, V., Carmichael, P., & Colizzi, M. (2015). Psychological support, puberty suppression, and psychosocial functioning in adolescents with gender dysphoria. *The Journal of Sexual Medicine, 12*(11), 2206–2214. https://doi.org/10.1111/jsm.13034

Delozier, A. M., Kamody, R. C., Rodgers, S., & Chen, D. (2020). Health disparities in transgender and gender expansive adolescents: A topical review from a minority stress framework. *Journal of Pediatric Psychology, 45*(8), 842–847. https://doi.org/10.1093/jpepsy/jsaa040

de Vries, A. L., McGuire, J. K., Steensma, T. D., Wagenaar, E. C., Doreleijers, T. A., & Cohen-Kettenis, P. T. (2014). Young adult psychological outcome after puberty suppression and gender reassignment. *Pediatrics, 134*(4), 696–704. https://doi.org/10.1542/peds.2013-2958

Dhanani, L. Y., & Totton, R. R. (2023). Have you heard the news? The effects of exposure to news about recent transgender legislation on transgender youth and young adults. *Sexuality Research & Social Policy, 20*, 1345–1359. https://doi.org/10.1007/s13178-023-00810-6

Doyle, D. M., Lewis, T. O. G., & Barreto, M. (2023). A systematic review of psychosocial functioning changes after gender-affirming hormone therapy among transgender people. *Nature Human Behaviour, 7*(8), 1320–1331. https://doi.org/10.1038/s41562-023-01605-w

Durwood, L., Kuvalanka, K. A., Kahn-Samuelson, S., Jordan, A. E., Rubin, J. D., Schnelzer, P., Devor, A. H., & Olson, K. R. (2022). Retransitioning: The experiences of youth who socially transition genders more than once. *International Journal of Transgender Health, 23*(4), 409–427. https://doi.org/10.1080/26895269.2022.2085224

Fish, J. N., & Russell, S. T. (2020). Sexual orientation and gender identity change efforts are unethical and harmful. *American Journal of Public Health, 110*(8), 1113–1114. https://doi.org/10.2105/AJPH.2020.305765

Gallagher, S., Smigelski, C., Luikenaar, R. A. C., & Dugi, D. (2022). Pelvic physical therapy for gender-affirming genital vaginoplasty. In M. van Trotsenburg, R. A. C. Luikenaar, & M. C. Meriggiola (Eds.), *Context, principles and practice of transgynecology* (pp. 261–266). Cambridge University Press. https://doi.org/10.1017/9781108899987.044

Geilhufe, B., Tripp, O., Silverstein, S., Birchfield, L., & Raimondo, M. (2021). Gender-affirmative eating disorder care: Clinical considerations for transgender and gender expansive children and youth. *Pediatric Annals, 50*(9), Article e371–e378. https://doi.org/10.3928/19382359-20210820-01

Glidden, D., Bouman, W. P., Jones, B. A., & Arcelus, J. (2016). Gender dysphoria and autism spectrum disorder: A systematic review of the literature. *Sexual Medicine Reviews, 4*(1), 3–14. https://doi.org/10.1016/j.sxmr.2015.10.003

Goldenberg, T., Gamarel, K. E., Reisner, S. L., Jadwin-Cakmak, L., & Harper, G. W. (2021). Gender affirmation as a source of resilience for addressing stigmatizing healthcare experiences of transgender youth of color. *Annals of Behavioral Medicine, 55*(12), 1168–1183. https://doi.org/10.1093/abm/kaab011

Holt, V., Skagerberg, E., & Dunsford, M. (2016). Young people with features of gender dysphoria: Demographics and associated difficulties. *Clinical Child Psychology and Psychiatry, 21*(1), 108–118. https://doi.org/10.1177/1359104514558431

Johns, M. M., Gordon, A. R., Andrzejewski, J., Harper, C. R., Michaels, S., Hansen, C., Fordyce, E., & Dunville, R. (2023). Differences in health care experiences among transgender and gender diverse youth by gender identity and race/ethnicity. *Prevention Science, 24*(6), 1128–1141. https://doi.org/10.1007/s11121-023-01521-5

Johns, M. M., Zamantakis, A., Andrzejewski, J., Boyce, L., Rasberry, C. N., & Jayne, P. E. (2021). Minority stress, coping, and transgender youth in schools—Results from the resilience and transgender youth study. *The Journal of School Health, 91*(11), 883–893. https://doi.org/10.1111/josh.13086

Kuper, L. E., Stewart, S., Preston, S., Lau, M., & Lopez, X. (2020). Body dissatisfaction and mental health outcomes of youth on gender-affirming hormone therapy. *Pediatrics, 145*(4), e20193006. Advance online publication. https://doi.org/10.1542/peds.2019-3006

Lee, J. Y., & Rosenthal, S. M. (2023). Gender-affirming care of transgender and gender-diverse youth: Current concepts. *Annual Review of Medicine, 74*(1), 107–116. https://doi.org/10.1146/annurev-med-043021-032007

Leggett-James, M. P., Faur, S., Kaniušonytė, G., Žukauskienė, R., & Laursen, B. (2023). The perils of not being attractive or athletic: Pathways to adolescent adjustment difficulties through escalating unpopularity. *Journal of Youth and Adolescence, 52*(11), 2231–2242. https://doi.org/10.1007/s10964-023-01835-1

Light, A. D., Obedin-Maliver, J., Sevelius, J. M., & Kerns, J. L. (2014). Transgender men who experienced pregnancy after female-to-male gender transitioning. *Obstetrics and Gynecology, 124*(6), 1120–1127. https://doi.org/10.1097/AOG.0000000000000540

Marinkovic, M., & Newfield, R. S. (2017). Chest reconstructive surgeries in transmasculine youth: Experience from one pediatric center. *International Journal of Transgenderism, 18*(4), 376–381. https://doi.org/10.1080/15532739.2017.1349706

McGuire, T. C., McCormick, K. C., Koch, M. K., & Mendle, J. (2019). Pubertal maturation and trajectories of depression during early adolescence. *Frontiers in Psychology, 10*(1362), 1362. Advance online publication. https://doi.org/10.3389/fpsyg.2019.01362

Morris, E. R., & Galupo, M. P. (2019). "Attempting to dull the dysphoria": Nonsuicidal self-injury among transgender individuals. *Psychology of Sexual Orientation and Gender Diversity, 6*(3), 296–307. https://doi.org/10.1037/sgd0000327

Mountz, S. (2020). Remapping pipelines and pathways: Listening to queer and transgender youth of color's trajectories through girls' juvenile justice facilities. *Affilia, 35*(2), 177–199. https://doi.org/10.1177/0886109919880517

Murano-Kinney, S. (2024). Banning puberty-pausing medications endangers transgender adolescents. *The American Journal of Bioethics, 24*(8), 4–8. https://doi.org/10.1080/15265161.2024.2371117

Newman, B. M., & Newman, P. R. (2021). *Theories of adolescent development*. Academic Press.

Olson, K. R., Durwood, L., Horton, R., Gallagher, N. M., & Devor, A. (2022). Gender identity 5 years after social transition. *Pediatrics, 150*(2), e2021056082. Advance online publication. https://doi.org/10.1542/peds.2021-056082

Olson, K. R., Raber, G. F., & Gallagher, N. M. (2024). Levels of satisfaction and regret with gender-affirming medical care in adolescence. *JAMA Pediatrics, 178*(12), 1354–1361. https://doi.org/10.1001/jamapediatrics.2024.4527

Olson-Kennedy, J., Warus, J., Okonta, V., Belzer, M., & Clark, L. F. (2018). Chest reconstruction and chest dysphoria in transmasculine minors and young adults: Comparisons of nonsurgical and postsurgical cohorts. *JAMA Pediatrics, 172*(5), 431–436. https://doi.org/10.1001/jamapediatrics.2017.5440

Pariseau, E. M., Chevalier, L., Long, K. A., Clapham, R., Edwards-Leeper, L., & Tishelman, A. C. (2019). The relationship between family acceptance-rejection and transgender youth psychosocial functioning. *Clinical Practice in Pediatric Psychology, 7*(3), 267–277. https://doi.org/10.1037/cpp0000291

Park, I. Y., Speer, R., Whitfield, D. L., Kattari, L., Walls, E. N., & Christensen, C. (2022). Predictors of bullying, depression, and suicide attempts among youth: The intersection of race/ethnicity by gender identity. *Children and Youth Services Review, 139*, 106536. Advance online publication. https://doi.org/10.1016/j.childyouth.2022.106536

Peitzmeier, S., Gardner, I., Weinand, J., Corbet, A., & Acevedo, K. (2017). Health impact of chest binding among transgender adults: A community-engaged, cross-sectional study. *Culture, Health & Sexuality, 19*(1), 64–75. https://doi.org/10.1080/13691058.2016.1191675

Pfeifer, J. H., & Allen, N. B. (2021). Puberty initiates cascading relationships between neurodevelopmental, social, and internalizing processes across adolescence. *Biological Psychiatry, 89*(2), 99–108. https://doi.org/10.1016/j.biopsych.2020.09.002

Pollitt, A. M., Ioverno, S., Russell, S. T., Li, G., & Grossman, A. H. (2019). Predictors and mental health benefits of chosen name use among transgender youth. *Youth & Society, 53*(2), 320–341. https://doi.org/10.1177/0044118X19855898

Poquiz, J. L., Coyne, C. A., Garofalo, R., & Chen, D. (2021). Comparison of gender minority stress and resilience among transmasculine, transfeminine, and nonbinary adolescents and young adults. *The Journal of Adolescent Health, 68*(3), 615–618. https://doi.org/10.1016/j.jadohealth.2020.06.014

Price-Feeney, M., Green, A. E., & Dorison, S. (2020). Understanding the mental health of transgender and nonbinary youth. *The Journal of Adolescent Health, 66*(6), 684–690. https://doi.org/10.1016/j.jadohealth.2019.11.314

Sorbara, J. C., Chiniara, L. N., Thompson, S., & Palmert, M. R. (2020). Mental health and timing of gender-affirming care. *Pediatrics, 146*(4), e20193600. Advance online publication. https://doi.org/10.1542/peds.2019-3600

Sorbara, J. C., Ngo, H. L., & Palmert, M. R. (2021). Factors associated with age of presentation to gender-affirming medical care. *Pediatrics, 147*(4), e2020026674. Advance online publication. https://doi.org/10.1542/peds.2020-026674

Strang, J. F., Anthony, L. G., Song, A., Lai, M. C., Knauss, M., Sadikova, E., Graham, E., Zaks, Z., Wimms, H., Willing, L., Call, D., Mancilla, M., Shakin, S., Vilain, E., Kim, D. Y., Maisashvili, T., Khawaja, A., & Kenworthy, L. (2023). In addition to stigma: Cognitive and autism-related predictors of mental health in transgender adolescents. *Journal of Clinical Child and Adolescent Psychology, 52*(2), 212–229. https://doi.org/10.1080/15374416.2021.1916940

Taliaferro, L. A., McMorris, B. J., Rider, G. N., & Eisenberg, M. E. (2019). Risk and protective factors for self-harm in a population-based sample of transgender youth. *Archives of Suicide Research, 23*(2), 203–221. https://doi.org/10.1080/13811118.2018.1430639

Tankersley, A. P., Grafsky, E. L., Dike, J., & Jones, R. T. (2021). Risk and resilience factors for mental health among transgender and gender nonconforming (TGNC) youth: A systematic review. *Clinical Child and Family Psychology Review, 24*(2), 183–206. https://doi.org/10.1007/s10567-021-00344-6

Testa, R. J., Coolhart, D., & Peta, J. L. (2015). *The gender quest workbook: A guide for teens and young adults exploring gender identity*. New Harbinger Publications.

Toomey, R. B., Syvertsen, A. K., & Shramko, M. (2018). Transgender adolescent suicide behavior. *Pediatrics, 142*(4), e20174218. Advance online publication. https://doi.org/10.1542/peds.2017-4218

Turban, J. L., King, D., Carswell, J. M., & Keuroghlian, A. S. (2020). Pubertal suppression for transgender youth and risk of suicidal ideation. *Pediatrics, 145*(2), e20191725. Advance online publication. https://doi.org/10.1542/peds.2019-1725

Turban, J. L., Loo, S. S., Almazan, A. N., & Keuroghlian, A. S. (2021). Factors leading to "detransition" among transgender and gender diverse people in the United States: A mixed-methods analysis. *LGBT Health, 8*(4), 273–280. https://doi.org/10.1089/lgbt.2020.0437

Vance, S. R., Jr., Boyer, C. B., Glidden, D. V., & Sevelius, J. (2021). Mental health and psychosocial risk and protective factors among Black and Latinx transgender youth compared with peers. *JAMA Network Open, 4*(3), e213256. Advance online publication. https://doi.org/10.1001/jamanetworkopen.2021.3256

Vance, S. R., Jr., Chen, D., Garofalo, R., Glidden, D. V., Ehrensaft, D., Hidalgo, M., Tishelman, A., Rosenthal, S. M., Chan, Y. M., Olson-Kennedy, J., & Sevelius, J. (2023). Mental health and gender affirmation of Black and Latine transgender/nonbinary youth compared to White peers prior to hormone initiation. *The Journal of Adolescent Health, 73*(5), 880–886. https://doi.org/10.1016/j.jadohealth.2023.06.022

van der Loos, M. A. T. C., Hannema, S. E., Klink, D. T., den Heijer, M., & Wiepjes, C. M. (2022). Continuation of gender-affirming hormones in transgender people starting puberty suppression in adolescence: A cohort study in the Netherlands. *The Lancet Child & Adolescent Health, 6*(12), 869–875. https://doi.org/10.1016/S2352-4642(22)00254-1

van der Loos, M. A. T. C., Klink, D. T., Hannema, S. E., Bruinsma, S., Steensma, T. D., Kreukels, B. P. C., Cohen-Kettenis, P. T., de Vries, A. L. C., den Heijer, M., & Wiepjes, C. M. (2023). Children and adolescents in the Amsterdam Cohort of Gender

Dysphoria: Trends in diagnostic- and treatment trajectories during the first 20 years of the Dutch Protocol. *The Journal of Sexual Medicine, 20*(3), 398–409. https://doi.org/10.1093/jsxmed/qdac029

Veale, J. F., Deutsch, M. B., Devor, A. H., Kuper, L. E., Motmans, J., Radix, A. E., & Amand, C. S. (2022). Setting a research agenda in trans health: An expert assessment of priorities and issues by trans and nonbinary researchers. *International Journal of Transgender Health, 23*(4), 392–408. https://doi.org/10.1080/26895269.2022.2044425

Verbeek, M. J. A., Hommes, M. A., Stutterheim, S. E., van Lankveld, J. J. D. M., & Bos, A. E. R. (2020). Experiences with stigmatization among transgender individuals after transition: A qualitative study in the Netherlands. *International Journal of Transgender Health, 21*(2), 220–233. https://doi.org/10.1080/26895269.2020.1750529

Wilson, C., & Cariola, L. A. (2020). LGBTQI+ youth and mental health: A systematic review of qualitative research. *Adolescent Research Review, 5*(2), 187–211. https://doi.org/10.1007/s40894-019-00118-w

11
AFFIRMATIVE CARE WITH TRANS AND NONBINARY OLDER ADULTS

KYLE L. BOWER AND MARY CHASE MIZE

Trans and nonbinary (TNB) older adults are continually shaping their identities, providing foundations, building legacies, and teaching self-acceptance to promote the betterment of future TNB generations (Bower, 2018). Of the nearly 1.4 million adults in the United States who identify as TNB, over 170,000 are over age 65 (Herman et al., 2022). This number is expected to increase rapidly; by 2050, the world's population of adults over 60 will double, and the number of older TNB adults will increase within the older population globally (World Health Organization, 2024). TNB communities have always existed in our world (Stryker, 2017); yet, despite this fact and the projected population growth among older TNB communities, there is a dearth of research on the specific needs of TNB older adults. Scholars (e.g., Adan et al., 2021; Fredriksen-Goldsen, 2023) are striving to close this gap. For instance, in a study about perspectives on aging as a TNB older adult, Adan et al. (2021) found themes and challenges within the aging TNB community, including both fears (mistreatment in elder care, isolation and loneliness that may be exacerbated by holding a TNB identity, and vulnerability related to financial stress and health care system inclusivity) and strengths (embracing one's self-truth as a TNB older adult, giving back to their community). In addition, in a study of 205 LGBTQ+ older adults, more than one-third of their sample identified as

---

https://doi.org/10.1037/0000471-012
Affirmative Counseling and Psychological Practice With Trans and Nonbinary Clients, Second Edition, A. Singh and R. McCullough (Editors)
Copyright © 2026 by the American Psychological Association. All rights reserved.

nonbinary, which challenges the preconceived notion of gender fluidity only being present among younger cohorts (Fredriksen-Goldsen et al., 2022).

In this chapter, we share challenges and opportunities in TNB aging, as well as mental health providers' (MHPs') efforts to address the social inequities TNB individuals experience in later life. We discuss unique aging experiences related to TNB identity including aging as a lifelong process, intersectional approaches to understanding and navigating mental health needs of TNB older adults, end-of-life care, death and grief experiences of TNB older adults, and affirmative counseling practices. We conclude the chapter with a review of an affirmative counseling model and recommendations for MHPs to better prepare them to meet the needs of older TNB persons. Case studies demonstrating issues that TNB older adults encounter are interspersed throughout the chapter.[1]

LIFE COURSE DEVELOPMENT FOR TRANS AND NONBINARY OLDER ADULTS

Gerontology is the scientific study of aging and older adulthood. The interdisciplinary nature of the study of aging is an opportunity to apply a gerontological focus to fields such as medicine, mental health care, sociology, psychology, career, and all other sectors involving the lives of older adults. For TNB older adults, a lifespan developmental theory may be especially useful for understanding the process of TNB aging as this perspective emphasizes that sociocultural, historical, biological, and social contexts critically influence aging and development (Antonucci et al., 2014; Schaie & Willis, 2021; Spencer et al., 2021). From a lifespan developmental theory perspective, the aging experiences of TNB older adults are nuanced and complex (Knochel & Seelman, 2020). The baby boomer generation (1946–1964) came of age during a period of significant social change, challenging traditional norms through movements like the Civil Rights Movement led by Dr. Martin Luther King Jr. and the resurgence of feminism (Bower, 2018). LGBTQ+ Boomers, often referred to as the "pride generation," are known for having greater visibility, reduced identity concealment, and increased advocacy for human rights compared to earlier age cohorts (Fredriksen-Goldsen et al., 2022). While this group played a key role in reshaping societal perceptions of homosexuality and gender identity, they also experience higher levels of internalized stigma and shame during later adulthood (Fredriksen-Goldsen et al., 2017). As clinicians, it is necessary to comprehensively explore our subjectivities that inform issues of diversity that span

---

[1]The case examples in this chapter have been modified to disguise the clients' identities and protect their confidentiality.

sociocultural perspectives and historical context, so we may forge intentional and lasting connections with clients (Lorusso et al., 2023).

Trans and Nonbinary Older Adult Identity Disclosure

Older TNB clients often have complex experiences of gender identity and gender expression that may have remained fluid throughout life and can influence TNB identity disclosure (Knauer, 2015). For instance, while some TNB persons pursue social or medical transition earlier in their lifespan, others wait until midlife or later life. Many older TNB adults may have begun their social and medical transitions after age 65 during their older adulthood, which yields very different aging experiences within the TNB community (e.g., those TNB older adults who began social and medical transition earlier in their lifespan, which was more uncommon among this age cohort, are likely to experience different physical, social, and emotional transitions and milestones than those who pursue social and medical transition in later life; Witten & Eyler, 2012). Older TNB adults who pursue gender-affirming surgery in later life will likely experience a longer postoperative recovery time due to aging-related risk factors such as fall risk, pressure sore risk, and joint problems, and may need more social support during recovery (Iwamoto et al., 2023). For older adults who undergo gender-affirming hormone therapy, it is critical for preventative screening for conditions such as cancer and osteoporosis to be available to the TNB aging community since the risk of these conditions increases with age (Cheung et al., 2023; Iwamoto et al., 2023).

Many older TNB adults experience identity disclosure as a life-long and deeply personal process that is also influenced by society and their social relationships (Witten, 2016). For example, Fabbre (2014) studied the intersection of existential and queer perspectives on aging across the life course and, despite the lack of literature on aging experiences among TNB older adults, found critical themes regarding the process of coming out in later life. First, regarding the pursuit social and medical transition in later life, researchers found the realization of "having only so much time left to live" (p. 166) was a strong motivation for coming out or completing social and medical transition among TNB older adults. Fabbre (2014) further explains there is an intersection between individual and societal factors when an older adult pursues gender identity disclosure; facing awareness of death may motivate older TNB adults to embrace their authentic selves with the time they have left to live.

Koller and Urbanski (2023) found age at time-of-transitioning as a major influence in the lived experience of TNB older adults. For example, TNB adults who come out earlier in their lifespan may experience more time living (and aging) in the TNB community. For older TNB adults who come out later in life, anticipating fear of loss of relationships, the complexity of health care, and finding acceptance in the LGBTQ+ community may be factors impacting their lived experiences (Koller & Urbanski, 2023). Fabbre (2014) also found that TNB older adults who came out in later life "did what they were supposed to do" or felt they "served time" conforming to social expectations during earlier stages of their lifespan (p. 166). The authors noted that through reflection, TNB older adults came to understand their life phases with a new perspective, easing their perceived frustration of not having as much time to embrace their true gender identity.

The age at which gender identity transition occurs for TNB older adults is an influential theme MHPs can explore with clients (Koller & Urbanski, 2023). Transitions earlier in the lifespan, whether socially or medically through affirmative care procedures, may present different experiences and challenges for TNB adults as they encounter the aging process. Older TNB adults who come out earlier in their lives may simply have more time to live fully in their identity—to build relationships and community as a TNB person. On the other hand, TNB adults who come out later in life may experience different physical challenges with affirmative health care practices (such as hormone therapy and osteoporosis risk), as well as social challenges (such as fear of loss of existing relationships and community). These experiences are different and crucial for MHPs to consider when providing care to older TNB clients.

Fear of discrimination may also contribute to coming out or pursuing social and medical transition in later life. Auldridge and colleagues (2012) found 70% of older TNB adults reported delaying their medical and social transition due to fears of being discriminated against in the workforce. Their fear is not unfounded, as many TNB older adults report having experienced discrimination in the workplace regarding hiring, promotions, and firing over their life course (Fredriksen-Goldsen et al., 2022). While some TNB older adults experience their full identity disclosure as resistance (such as participating in public demonstrations of activism and advocacy as a fully visible TNB person; Fabbre, 2017; Fredriksen-Goldsen et al., 2022), others may not disclose their TNB identities for fear of discrimination from formal care institutions, health aids, and even physicians (Services and Advocacy for Gay, Lesbian, Bisexual, and Transgender Elders [SAGE], 2014; see also Ippolito & Witten, 2014; Maddux, 2011). Fear of mistreatment in elder care is a primary concern among TNB older adults (Adan et al., 2021); many may adhere to social norms of their sex assigned at birth while navigating care settings.

Furthermore, SAGE and the National Center for Transgender Equality (NCTE; 2012) report that people of color access health care less frequently and thus are at higher risk for health complications in older adulthood (Kim, 2017). Scholars have found that implicit bias among health care providers impacts health disparities based on gender, race, ethnicity, and sexual orientation (Casanova-Perez et al., 2022; Maina et al., 2018). TNB older adults who also identify as people of color may experience heightened disparities in care and detrimental care outcomes due to provider bias and discrimination at the intersection of their TNB and people of color identities (Casanova-Perez et al., 2022). TNB adults who identify as people of color are at heightened risk for experiencing discrimination in health care settings, such as name and gender misidentification, overt insensitivity from staff, and providers making harmful and inaccurate assumptions about their medical history (Smart et al., 2020). The intersection of these two identities—TNB and people of color—impacts health care seeking behavior as well, whereas experiences of distrust of medical systems in people of color communities (Musa et al., 2009) may also impact health care avoidance in TNB communities due to anticipated discrimination (Kcomt et al., 2020).

Trans Identity Disclosure Case Study 1: Tina
Tina is a 68-year-old Black trans woman. Tina began her social and medical transition 10 years ago, after she retired early from her career in the military. After hours of intense abdominal pain, Tina finally agreed to let her wife, Ruby, take her to the emergency room for treatment in the middle of the night. Tina was adamant to "get through it" so she could see her primary care doctor in the morning, with whom she feels safe and respected. During the emergency room triage, Tina said her pain was 10/10, and Ruby asked if there was anything at all she could have to feel better. The nurse responded in a kind but condescending tone, "Okay young lady, I'll see what I can do, okay?" but did not follow up, nor was any pain medicine administered. During the doctor's assessment, Tina disclosed she was trans. The doctor responded with surprise, saying "huh, wow, you look like a woman." During a physical examination of her abdomen, Tina cried out in anguish and vomited on the table. The doctor ordered a CT scan and discovered her appendix had ruptured. She was rushed to emergency surgery and spent 4 days recovering from sepsis.

Mental Health Provider Response. In this case study, Tina experiences the intersection of ageism, racism, sexism, and genderism from this health care setting. The ageist, infantilizing language of being called "young lady" and the dismissive concern of Tina's pain led providers to essentially ignore her pain level. Black patients, especially Black women, are less likely to receive painkillers for acute pain compared to White patients (Lee et al., 2019). Tina may have felt pressure to disclose her TNB identity prior to her physical exam and experienced a harmful microaggression from the doctor's response. All these intersecting oppressions led to a severe health crisis that could have likely been avoided if Tina received appropriate pain management and earlier intervention. Instead, Tina's reluctance to seek treatment was met with a traumatic medical experience, which may decrease her likelihood of seeking future emergency care.

MHPs in hospital settings, such as clinical social workers and behavioral health assessment counselors, can advocate for both TNB and age-inclusive practices within emergency care settings. At the time of writing this chapter, we acknowledge the hostility and erasure of programs prioritizing diversity, equity, and inclusion across multiple sectors of public life. TNB identity disclosure may likely continue to pose additional risks of harm by stripping some of the protections that diversity, equity, and inclusion initiatives may provide. While formal sensitivity training for all hospital staff addressing ageism and promoting TNB inclusive education may be a preferred method of advocacy, the work of MHPs in this current political climate requires learning and modeling TNB and age-inclusive practices in the workplace. For example, MHPs in emergency care settings can prioritize interdisciplinary discussions with providers to affirm the dignity of older trans patients by modeling language, such as continuing inclusion of pronouns in intake procedures, continually using correct pronouns in interdisciplinary care settings, and refraining from infantilizing speech. Intersectional approaches will continue to serve as the foundation for navigating mental health needs of older TNB adults as we discuss changes in health status, health care systems, federal services, long-term care, and end-of-life care.

AN INTERSECTIONAL APPROACH TO NAVIGATING MENTAL HEALTH NEEDS OF TRANS AND NONBINARY OLDER ADULTS

As older adulthood presents new experiences and challenges, MHPs should consider how best to support the quality of life of TNB older adult clients during their later years. It is well documented that LGBTQ+ communities experience higher rates of mental health distress, crisis, and trauma throughout their life course (Fredriksen-Goldsen et al., 2014). Recently, organizations serving TNB older adults collaborated to create a resource centering the generational trauma they may experience and using it to outline two models of care: person-centered care (PCC) and trauma-informed care (TIC; FORGE & SAGE, 2023). PCC originated from a need for compassionate and culturally responsive care practices that respond to the diversifying elder population (FORGE & SAGE, 2023). For instance, the Pioneer Network (2023) is a national organization that focuses on providing culturally responsive care to older adults and educating practitioners on transformative practices that endorse a PCC model (Pioneer Network, 2023). Through this network, states have formed coalitions to serve older adults more effectively on a more local level (Pioneer Network, 2023). In connection with PCC, TIC recognizes how past experiences are internalized, not only psychologically but also physiologically. Together, PCC and TIC provide a care framework that "creates safety, is based on shared decision making, empowers older adults, promotes healing, addresses clients' emotional as well as physical needs, and provides care in line with clients' care preferences" (FORGE & SAGE, 2023, p. 6). Later in the chapter, we summarize affirmative counseling practices informed by this framework.

NAVIGATING HEALTH CARE AND OTHER SOCIAL SERVICES SYSTEMS IN LATER ADULTHOOD

Prior to the turn of the century, TNB older adults were often less visible to all but their close circles. In addition, MHPs should be aware that health care and other social service systems that serve older adults often lack the necessary training and supervision to understand what TNB-affirming care looks like (Witten, 2016). As TNB people continue to enter later adulthood, researchers and health professionals are actively learning more about how to support older TNB adults as their overall health changes (and resulting medical needs; Iwamoto et al., 2023). Deepening MHP understanding of these changes is important, as older TNB adults are more likely to experience higher levels of trauma related to their physical and mental health within health care and other social services systems (Cook-Daniels, 2016; Grassau et al., 2021). For instance, the impact of the history of gatekeeping and pathologizing of TNB people has been detrimental, and older adults who identify as TNB are more likely to experience victimization, internalized stigma, and verbal and physical abuse (Fredriksen-Goldsen et al., 2022). Therefore, it is important for MHPs to understand the ways that mental health care intersects with existing health care systems, social services systems, and overall physical health for older TNB clients.

Health Care Systems

During later life, older adults typically rely on health care systems more regularly for physical and mental health needs. While diseases and disorders are not necessarily considered to be a part of the normal aging process, we do know that 95% of persons over the age of 65 are living with at least one chronic condition, and 80% have two or more chronic conditions (National Council on Aging, 2023). Furthermore, LGBTQ+ older adults are more likely to experience *compression of morbidity*, which refers to the earlier onset of functional limitations that are correlated with minoritized social and economic positions throughout life (Fredriksen-Goldsen & Kim, 2017). Although health care systems are becoming more inclusive, there is still much to be accomplished to meet the needs of TNB older adults and provide spaces where they feel safe and supported. This becomes especially important in later life when age adds another layer of vulnerability to their identity.

As previously discussed, it is not always easy for TNB people to find gender-affirming health care providers who support their potential social and medical transition needs. If they are able to find these providers, they may feel significant distrust as they are somewhat dependent upon them as gatekeepers to approve such treatment (e.g., referral to hormone therapy and gender-affirming surgery). What is exacerbating this issue is that, although there are policies in practice, personnel are not always accommodating, and, at times, people working for these social services often actively discriminate against TNB people (NCTE, 2023). To combat these prejudices, the NCTE consistently monitors federal policies and provides information to educate people on how to contest perceived maltreatment. For instance, as of 2018, gender markers are no longer printed on Medicare cards, which makes services more universally available, and TNB older adults are not as easily denied in the case their gender markers do not match the gender they identify as (NCTE, 2023).

Federal Services

MHPs should be aware that, in the United States, the Older Americans Act funds programs and services for older Americans and their caregivers through a national network of state units on aging, area agencies on aging, and over 20,000 service providers (Administration for Community Living [ACL], 2023). Congregate and home-delivered meals, information and referral services, elder abuse prevention, caregiver support, health and wellness programs, in-home care, and other services to enable older adults to age well in their community encompass this aging services network. The Older Americans Act identifies some groups as populations of older adults with greatest social need (ACL,

2023). This distinction allows funded organizations to direct resources specifically to older adults in these communities, particularly older adults who are Black, Latinx, Indigenous and Native American Persons, Asian and Pacific Islanders, and other persons of color, as well as members of religious minoritized communities, LGBTQ+ persons, those with disabilities, and those who live in rural areas (ACL, 2023). The designation of LGBTQ+ older adults was applied to all state plans within the aging services network in 2022 (ACL, 2023).

Another critical federal service that impacts and interacts with existing health systems is Medicare, the federal health insurance program in the United States for people over 65. Recent legislation enhanced accessibility for TNB older adults to utilize their Medicare benefits for mental health care. As of January 1, 2024, for the first time ever, licensed professional counselors and licensed marriage and family therapists are recognized as Medicare providers. However, federal funding for Medicare is currently under political scrutiny and although progress was made to provide more comprehensive coverage to elders, the polarized political climate generates additional fear among LGBTQ+ older adults (Flatt, 2025).

Long-Term Care

Without informal caregiving support from family and friends, some TNB older adults must rely on institutional care. With these decisions come repercussions that may further impact their health. Federal Regulation 42, Code of Federal Regulations 483.10 states that residents have the right to dignity in their existence, self-determination, communication, and access to people and services both inside and outside of the facility (National Archives and Records Administration, 2023); this provides protection for TNB residents from the discrimination and prejudice they face. TNB adults fear they will experience bias and mistreatment—not only from long-term care services—but also from other residents (Kortes-Miller et al., 2018; Pang et al., 2019; Putney et al., 2018). While some find they need to "return to the closet" to protect themselves (Maddux, 2011), others are propelled to complete their physical transition to pass as cisgender (de Vries et al., 2019; Witten, 2016), meaning one's gendered characteristics (such as facial hair or appearance of breasts) align with how others perceive their natal sex. Furthermore, discrimination and fear are correlated with negative health outcomes (Fredriksen-Goldsen et al., 2014; Knochel & Flunker, 2021; White Hughto & Reisner, 2018). For instance, an alarming finding across multiple studies raises awareness that, in the face of increased dependency, TNB older adults will contemplate suicide rather than access long-term care (Knochel & Flunker, 2021; Progovac et al., 2020).

Although receiving support from long-term care seems bleak, recent research underscores narratives of resilience. Even through perceived fear, TNB older adults are choosing to live more authentically in their environment, knowing that there are fewer years ahead of them than at prior life stages (Fabbre, 2016; Knochel & Flunker, 2021). Considering these adults have confined themselves to a gender binary or performing gender in a way that meets the standards of cisnormativity, MHPs should explore gender transition with TNB older adults while normalizing gender affirmation as a right for all people, in any setting, at any age.

End-of-Life Care, Death, and Grief Experiences of Trans and Nonbinary Older Adults

Identity development is an ongoing process throughout the lifespan for all people. According to Erikson's theory of psychological development, at the end of life, people are more likely to interpret their age as a representation of life nearly completed rather than one that is yet to be lived (Erikson, 1963). Awareness of mortality may yield personal growth at any age of the lifespan and is an important developmental task of older adulthood (Erikson, 1963; Schippers & Ziegler, 2019). The intersection of mortality and TNB identity in older adulthood is important to consider. Researchers have found TNB persons have a lower life expectancy than non-TNB communities. For instance, in a 2022 cohort comparison study, 25% of TNB persons in the United States died by age 69 while 25% of non-TNB persons died by age 75; 50% of the TNB cohort died by age 77 while 50% of the non-TNB cohort died by age 84 (L. D. Hughes et al., 2022). Another cohort study found elevated overall mortality of TNB people compared to cisgender people, particularly among deaths from external causes such as suicide (Jackson et al., 2023).

The impact of anti-TNB discrimination is evident in many TNB older adults' experiences with navigating end-of-life care; like navigating other health care systems, fear of mistreatment alongside fears of loss of autonomy in meeting personal care needs is a persistent theme (Catlett et al., 2023; Lowers, 2017). Loss of autonomy is one of many situations that may occur with old age; with older adulthood comes increased likelihood of experiencing the deaths of friends and family. It is normal to experience *grief*—the widespread response to loss—as it relates to cumulative losses in the aging process. Maintaining intimate relationships at the end of life is an important way TNB older adults can cope with loss accumulation. Recent research emphasizes the importance of sexual health as being inclusive of end of life, as intimacy can be experienced in a variety of ways including physical, emotional, and spiritual means (Acquaviva, 2017; Bower, Stahl, et al., 2021). Listening and following the direction of TNB older adults is recommended, as they have a strong knowledge of their health and well-being and may have ideas of their own on how they want to maintain intimacy during their end of life (Bower, Stahl, et al., 2021; SAGE, 2018).

Planning for end-of-life decisions can be difficult, yet a helpful and reassuring experience. TNB identities intersect with aging challenges and opportunities in a specific way regarding end-of-life planning. TNB adults and older adults often do not create wills, have a durable power of attorney for health care, or participate in informal conversations about their wishes (Henry et al., 2019; Witten, 2014). Challenges such as discrepancies in names on legal documents, access to resources to prepare such documents, cumulative experiences of barriers to health care services, and fear of discrimination may further complicate the process and decisions TNB older adults make regarding end-of-life care (Henry et al., 2019). For some TNB older adults, this can be overwhelming, and MHPs should remain aware of the increased risk of suicide among TNB older adults (Progovac et al., 2020), noting possible triggers before, during, or after these conversations (FORGE & SAGE, 2023). MHPs are encouraged to explore this important issue with TNB older adults to assist them in making end-of-life decisions that are culturally responsive and uphold their right to dignity, such as understanding cultural beliefs regarding the origin and meaning of pain and pain management and religious and spiritual beliefs regarding death (Givler et al., 2023; see also Chapter 14 on religion and spirituality).

End-of-Life Case Study 2: Dani
Dani is 66 years old and identifies as nonbinary and biracial. Dani has been pacemaker-dependent since they suffered a massive heart attack at 48 years old, reducing their heart functioning to only 30%. Dani was diagnosed with congestive heart failure three years ago and was recently discharged from the hospital after a severe episode of shortness of breath and fluid buildup in their lungs. Upon discharge, they were admitted to home hospice care because Dani's cardiologist said their prognosis was less than 6 months left to live. Since arriving home, Dani has been experiencing relational conflict with their wife, Lynne.

Lynne met with the hospice counselor and nurse to discuss Dani's treatment and is very concerned about Dani's pacemaker. According to the hospice nurse, if Dani's heart moves into an irregular rhythm during the process of dying, they could be shocked repeatedly; this may result in a physically and emotionally painful experience for both Dani and Lynne. Lynne has broached turning the shocking-sensor feature off their pacemaker, but Dani feels like Lynne is giving up on them. Dani is also hesitant to take morphine; they understand on one level that it will not speed up the dying process, but at the same time, Dani's Catholic upbringing and strong religious influence from their mother conflicts with the pacemaker and hospice drug options. Dani has an uncomfortable feeling that they are "playing God." At the same time, Dani is afraid and sad to accept they are dying. Dani doesn't want to experience painful shocks at the time of death, and they also want to keep trying to find ways to manage their illness.

Mental Health Provider Response. Dani's hospice counselor is positioned to support Dani's mental health at the end of their life by holding a space to process the deep conflict of their religious convictions as well as awareness of their impending death. Reminiscent therapy (RT) may be an effective intervention for this work. RT has early traces to Butler (1963)'s work regarding life review, in which an individual reflects on their life experiences, relationships, and unfinished business (Woods et al., 2018). Within an RT framework, Dani's counselor can process and explore their upbringing and the religious influence of their mother as they relate to their health care decision making. RT may also serve as a background for processing meaning in life across Dani's profession, relationships, and TNB identity. Drawing from Erikson's Stages of Psychosocial Development (van der Kaap-Deeder et al., 2020), RT may be a vehicle for Dani to strengthen virtue at the end of their life; it will allow them to look back on their life and feel satisfaction with all aspects—both good and bad—revisit and resolve other developmental tasks, and strengthen their systems of support.

SYSTEMS OF SUPPORT FOR TRANS AND NONBINARY OLDER ADULTS

The meaning of social relationships shifts over time and in tandem with certain milestones. In midlife and later life, caregiving roles and responsibilities become more salient as health concerns change in severity and frequency. Without adequate care planning, TNB older adult clients may consider the transition to becoming a caregiver or care recipient to be another significant change in their lives. Once again, their relationships within their social network change and their roles within that network may also need to be redefined. While this can be a meaningful transition for many adults, it can also be challenging. If TNB older adults experience fear of being denied care and are concerned about being a burden to their loved ones, care planning can become more difficult (Ippolito & Witten, 2014). The cumulative fear of discrimination across existing systems of care impacts care planning decisions for 61% of TNB older adults (Flatt et al., 2025).

Family Support

Caregiving can be a challenging time for families as roles and responsibilities are reorganized and redistributed. Furthermore, the shift in identity and reconceptualizing one's purpose is a new experience for many adults, including those who identify as TNB. For example, a parental figure who enjoys managing family gatherings and sustaining family connectedness may no longer be able to serve that same role once they become reliant on a spouse or adult children to manage their physical care and maintain their socioemotional connections. Although this scenario places the older adult as the care recipient, it may also be that the TNB client is acting as a primary caregiver to someone else. Fredriksen-Goldsen et al. (2022) surveyed LGBTQ+ older adults (median age of 59.9) and found that more than a fourth of TNB older adults were receiving care from an informal caregiver, and over a third were caregivers themselves. It is common for TNB people to have at least one living child within their social network (Fredriksen-Goldsen et al., 2022; Kim et al., 2017). MHPs should be mindful of the range of tension (from mild indifference to outright shunning) that TNB people may face in relation to their family of origin. Adult children can be a beneficial resource for their parents in later life; however, the quality of those relationships range considerably. At worst, TNB people lose connections due to lost custody in an acrimonious divorce proceeding (Minter & Wald, 2012); and, at best, children are supportive of their parent's transition process.

Peer Groups

In response to nonaccepting family members, many TNB people turn to their peers and develop what has become known as a *family of choice* (Greene, 2021; M. Hughes & Kentlyn, 2011). Families of choice can help provide basic care for TNB elders as they face health concerns and end-of-life issues. Finding peers to build a support community can be an important part of developing a support system. A 2011 study found the majority (82%) of TNB respondents report a positive sense of belonging to the LGBTQ+ community, adequate levels of perceived social support, and involvement in religious or spiritual practices (Fredriksen-Goldsen, 2011). More recent research has found that cultural factors such as race and ethnicity inform the experiences TNB adults have in seeking community and TNB people "connected more with communities that resonated with the multiplicity of their own lives" (Stone et al., 2020, p. 226). Further, Hagai et al. (2020) found that White LGBTQ+ older adults saw their gender and sexual orientation as primary to their identities, whereas LGBTQ+ older adults of color were more likely to view their identities from an intersectional lens. Thus, the intersection of TNB identity and other dimensions of identity may be important for older TNB adults to develop and maintain resilience in the aging process.

Research has also suggested that forming intergenerational relationships may uniquely affect older TNB people (Bower, Lewis, et al., 2021). Flatt et al. (2025) reported that 84% of LGBTQ+ older adults are friends with others outside of their age cohort and 79% are interested in developing intergenerational friendships. MHPs can help TNB older adults build strong, affirming, multigenerational support networks (Knochel & Flunker, 2021). Knochel & Flunker (2021) explain how TNB people who solely rely on a same-age spouse or peers should also consider their spouse's health and mortality. They advise practitioners to help clients identify potential caregivers within different age cohorts. An added benefit is that there is a reciprocity to these relationships, as older adults have valuable experiences they can share with younger cohorts (Bower, Lewis, et al., 2021; Knochel & Flunker, 2021). More research in this area will assist in developing an understanding of reciprocity between members of varying generations.

AFFIRMATIVE COUNSELING WITH TRANS AND NONBINARY OLDER ADULTS

We conclude this chapter by summarizing themes and elaborating on additional actionable steps MHPs can take to provide TNB older adults affirming and compassionate care, take a holistic approach to mental health into consideration, and support the call for effective PCC models that integrate culturally responsive care strategies.

Taking a Life Course Perspective

Adopting a life course perspective can better engage TNB older adult clients in honoring how their current identity has been shaped through various life experiences. This emphasis on life course perspective is especially pertinent to understanding the complex meaning of gender identity given one's sociohistorical experiences of harassment, prejudice, and discrimination (Porter et al., 2016). For instance, Fredriksen-Goldsen et al. (2022) proposed the *Iridescent Life Course Perspective* which further questions normative life events and trajectories to better conceptualize how older adults came to be the person they are today. When applied to the older TNB population, practitioners should seek to familiarize themselves with how particular decisions in early adulthood (e.g., timing of transition, choice to pass as cisgender, or signal to others in their community) affect them later in life. As MHPs, it is crucial to empower TNB older adults to maintain social networks supporting their well-being.

Exploring Social Support

For older adults, family acceptance is an important factor in determining access to and utilization of health care by TNB people. The Family Resilience Framework (Walsh, 2016) or Convoy Model of Social Relations (Antonucci et al., 2014) may be helpful in this regard to assist clients in assessing risk and forming positive adaptation strategies. Building strong, multigenerational support networks is beneficial for both older and younger age cohorts. However, ageism is pervasive and stifles connection. There has been considerable focus on the generational trauma experienced by older TNB people. This is not to say that today's youth are privileged in comparison to their elders. To compare age cohorts is unjust. It is more accurate and beneficial to acknowledge how current stressors differ from those experienced in earlier decades and how older adults may internalize accumulated stress in relation to their gender identity. MHPs are encouraged to advocate for intergenerational connectedness and support meaningful relationships that facilitate TNB people's ability to live openly if they so choose. As MHPs, advocates, and coconspirators, we need to unpack the many complicated issues of social injustice as experienced by TNB persons in later life. Therefore, MHPs working with TNB older adults must consider the impact of interlocking oppressions on older TNB adult mental health.

Addressing Intersectional Discrimination and Oppression

Throughout the chapter, we have discussed a persistent theme of fear of oppression and discrimination among TNB older adults who navigate multifaceted systems of care in older adulthood. It is critical for MHPs to understand the interlocking systems of genderism, sexism, racism, ageism, ableism, and other forms of oppression on the health and well-being of TNB older adults. There is much to learn from older adults by listening to their life narratives. Research suggests that, when faced with adversity, TNB people can demonstrate extraordinary resilience as they navigate oppressive systems (Bower, Lewis, et al., 2021; Singh et al., 2011; Singh & McKleroy, 2011; Witten, 2014). Although advocacy should continue to make general society aware of the inadequacy of the gender binary, advancement of TNB rights has occurred because TNB older people made space for change and younger generations are now utilizing the space that was created. MHPs have an important role in helping TNB older adult clients navigate the complexities of their lived experiences. Although often overlooked, language—which may be different for older TNB adults—is significant in affirming one's identity in relation to their race, ethnicity, sexual orientation, socioeconomic status, and age (Coleman et al., 2022).

Consistently Evaluating Affirmative Care and Supporting Client Empowerment

The National Resource Center on LGBTQ+ Aging (2012) published a guidebook that recommends that clinicians not assume clients' identities based on their appearance or experiences, as sexual orientation and gender identity are only two aspects of who they are as a person. While visibility of their TNB identity is important in later life, it should also be considered in the context of personal safety, as no one should be forced or coerced into sharing personal information about their identity. Therefore, MHPs should specifically address the lived experiences of older adults and observe triggers that may impact the quality of care (FORGE & SAGE, 2023). MHPs can support individual agency for TNB older adults, concerning how much information they share, to whom, and within what context. It is equally important to further empower TNB older adults through shared resources and reliable information so they can advocate for themselves beyond the safe space of the MHP's office.

CHAPTER SUMMARY

TNB older adults are making bold decisions about who they are and who they want to be in later life; yet, MHPs should be mindful that there is considerable fluidity in how TNB older adults self-identify and in their lived experiences depending on the historical context in which they age (e.g., TNB identity development, TNB-affirming health care, online and in-person social support for TNB aging, experiences of interlocking oppressions such as racism). We encourage you to review the references available at the end of this chapter, as the publications embed lists, tables, and visuals that will hopefully enrich meaningful conversations that promote a holistic approach to clinical care in later adulthood for TNB adults. Through our experiences as gerontologists and MHPs, TNB older adults have taught us about the necessity of learning from one another. MHPs are encouraged to continue building a network of coonspirators, offer inclusive and affirmative therapeutic spaces, and assist TNB older adults in exploring their own gender trajectories that can be an expression of human agency, resistance, and radical self-love.

REFERENCES

Acquaviva, K. D. (2017). *LGBTQ-inclusive hospice and palliative care: A practical guide to transforming professional practice.* Columbia University Press. https://doi.org/10.17312/harringtonparkpress/2017.03lgbtqihpc

Adan, M., Scribani, M., Tallman, N., Wolf-Gould, C., Campo-Engelstein, L., & Gadomski, A. (2021). Worry and wisdom: A qualitative study of transgender elders' perspectives on aging. *Transgender Health, 6*(6), 332–342. https://doi.org/10.1089/trgh.2020.0098

Administration for Community Living. (2023, October 18). *Older Americans Act.* https://acl.gov/about-acl/older-americans-act-oaa

Antonucci, T. C., Ajrouch, K. J., & Birditt, K. S. (2014). The convoy model: Explaining social relations from a multidisciplinary perspective. *The Gerontologist, 54*(1), 82–92. https://doi.org/10.1093/geront/gnt118

Auldridge, A., Tamar-Mattis, A., Kennedy, S., Ames, E., & Tobin, H. J. (2012). *Improving the lives of transgender older adults: Recommendations for policy and practice.* Retrieved from https://www.lgbtagingcenter.org/resources/resource.cfm?r=520

Bower, K. L. (2018). Generativity among LGBT older adults [Doctoral dissertation, University of Georgia]. https://getd.libs.uga.edu/pdfs/bower_kyle_l_201805_phd.pdf

Bower, K. L., Lewis, D. C., Bermúdez, J. M., & Singh, A. A. (2021). Narratives of generativity and resilience among LGBT older adults: Leaving positive legacies despite social stigma and collective trauma. *Journal of Homosexuality, 68*(2), 230–251. https://doi.org/10.1080/00918369.2019.1648082

Bower, K. L., Stahl, K. A. M., Seponski, D., & Lewis, D. C. (2021). Intimate expression during the end of life: Considerations for Practitioners working with sexual and gender minority older adults. In S. J. Dodd (Ed.), *The Routledge international handbook of social work and sexualities* (pp. 217–230). Routledge. https://doi.org/10.4324/9780429342912-19

Butler, R. (1963). The life review: An interpretation of reminiscence in the aged. *Psychiatry, 26*, 65–76. https://doi.org/10.1080/00332747.1963.11023339

Casanova-Perez, R., Apodaca, C., Bascom, E., Mohanraj, D., Lane, C., Vidyarthi, D., Beneteau, E., Sabin, J., Pratt, W., Weibel, N., & Hartzler, A. L. (2022). Broken down by bias: Healthcare biases experienced by BIPOC and LGBTQ+ patients. *AMIA Annual Symposium Proceedings, 2021*, 275–284. https://pubmed.ncbi.nlm.nih.gov/35308990/

Catlett, L., Acquaviva, K. D., Campbell, L., Ducar, D., Page, E. H., Patton, J., & Campbell, C. (2023). End-of-life care for transgender older adults. *Global Qualitative Nursing Research, 10*, 1–13. https://doi.org/10.1177/23333936231161128

Cheung, A. S., Nolan, B. J., & Zwickl, S. (2023). Transgender health and the impact of aging and menopause. *Climacteric, 26*(3), 256–262. https://doi.org/10.1080/13697137.2023.2176217

Coleman, E., Radix, A. E., Bouman, W. P., Brown, G. R., de Vries, A. L. C., Deutsch, M. B., Ettner, R., Fraser, L., Goodman, M., Green, J., Hancock, A. B., Johnson, T. W., Karasic, D. H., Knudson, G. A., Leibowitz, S. F., Meyer-Bahlburg, H. F. L., Monstrey, S. J., Motmans, J., Nahata, L., . . . Arcelus, J. (2022). Standards of care for the health of transgender and gender diverse people, version 8. *International Journal of*

Transgender Health, 23(Suppl. 1), S1–S259. https://doi.org/10.1080/26895269.20 22.2100644

Cook-Daniels, L. (2016). Understanding transgender elders. In D. A. Hurley & P. B. Teaster (Eds.), *Handbook of LGBT elders: An interdisciplinary approach to principles, practices, and policies* (pp. 285–308). Springer. https://doi.org/10.1007/978-3-319-03623-6_14

de Vries, B., Gutman, G., Humble, Á., Gahagan, J., Chamberland, L., Aubert, P., Fast, J., & Mock, S. (2019). End-of-life preparations among LGBT older Canadian adults: The missing conversations. *International Journal of Aging & Human Development, 88*(4), 358–379. https://doi.org/10.1177/0091415019836738

Erikson, E. H. (1963). *Childhood and society* (2nd ed.). W. W. Norton.

Fabbre, V. D. (2014). Gender transitions in later life: The significance of time in queer aging. *Journal of Gerontological Social Work, 57*(2-4), 161–175. https://doi.org/10.1080/01634372.2013.855287

Fabbre, V. D. (2016). Agency and social forces in the life course: The case of gender transitions in later life. *The Journals of Gerontology: Series B, 72*(3), 479–487. https://doi.org/10.1093/geronb/gbw109

Flatt, J., Klenczar, B., Uddin, J., OHala, M., Rook, E., & SAGE. (2025). *State of LGBTQ+ aging: Brief report*. SAGE USA. https://lgbtagingcenter.org/library/item/state-of-lgbtq-aging-survey-brief-report/

FORGE, & Advocacy for Gay, Lesbian, Bisexual, and Transgender Elders. (2023, January 23). *Person-centered, trauma-informed care of transgender older adults*. National Resource Center on LGBT Aging. https://lgbtagingcenter.org/wp-content/uploads/2024/06/SAGE-Trans-TIC-Final.pdf

Fredriksen-Goldsen, K. I. (2011). Resilience and disparities among lesbian, gay, bisexual, and transgender older adults. *The Public Policy and Aging Report, 21*(3), 3–7. https://doi.org/10.1093/ppar/21.3.3

Fredriksen-Goldsen, K. I. (2023). Blueprint for future research advancing the study of sexuality, gender, and equity in later life: Lessons learned from aging with pride, the national health, aging, and sexuality/gender study (NHAS). *The Gerontologist, 63*(2), 373–381. https://doi.org/10.1093/geront/gnac146

Fredriksen-Goldsen, K. I., Cook-Daniels, L., Kim, H. J., Erosheva, E. A., Emlet, C. A., Hoy-Ellis, C. P., Goldsen, J., & Muraco, A. (2014). Physical and mental health of transgender older adults: An at-risk and underserved population. *The Gerontologist, 54*(3), 488–500. https://doi.org/10.1093/geront/gnt021

Fredriksen-Goldsen, K. I., Emlet, C. A., Fabbre, V. D., Kim, H. J., Lerner, J., Jung, H. H., Harner, V., Goldsen, J. (2022). Historical and social forces in the Iridescent Life Course: Key life events and experiences of transgender older adults. *Ageing & Society, 44*(7), 1700–1722. 10.1017/s0144686x22000563

Fredriksen-Goldsen, K. I., & Kim, H. J. (2017). The science of conducting research with LGBT older adults—an introduction to aging with pride: National health, aging, and sexuality/gender study (NHAS). *The Gerontologist, 57*(Suppl. 1), S1–S14. https://doi.org/10.1093/geront/gnw212

Fredriksen-Goldsen, K. I., Kim, H. J., Bryan, A. E. B., Shiu, C., & Emlet, C. A. (2017). The cascading effects of marginalization and pathways of resilience in attaining good health among LGBT older adults. *The Gerontologist, 57*(Suppl. 1), S72–S83. https://doi.org/10.1093/geront/gnw170

Givler, A., Bhatt, H., & Maani-Fogelman, P. A. (2023, May 22). *The importance of cultural competence in pain and palliative care.* StatPearls. https://www.ncbi.nlm.nih.gov/books/NBK493154/

Grassau, P., Stinchcombe, A., Thomas, R., & Wright, D. K. (2021). Centering sexual and gender diversity within Compassionate Communities: Insights from a community network of LGBTQ2S+ older adults. *Palliative Care and Social Practice, 15*, 26323524211042630. https://doi.org/10.1177/26323524211042630

Greene, J. (2021). Labor of love: The formalization of care in transgender kinship organizations. *Organization, 28*(6), 930–948. https://doi.org/10.1177/1350508421995763

Hagai, E. B., Annechino, R., Young, N., & Antin, T. (2020). Intersecting sexual identities, oppressions, and social justice work: Comparing LGBTQ baby boomers to millennials who came of age after the 1980s AIDS epidemic. *Journal of Social Issues, 76*(4), 971–992. https://doi.org/10.1111/josi.12405

Henry, R. S., Perrin, P. B., Coston, B. M., & Witten, T. M. (2019). Transgender and gender non-conforming adult preparedness for aging: Concerns for aging, and familiarity with and engagement in planning behaviors. *International Journal of Transgender Health, 21*(1), 58–69. https://doi.org/10.1080/15532739.2019.1690612

Herman, J., Flores, A., & O'Neill, K. (2022, June 10). *How many adults and youth identify as transgender in the United States?* School of Law Williams Institute, UCLA. https://escholarship.org/uc/item/4xs990ws

Hughes, L. D., King, W. M., Gamarel, K. E., Geronimus, A. T., Panagiotou, O. A., & Hughto, J. M. (2022). Differences in all-cause mortality among transgender and non-transgender people enrolled in private insurance. *Demography, 59*(3), 1023–1043. https://doi.org/10.1215/00703370-9942002

Hughes, M., & Kentlyn, S. (2011). Older LGBT people's care networks and communities of practice: A brief note. *International Social Work, 54*(3), 436–444. https://doi.org/10.1177/0020872810396254

Ippolito, J., & Witten, T. M. (2014). Aging. In L. Erickson-Schroth (Ed.), *Trans bodies, trans selves: A resource for the transgender community* (pp. 476–497). Oxford University.

Iwamoto, S. J., Defreyne, J., Kaoutzanis, C., Davies, R. D., Moreau, K. L., & Rothman, M. S. (2023). Gender-affirming hormone therapy, mental health, and surgical considerations for aging transgender and gender diverse adults. *Therapeutic Advances in Endocrinology and Metabolism, 14*, 20420188231166494. https://doi.org/10.1177/20420188231166494

Jackson, S. S., Brown, J., Pfeiffer, R. M., Shrewsbury, D., O'Callaghan, S., Berner, A. M., Gadalla, S. M., & Shiels, M. S. (2023). Analysis of mortality among transgender and gender diverse adults in England. *JAMA Network Open, 6*(1), e2253687. Advance online publication. https://doi.org/10.1001/jamanetworkopen.2022.53687

Kcomt, L., Gorey, K. M., Barrett, B. J., & McCabe, S. E. (2020). Healthcare avoidance due to anticipated discrimination among transgender people: A call to create trans-affirmative environments. *SSM–Population Health, 11*, 100608. https://doi.org/10.1016/j.ssmph.2020.100608

Kim, H. J., Fredriksen-Goldsen, K. I., Bryan, A. E. B., & Muraco, A. (2017). Social network types and mental health among LGBT older adults. *The Gerontologist, 57*(Suppl. 1), S84–S94. https://doi.org/10.1093/geront/gnw169

Kim, H. J., Jen, S., & Fredriksen-Goldsen, K. I. (2017). Race/ethnicity and health-related quality of life among LGBT older adults. *The Gerontologist, 57*(Suppl. 1), S30-S39. https://doi.org/10.1093/geront/gnw172

Knauer, N. J. (2015). LGBT older adults: Chosen family and caregiving. *Journal of Law and Religion, 31*, 1–30. https://doi.org/10.2139/ssrn.2721451

Knochel, K. A., & Flunker, D. (2021). Long-term care expectations and plans of transgender and nonbinary older adults. *Journal of Applied Gerontology, 40*(11), 1542–1550. https://doi.org/10.1177/0733464821992919

Knochel, K. A., & Seelman, K. L. (2020). Understanding and working with transgender/nonbinary older adults. In S. K. Kattari, M. K. Kinney, L. Kattari, & N. E. Walls (Eds.), *Social work and health care practice with transgender and nonbinary individuals and communities* (pp. 120–133). Routledge. https://doi.org/10.4324/9780429443176-11

Koller, J., & Urbanski, P. (2023). Aging and the lived experiences of transgender and gender nonconforming older adults. *Innovation in Aging, 7*(Suppl. 1), 796. https://doi.org/10.1093/geroni/igad104.2569

Kortes-Miller, K., Boulé, J., Wilson, K., & Stinchcombe, A. (2018). Dying in long-term care: Perspectives from sexual and gender minority older adults about their fears and hopes for end of life. *Journal of Social Work in End-of-Life & Palliative Care, 14*(2-3), 209–224. https://doi.org/10.1080/15524256.2018.1487364

Lee, P., Le Saux, M., Siegel, R., Goyal, M., Chen, C., Ma, Y., & Meltzer, A. C. (2019). Racial and ethnic disparities in the management of acute pain in US emergency departments: Meta-analysis and systematic review. *The American Journal of Emergency Medicine, 37*(9), 1770–1777. https://doi.org/10.1016/j.ajem.2019.06.014

Lorusso, M. M., Compare, C., & Albanesi, C. (2025). Current vs. desired: Transforming the gender-affirming path through the work of trans, non-binary, and gender-questioning activists within an ecological framework. *Sexuality Research and Social Policy, 22*(1), 176–190. https://doi.org/10.1007/s13178-023-00905-0

Lowers, J. (2017). End-of-life care planning for lesbian, gay, bisexual, and transgender individuals. *Journal of Hospice & Palliative Nursing, 19*(6), 526–533. https://doi.org/10.1097/NJH.0000000000000377

Maddux, S. (Producer & Director). (2011). *Gen silent* [Film]. Interrobang Productions.

Maina, I. W., Belton, T. D., Ginzberg, S., Singh, A., & Johnson, T. J. (2018). A decade of studying implicit racial/ethnic bias in healthcare providers using the implicit association test. *Social Science & Medicine, 199*, 219–229. https://doi.org/10.1016/j.socscimed.2017.05.009

Minter, S. P., & Wald, D. H. (2012). Protecting parental rights. In J. L. Levi & E. E. Monnin-Browder (Eds.), *Transgender family law: A guide to effective advocacy* (pp. 63–85). AuthorHouse.

Musa, D., Schulz, R., Harris, R., Silverman, M., & Thomas, S. B. (2009). Trust in the health care system and the use of preventive health services by older Black and White adults. *American Journal of Public Health, 99*(7), 1293–1299. https://doi.org/10.2105/AJPH.2007.123927

National Archives and Records Administration. (2023, March 15). *Code of Federal Regulations Title 42 Part 483*. https://www.ecfr.gov/current/title-42/chapter-IV/subchapter-G/part-483

National Center for Transgender Equality. (2023). *Know your rights: Medicare.* Retrieved from https://transequality.org/know-your-rights/medicare

National Council on Aging. (2023, October 20). *Get the facts on health aging.* https://www.ncoa.org/article/get-the-facts-on-healthy-aging

National Resource Center on LGBT Aging. (2012). *Inclusive services for LGBT older adults: A practical guide to creating welcoming agencies.* https://www.lgbtagingcenter.org/resources/resource.cfm?r=487

Pang, C., Gutman, G., & de Vries, B. (2019). Later life care planning and concerns of transgender older adults in Canada. *International Journal of Aging & Human Development, 89*(1), 39–56. https://doi.org/10.1177/0091415019843520

Pioneer Network. (2023). *Pioneers in culture change and person-directed care.* https://www.pioneernetwork.net/about-us/overview/

Porter, K. E., Brennan-Ing, M., Chang, S. C., Dickey, L. M., Singh, A. A., Bower, K. L., & Witten, T. M. (2016). Providing competent and affirming services for transgender and gender nonconforming older adults. *Clinical Gerontologist, 39*(5), 366–388. https://doi.org/10.1080/07317115.2016.1203383

Progovac, A. M., Mullin, B. O., Dunham, E., Reisner, S. L., McDowell, A., Sanchez Roman, M. J., Dunn, M., Telingator, C. J., Lu, F. Q., Breslow, A. S., Forstein, M., & Cook, B. L. (2020). Disparities in suicidality by gender identity among Medicare beneficiaries. *American Journal of Preventive Medicine, 58*(6), 789–798. https://doi.org/10.1016/j.amepre.2020.01.004

Putney, J. M., Keary, S., Hebert, N., Krinsky, L., & Halmo, R. (2018). "Fear runs deep:" The anticipated needs of LGBT older adults in long-term care. *Journal of Gerontological Social Work, 61*(8), 887–907. https://doi.org/10.1080/01634372.2018.1508109

Schaie, K. W., & Willis, S. L. (2021). *Handbook of the psychology of aging.* Academic Press.

Schippers, M. C., & Ziegler, N. (2019). Life crafting as a way to find purpose and meaning in life. *Frontiers in Psychology, 10,* 2778. https://doi.org/10.3389/fpsyg.2019.02778

Services and Advocacy for Gay, Lesbian, Bisexual, and Transgender Elders. (2018). *The facts on LGBT aging.* https://www.sageusa.org/wp-content/uploads/2018/05/sageusa-the-facts-on-lgbt-aging.pdf

Services and Advocacy for Gay, Lesbian, Bisexual, and Transgender Elders, & National Center for Transgender Equality. (2012). *Improving the lives of transgender older adults: Recommendations for policy and practice.* http://transequality.org/sites/default/files/docs/resources/TransAgingPolicyreportFull.pdf

Singh, A. A., Hays, D. G., & Watson, L. S. (2011). Strength in the face of adversity: Resilience strategies of transgender individuals. *Journal of Counseling and Development, 89*(1), 20–27. https://doi.org/10.1002/j.1556-6678.2011.tb00057.x

Singh, A. A., & McKleroy, V. S. (2011). "Just getting out of bed is a revolutionary act": The resilience of transgender people of color who have survived traumatic life events. *Traumatology, 17*(2), 34–44. https://doi.org/10.1177/1534765610369261

Smart, B. D., Mann-Jackson, L., Alonzo, J., Tanner, A. E., Garcia, M., Refugio Aviles, L., & Rhodes, S. D. (2020). Transgender women of color in the U.S. South: A qualitative study of social determinants of health and healthcare perspectives. *International Journal of Transgender Health, 23*(1–2), 164–177. https://doi.org/10.1080/26895269.2020.1848691

Spencer, K. G., Berg, D. R., Bradford, N. J., Vencill, J. A., Tellawi, G., & Rider, G. N. (2021). The gender-affirmative life span approach: A developmental model for clinical work with transgender and gender-diverse children, adolescents, and adults. *Psychotherapy, 58*(1), 37–49. https://doi.org/10.1037/pst0000363

Stone, A. L., Nimmons, E. A., Salcido, R., Jr., & Schnarrs, P. W. (2020). Multiplicity, race, and resilience: Transgender and non-binary people building community. *Sociological Inquiry, 90*(2), 226–248. https://doi.org/10.1111/soin.12341

Stryker, S. (2017). *Transgender histories: The roots of today's revolution*. Seal Studies.

van der Kaap-Deeder, J., Soenens, B., Van Petegem, S., Neyrinck, B., De Pauw, S., Raemdonck, E., & Vansteenkiste, M. (2020). Live well and die with inner peace: The importance of retrospective need-based experiences, ego integrity and despair for late adults' death attitudes. *Archives of Gerontology and Geriatrics, 91*, 104184. https://doi.org/10.1016/j.archger.2020.104184

Walsh, F. (2016). Family resilience: A developmental systems framework. *European Journal of Developmental Psychology, 13*(3), 313–324. https://doi.org/10.1080/17405629.2016.1154035

White Hughto, J. M., & Reisner, S. L. (2018). Social context of depressive distress in aging transgender adults. *Journal of Applied Gerontology, 37*(12), 1517–1539. https://doi.org/10.1177/0733464816675819

Witten, T. M. (2014). It's not all darkness: Robustness, resilience, and successful transgender aging. *LGBT Health, 1*(1), 24–33. https://doi.org/10.1089/lgbt.2013.0017

Witten, T. M. (2016). The intersectional challenging of aging and being a gender nonconforming adult. *Generations, 40*(2), 63–70. https://www.jstor.org/stable/10.2307/26556204

Witten, T. M., & Eyler, A. E. (2012). *Gay, lesbian, bisexual, and transgender aging: Challenges in research, practice, and policy*. Johns Hopkins University Press. https://doi.org/10.1353/book.16339

Woods, B., O'Philbin, L., Farrell, E. M., Spector, A. E., & Orrell, M. (2018). Reminiscence therapy for dementia. *Cochrane Database of Systematic Reviews, 3*(3), CD001120. Advance online publication. https://doi.org/10.1002/14651858.CD001120.pub3

World Health Organization. (2024, October 1). *Aging and health*. https://www.who.int/news-room/fact-sheets/detail/ageing-and-health

PART III
CLINICAL SKILLS AND INTERVENTIONS

12

GENDER-AFFIRMING ASSESSMENT AND TREATMENT OF TRAUMA WITH TRANS AND NONBINARY CLIENTS

THEODORE R. BURNES, JAN E. ESTRELLADO, AND ANNELIESE SINGH

In practicing affirmative counseling and psychological practice with trans and nonbinary (TNB) clients, it is regrettably paramount that mental health professionals (MHPs) are well-versed in working with multiple forms of trauma in order to achieve successful treatment outcomes. In the last forty years, interdisciplinary understandings of trauma have resulted in multiple definitions (Cross & O'Donnell, 2022). Embedded in these multiple understandings are common threads that trauma originates from "an event, series of events, or set of circumstances that is experienced by an individual as physically or emotionally harmful or threatening and that has lasting adverse effects on the individual's functioning and physical, social, emotional, or spiritual wellbeing" (Substance Abuse and Mental Health Services Administration, Trauma and Justice Strategic Initiative, 2014, p. 7).

These clinical definitions often fail to reflect the impact of social location and identities for many TNB survivors of trauma, which are key factors in the assessment and treatment of clients by MHPs. As reflected by Rae in the following case study, intersectional frameworks that are necessary for psychological practice are often absent from discussions of trauma (Cross & O'Donnell, 2022). For example, definitions of event-based trauma often fail to incorporate

https://doi.org/10.1037/0000471-013
Affirmative Counseling and Psychological Practice With Trans and Nonbinary Clients, Second Edition, A. Singh and R. McCullough (Editors)
Copyright © 2026 by the American Psychological Association. All rights reserved.

intergenerational trauma that many TNB consumers of mental health services who are also people of color experience.

CASE STUDY: RAE

Rae (they/them) identifies as a 24-year-old Black nonbinary queer person. Rae and their boyfriend (who identifies as a Black cisgender queer man) have been dating for approximately three months, and they have been in a sexually active relationship for the last two months. Rae has just discovered that they are pregnant. Not having been pregnant before, Rae has some fears about it and is especially worried that certain attributes of pregnancy may accentuate parts of their biological sex that may not be congruent with their nonbinary gender. Rae is also worried that neither they nor their boyfriend have the economic resources to support a child, because they have both just graduated from school, and neither of them yet have a job. Rae's boyfriend does not want to have a baby and suggests that Rae think about having an abortion. During the conversation, Rae's boyfriend makes several offensive comments about Rae's gender and their prospective ability to parent. The conversation results in Rae feeling confused, embarrassed, and experiencing an increase in gender dysphoria (which they experience periodically in unsafe situations). Rae knows little about the abortion process but has heard many negative things about it from both media and people in their life. As Rae begins to contemplate the upcoming months, they grow more nervous, scared, and experience feelings of isolation. Although they have not engaged in self-harming behavior since high school, when they experienced extreme bullying, they start to feel certain triggers for self-harm again.

RATES OF TRAUMA

In the first edition of this book, authors noted that trauma was experienced at higher rates for TNB individuals than many other groups of people who access psychological services (Richmond et al., 2017). Unfortunately, these data has remained consistent for many TNB people, including the recent documentation of experiences in health care (Cicero et al., 2019; Romanelli & Lindsay, 2020), family rejection (Gamio Cuervo et al., 2022; Keeley, 2022), rejection from one or multiple intimate partners (Gunby & Butler, 2022), and workplace discrimination (Viehl et al., 2022). These experiences range in the type of trauma experienced, including daily microaggressions and insults, verbal harassment, and physical discrimination (Morris et al., 2020). Multiple forms of violence—including murder, physical and emotional abuse, rape, childhood sexual abuse, and hate-oriented neglect—against TNB people is prevalent but continues to be understudied (Grocott et al., 2022). Further, such violence has been a prevalent phenomenon that has received little scholastic attention (Burnes et al., 2016) since the first edition of this text (Richmond et al., 2017). Although not the focus of this chapter, these trauma experiences are largely driven by toxic and hostile cisheteronormativity and cisgender people themselves, and there is a dire need for research, practice, and advocacy interventions with cisgender people to shift societal culture and climate towards TNB-affirming attitudes and societal practices.

In addition, MHPs should be aware that many researchers suggest that rates of violence against TNB people are underreported due to a variety of factors, including fear of further retaliation and the outing of gender identity in unsafe environments (Flores et al., 2021). Nonetheless, TNB adults survive traumatic experiences (including violence and victimization) at a rate that is at least four times higher than their cisgender peers (Flores et al., 2021). Data about nonbinary people's experiences of trauma are still nascent in psychological research (see Chapter 7, this volume, for more on this), but reports are increasingly common within health care practice (Barbee & Schrock, 2019).

As exemplified by Rae, these data are different when examining rates in specific groups of TNB people, such as trans women and trans people of color. TNB people of color are at increased risk for adult sexual assault when compared to their white TNB counterparts (Staples & Fuller, 2021). While a significant number of TNB individuals across race experience anti-TNB discrimination, TNB people of color reported higher levels of anti-TNB discrimination when accessing medical services, including in emergency rooms, with doctors and hospitals, and with ambulances and emergency medical technicians (Alizaga et al., 2022). Black TNB women are at higher risk of interaction with law enforcement and report not just verbal harassment and physical violence from law enforcement officers, but sexual violence as well (LaMartine et al., 2023). Readers should see Chapter 6 for further discussion of the experiences of TNB people and communities of color.

To address systems and experiences of trauma with their TNB clients from an affirmative lens, we will use an intersectional gender liberation framework that centers the experiences of TNB people. As we begin to describe and critique the evolution of trauma-informed care for TNB clients, our hope is to increase the quality of mental health services in these communities and to dismantle oppressive systems that do not address trauma experienced by TNB individuals.

THEORETICAL PERSPECTIVES OF TRAUMA

The progression of more recent trauma conceptualization can be seen from the fourth edition of the *Diagnostic and Statistical Manual of Mental Disorders* (*DSM-IV*; American Psychiatric Association, 1994). The removal of posttraumatic stress disorder (PTSD) from anxiety disorders to its own umbrella group of trauma disorders signaled the growing body of research and increased depth of understanding about trauma in the fifth edition (*DSM-5*; American Psychiatric Association, 2013). In the text revision of the *DSM-5* (*DSM-5-TR*; American Psychiatric Association, 2022), there were no changes to the PTSD diagnostic criteria, but members of the Ethnoracial Equity and Inclusion Work Group and Cross-Cutting Culture Review Group incorporated research on the impact of race on mental health disorders, including trauma disorders (Moran, 2022).

While the scholarship examining the relationship between sociopolitical stressors and trauma is developing, traditional conceptualizations of trauma continue to focus mostly on Western notions related to the individual (internal thoughts and feelings and external behaviors) and a discrete categorization defining the traumatic event. The diagnostic criteria for PTSD in the *DSM-5-TR* (American Psychiatric Association, 2022) reflects these conceptualizations (e.g., exposure to the threat to bodily harm, intrusive thoughts or feelings, avoidance, changes in cognitions and mood, arousal).

One limitation of the conceptualization of trauma defined by the *DSM-5-TR*'s PTSD diagnosis is its inability to address the effects of long-term exposure to trauma (American Psychiatric Association, 2022). The World Health Organization (2019) has chosen to acknowledge the impact of long-term exposure to trauma by including a complex PTSD diagnosis in the 11th revision of the International Disease Classification, in addition to a PTSD diagnosis. In her analysis of complex PTSD, Judith Herman (1992, 1992/2015) discussed the importance of seeing one's self reflected in others as an aspect of trauma recovery.

The American Psychological Association (2017) published its guidelines for treating PTSD, recommending psychotherapeutic and psychotropic interventions based on the most recent and strongest scientific evidence. One noted limitation of the guidelines is their ability to account for identity differences or environment (American Psychological Association, n.d.). This acknowledgment suggests that the recommended guidelines for treating PTSD have no explicit analysis of the sociopolitical context in which trauma occurs for people who experience oppression. Beyond the lack of acknowledgment of sociopolitical consequences, the guidelines provide no recommendations about how to address intersectionality and cultural contexts in trauma treatment (Bryant-Davis, 2019).

Scholars of color have been particularly influential in the incorporation of sociopolitical and intergenerational stressors in trauma conceptualization. Brave Heart's (1999) seminal work highlights the role of historical trauma and traditional protective factors among the Lakota. DeGruy's (2017) scholarship focuses on the intergenerational impact of trauma among descendants of enslaved people from Africa. Bryant-Davis's trauma research highlights both historical and sociocultural contexts (2010) needed to address trauma recovery with diverse populations (2019). Foo (2022) examines the effects of immigration trauma on complex PTSD. Carter and Pieterse (2020) investigate the consequences of racism as they manifest in traumatic stress symptoms. Menakem (2017) describes the pervasive experience of trauma among people in the United States due to its history of racism. For example, Menakem's (2017) conceptualization of the *soul wound* is an intergenerational trauma that is not only perpetuated between abusive family members and biological aspects of trauma transmission, but also through ". . . unsafe or abusive systems, structures, institutions, and/or cultural norms" (p. 10). These examples of the roles of social, historical, and political contexts in the experience of trauma are directly relevant to TNB people.

The effects of anti-TNB bias on trauma-related symptoms have been examined more recently. Richmond and colleagues (2012) describe a trauma conceptualization framework acknowledging the effects of anti-TNB violence. TNB people who encountered anti-TNB bias and nonaffirmation experiences, such as not seeing one's gender represented in day-to-day life, experienced greater PTSD symptom severity, even while controlling for exposure to other types of trauma (Barr et al., 2021).

Some of the complexities regarding conceptualization of trauma among TNB people include the following:

- What role do sociopolitical stressors, including transprejudice in daily living and intense anti-TNB legislation, play in the trauma presentation among TNB people?
- How does long-term exposure to traumatic events, including but not limited to anti-TNB–based threats to bodily harm, affect TNB people?
- How do interpersonal and systemic transprejudice affect trauma symptoms among TNB people who have experienced Criterion A traumatic events, such as witnessing violence, being repeatedly exposed to child abuse, or experiencing an assault?

While many of the answers to these questions require further examination, the following analyses will contextualize how current trauma models may be helpful or limiting when working with TNB people.

THE TRAUMA-INFORMED PARADIGM

There are many aspects to the traditional conceptualization of trauma that are relevant when working clinically with TNB people; however, increasing numbers of MHPs also incorporate aspects of trauma-focused work into their conceptualization and treatment without focusing on trauma in depth. As Knight (2020) reminds,

> Trauma-informed care is not trauma therapy. The focus of treatment is not necessarily on the trauma and its aftermath. Trauma-informed practitioners are attuned to the multifaceted treatment needs of their clients and recognize the connection between present-day challenges and past trauma. (p. 7)

With this differentiation, trauma-informed practice can address the differing contexts in which clients' trauma may surface, addressing themes such as safety, choice, empowerment, and diverse perspectives in healing.

One of the core elements of the trauma-informed paradigm is the assessment of safety. Encounters with threats to bodily harm and their sequelae can result in the need for safety on both interpersonal (Shalka & Leal, 2022) and intrapersonal levels (Gold, 2020). However, if the threat of safety continues to exist, it is difficult for successful trauma recovery to occur (Courtois & Ford, 2013). Given the ongoing dangers that exist for TNB people, efforts toward safety assessment (and trauma recovery) might be hampered by continued exposure to trauma.

Another component of traditional trauma conceptualization is interpersonal functioning. Mistrust of others (Staples & Fuller, 2021) and, in some cases, being unhelpfully trusting of others (i.e., the "excessive dependency, passivity, and superficial compliance with the wishes of others" [Courtois & Ford, 2013, p. 24]) are two ways trauma survivors might respond in relationships. Healthy relationships with others and reintegration with communities are important aspects of trauma recovery (Briere and Scott, 2014); however, trusting others may be difficult to do when the environment surrounding oneself is not affirming of TNB people and their experiences. Therefore, MHPs need to thoroughly assess the function and context of mistrust of others as either adaptive and appropriate (given anti-TNB environments) or limiting to their clients.

Trauma affects what one thinks and how one feels. Whether a person believes they are worthy of love, for example, might fundamentally shift after experiencing trauma. The corresponding feelings (i.e., shame, anger, sadness) related to those beliefs can often become overwhelming and sometimes lead to depression and anxiety (Ouhmad et al., 2023), as well as suicidality (McGrew et al., 2023). However, what if those thoughts and feelings are already influenced by a social and political context that communicates a TNB person's unworthiness on a daily basis? Suyemoto and Roemer (2018) discussed the limitation of talk therapy modalities that tend to focus on the internal experience, without the environments in which those internal experiences occur. By focusing only on the thoughts and feelings and not acknowledging their socio-environmental causes, TNB trauma survivors might inadvertently leave with the message that they (and not transprejudice) are the problem.

The need for TNB-specific models of trauma recovery is clear, given both the helpful and limited ways traditional trauma-related approaches address the experiences of TNB people. *The Trauma Recovery Model for Transgender, Nonbinary and Gender Expansive People of Color* (Estrellado, 2022), for example, identifies four aspects of trauma recovery that are particularly relevant to these communities: empowerment, affirmation, safety, and connection. Estrellado's model is informed by current knowledge about trauma recovery, including from Herman (1992, 1992/2015), and can offer considerations when using various forms of trauma recovery treatment. While the original model includes various examples related to transgender, nonbinary, and gender expansive people of color specifically, the model will be discussed here in relevance to TNB communities broadly.

Empowerment

Various forms of power are likely necessary for a successful trauma recovery, including the power to choose how, when, and which type of treatment a person wishes to engage with on their road to trauma recovery. In Estrellado's (2022) model, the conceptualization of a person's choice not to engage in gold-standard treatments (i.e., cognitive processing therapy or prolonged exposure) might not necessarily mean avoidance. Rather, the choice to seek other treatment modalities might be an acknowledgment that these treatments were not designed with the intersections of oppression-based experiences and different kinds of traumatic exposure in mind. Culturally responsive MHPs, then, might include this acknowledgment when discussing informed consent with TNB clients. Rather than seeing the choice to engage another modality or treatment attrition as avoidance, MHPs might view these outcomes as lack of fit with the client and their experiences.

Another form of empowerment in the clinical setting according to Estrellado's (2022) model is when TNB clients' perspectives and experiences are believed and affirmed. In a qualitative study examining TNB people's experiences in psychotherapy, Mizock and Lundquist (2016) found a number of missteps among MHPs, including overfocusing or underfocusing on gender identity, as well as having restrictive views on gender. These experiences might be effectively addressed by hearing the TNB client's perspectives on their own experiences, including their presenting problems and the role of gender identity in them ("To what degree do you think your experiences as a transmasc person play a part here?" "How was the response to your sexual assault layered with your experiences as a nonbinary person?"). By *facilitating* TNB clients' experiences as they may intersect with aspects of their trauma recovery, rather than *dictating* their experiences, trauma therapists might become more supportive of their clients.

Affirmation

Judith Herman (1992, 1992/2015) discussed the importance of seeing oneself reflected in others as an aspect of trauma recovery. Many TNB people, however, may not have had the experience of available models that reflect themselves, with or without exposure to traumatic events. When considering that the experience alone of being a TNB person may produce its own traumatic stress symptoms (Barr et al., 2021), affirming experiences become even more central to the trauma recovery of TNB people.

There are a number of ways that trauma therapists can provide an affirming environment for TNB people. One is to acknowledge the reality that there are not enough models reflecting TNB people's experiences and that this lack of accessible self-reflection likely has costs to the individual. Another affirming step is to help TNB people try to access the models that capture aspects of themselves they want to see. These can be personal qualities, a way of expressing gender, a quote, or a TV character that embodies aspects of themselves that reflect who they are or how they would like to engage with the world.

Treatment using this approach needs to be tailored to the client. Using what Lynn Northrop (personal communication, August 15, 2014) calls "little 'e' empiricism," trauma therapists can find what is effective with their clients to help them meet their treatment goals. Trauma therapists working successfully with TNB clients will find ways to address important aspects of trauma recovery more flexibly by using some of these strategies.

Safety

As mentioned previously in the chapter, a necessary ingredient of trauma recovery is safety. Trauma recovery among TNB people may be challenging given the exposure to danger TNB people in the United States face. There are a number of aspects related to safety in Estrellado's (2022) model worth considering in trauma therapy with TNB people.

Safety should be thought of in at least a few different contexts. While traditional trauma conceptualization would suggest that feeling safe in one's body is difficult due to the threat of bodily harm, a culturally responsive conceptualization would also acknowledge that TNB people's bodies may not have felt safe already due to dysphoria. For example, how might a *transmasc* person—a trans person who identifies with or expresses masculine gender—experience having their chests groped as part of a sexual assault when they already had dysphoria about their chest? The trauma therapist's willingness to acknowledge that one's body might not feel safe due to gender dysphoria and see the complexity that trauma might add to this experience is an important safety consideration among TNB people.

Effective MHPs acknowledge the realities of danger facing TNB people in their daily lives. Race, geographical location, socioeconomic status, and transmisogyny are some important aspects to consider when assessing the current level of danger TNB people might face. MHPs might provide psychoeducation on the challenge of establishing an internal sense of safety when the external threat to safety continues to exist. Using strategies to survive should not be viewed as avoidance and may be subjectively defined based on the TNB person's own assessment of their safety. For example, a young TNB person might choose to express their gender in a way that is more palatable to their family if they were worried about their family members responding in harmful or violent ways. This might be seen as a survival strategy rather than as avoidance.

Connection

Given the risk of exposure to violence TNB people face, the relational stakes are likely higher. This can happen in at least two notable ways. First, the investment in social connection might be stronger once relationships are deemed safe by the TNB person. Second, given the different kinds of social injustice TNB people face, the negotiation of power differentials in daily living is ongoing. Social support and community engagement were found to be protective factors that promoted a sense of belonging and connection among TNB people and communities of color (Farvid et al., 2021).

These contexts offer relevant opportunities for trauma recovery work. The culturally responsive MHP might contextualize the higher stakes involved with TNB people's social support networks. A strong investment in the outcomes of a TNB person's social relationships might be viewed through the lens of a potentially limited access to a broad support network. For example, rather than conceptualizing a TNB person's strong investment in a social support relationship as a "lack of boundaries," the MHP might validate the importance of the relationship as a crucial and meaningful aspect of the TNB person's life. Therefore, the therapeutic strategy might be how to honor oneself *and* the relationship, versus choosing self over other.

The other connection-focused element of trauma recovery among TNB people is the therapeutic relationship. The negotiation of power differentials in the therapeutic relationship are well-framed by feminist therapy, including feminist therapy with TNB people (Estrellado & Balsam, 2023). MHPs, especially cisgender MHPs, can promote egalitarianism and intersectionality through the use of appropriate self-disclosure and power-sharing with TNB clients (Conlin & Douglass, 2023). The use of these therapeutic strategies to strengthen connection is necessary for trauma recovery among TNB people in clinical settings.

FROM THEORY TO FIRE TO BACK IN THE FRYING PAN

Given the therapeutic strategies when working with TNB people in trauma recovery, it may be helpful to revisit the current "socio-cultural realities" (Bryant-Davis, 2010, p. 263) TNB people face. The context of the current sociopolitical environment for TNB people requires that trauma recovery theoretical frameworks be put into action to improve the quality of life for TNB people. Despite the increasing visibility of TNB people, violence continues to be an ongoing threat. The National Center for Transgender Equality (2022) reported 47 TNB people were murdered due to anti-TNB bias, the vast majority of whom were Black and Brown TNB women. In 2020, then presidential nominee Joe Biden labeled anti-TNB violence as an "epidemic that needs national leadership" (Taylor, 2020, p. 4).

While the threat of violence is real and continues to be associated with the experiences of many TNB people, the focus on violence tends to obscure other important aspects of TNB people's lives. These aspects, including finding strength and joy in one's TNB gender identity, are also important to acknowledge as part of the trauma recovery process. Holding both the realities of sociopolitical violence, as well as the ways that TNB people can continue to find strength and joy in the presence of violence, are essential to trauma recovery.

TRAUMATIC EXPERIENCES OF TRANS AND NONBINARY COMMUNITIES ACROSS THE LIFESPAN

Although "Part II: Working With Diverse Client Identities and Life Stages" has chapters specifically exploring developmental experiences for TNB communities across the lifespan, given the evolution of theoretical perspectives related to trauma, we also use a lifespan perspective in this chapter, as it is imperative that MHPs consider developmental factors when using a trauma-informed lens to work with TNB clients.

Prenatal and Infancy

Historically pathologized as "disorders of sexual development," *intersex* is an umbrella term for differences in our reproductive anatomies or sex-focused biological traits (interACT, 2021). TNB people who also identify as intersex often undergo coercive interactions with medical providers early in their lives (Richmond et al., 2017). Although some intersex traits are noticed using technology before birth or during infancy, others may not reflect until later in life. Surgeries on intersex infants are not lifesaving and therefore are not necessary during infancy. Such surgeries, combined with misinformation and inaccuracy about intersex people, often result in complex traumatic experiences for many intersex people, including the impact of violent surgeries and systemic erasure (Khanna, 2021). Much of this trauma occurs in part due to the systemic oppression of people who fall outside of sex and gender binaries. Many MHPs working with intersex children (or intersex adults who were met with medical interventions as children without their consent) focus on how such interventions negatively impact sense of self, posttraumatic growth through systemic justice, finding social connection, and developing acceptance (Hart & Shakespeare-Finch, 2022, p. 912).

Childhood

As scholars continue to document the victimization of TNB young children in schools (Mangin, 2020), MHPs often fail to consider that TNB clients first experience trauma in the form of child abuse, sometimes before the child enters traditional school environments. Researchers continue to explore and describe the ways in which trauma can negatively influence many facets of growth and development in young TNB children, including social (Burnes et al., 2016), neurological (Gill-Peterson, 2018), cognitive (Tishelman & Neumann-Mascis, 2018), and emotional (Sherman et al., 2020) development. As young children begin to exhibit a capability to differentiate between genders, they simultaneously begin to internalize systemic gender stereotypes and complex traumas. Many of these experiences of trauma are compounded by experiences of intersecting oppressions for TNB youth of color (Rusow et al., 2022), TNB youth of diverse sexual orientation identities (Hereth et al., 2020), and TNB youth with different neurological experiences (Oswald et al., 2022). In particular, researchers continue to explore the overlap between diagnoses related to neurodivergence and gender identity, with particular attention that the role of trauma may play for children who are both TNB and autistic (Gratton, 2019).

Adolescence

As addressed specifically in Chapter 3 in this text, advocacy is a crucial role of MHPs as anti-TNB legislation across multiple states will translate to increased risk of victimization that TNB adolescents experience (Viehl et al., 2022). As adolescents are forming their intersecting identities as a primary developmental task, their encounters with large pieces of hateful legislation often thwart these developmental experiences, resulting in trauma. At the time of this writing, multiple states have enacted restrictions that block adolescents from receiving care and affirming medical interventions (Dawson & Kates, 2022). Further, additional states are considering equally problematic laws. These compounded traumas at various systemic levels result in TNB adolescents engaging in many negative health-related behaviors and disconnecting from many of their sources of resilience and empowerment. As adolescents also engage in developmentally appropriate creation of peer relationships and age-appropriate social skills, TNB adolescents may struggle with such relational tasks for fear of ridicule and rejection, lack of self-efficacy, or fear of being outed if they have not yet disclosed their identity. TNB adolescents who are engaging in intimate relationships for the first time often halt such relationships due to these same fears (Fuller & Riggs, 2021).

TNB adolescents, particularly TNB people and communities of color, experience numerous forms of harassment and victimization (Zongrone et al., 2022). Such experiences of harassment and victimization may result in certain behaviors used to cope with such experiences that many MHPs unfortunately decontextualize and label as mood disturbances, characterological features, anxiety, dissociation, or conduct problems (Spivey & Edwards-Leeper, 2019). Although many MHPs are trained to treat symptoms from a lens of evidence-based practice, numerous scholars (Chen et al., 2023) name the difficulty of separating the symptoms from the larger context of hatred and gender bias that TNB adolescents face; thus, there is high demand for these adapting treatments meant for specific mental health sequelae that are focused on the experiences of TNB adolescents.

In coping with these traumatic experiences, TNB adolescents will engage trauma through self-injury, accelerated sexual behavior, or avoiding health care providers (e.g., MHPs, physicians, school counselors) who may further cause them suffering through uninformed, hurtful interactions (Ramos & Marr, 2023). There is a growing amount of literature reflecting the resilience of TNB youth (Tankersley et al., 2021) in finding social support through online communities (communities that support them in their gender identity) and reframing mental health challenges as they navigate relationships with family and friends (Burnes et al., 2016).

Midlife and Older Adulthood

The transition from adolescence to adulthood is often marked by a myriad of shifts in intimacy, perspective, and desire for larger contribution into society (Burnes et al., 2016). Like Rae in the case study, it is often a primary developmental task for individuals in their adult years to think about gaining intimacy. As noted previously, such intimacy can be difficult for TNB individuals who have encountered varying experiences of trauma or who are experiencing ongoing victimization and harassment. These experiences, as noted by Estrellado (2022), have an adverse impact on the experiences of intimacy and sexual expression for TNB people (Fielding, 2021). In addition, employment discrimination for TNB people continues to increase (Ciprikis et al., 2024). These various experiences create unique instances of trauma for TNB clients that add distressing complexity to their developmental experiences.

Midlife is also a time in which family planning and experiences of generativity within the family life cycle often prevail. Many TNB adults are engaging in a variety of gender-affirming surgeries in which they have difficult experiences with medical professionals, resulting in a fear of family planning that involves further engagement with medical professionals (Francis et al., 2018). Despite this fear, scholars suggest that TNB clients are consistently naming family planning as a topic that enters into clinical process, necessitating that MHPs have resources (TNB-affirming clinics, providers, doulas, and birthing centers) that can assist TNB people in reaching their goals to have a family. In addition, other TNB adults who have children may survive ongoing and complex trauma symptoms related to the discrimination that they and their family members may experience in various work, education, and community spaces. MHPs should have a contextual understanding of these varied ecological sources of traumatic stress, encouraging clients to engage in social support and regulation strategies whenever possible while also engaging in advocacy efforts to remove such bias and discrimination.

As TNB clients enter older adulthood, sources of developmental and cultural trauma unfortunately continue. Like many of their cisgender peers, TNB older adults are not immune to unfortunate incidents of elder and dependent adult abuse (Bloemen et al., 2019) that often intersect with gender-related violence. These intersectional sources of traumatic stress can have a compounded impact on TNB older adults (Fabbre & Gaveras, 2020). In particular, as older adults may engage with a higher rate of medical care services in comparison to people of younger developmental stages, TNB older adult clients may undergo increased experiences of interpersonal violence from medical providers, particularly in countries such as the United States where there is large political backlash (Perone, 2020).

As these various developmental stages imply, traumatic experiences of TNB people occur within a developmental context, and it is critical for MHPs to use not only theoretical understandings of trauma, but also developmental contextualism as part of their diagnostic and theoretical conceptualizations of TNB clients. Using a theoretical framework that grounds trauma in intersectional and developmental context ensures that MHPs are carefully considering diagnostic criteria within relevant cultural experiences. It is these comprehensive frameworks that provide strong rationale and grounding for assessment, treatment planning, and interventions with TNB clients who have survived traumatic experiences.

ASSESSMENT OF TRAUMA WITH TRANS AND NONBINARY CLIENTS

Because experiences of trauma can be prevalent throughout the lifespan for TNB people (Merrick et al., 2018), MHPs need to have strong awareness, knowledge, and skills in trauma assessment. In addition, this trauma assessment must have integrated attention to TNB clients' multiple identities, as we have noted earlier, because they also experience interlocking oppressions in addition to anti-TNB societal bias (e.g., racism, sexism, heterosexism, ableism, classism, Islamophobia, antisemitism, etc.). We discuss affirming approaches to trauma assessment with TNB communities next.

Posttraumatic Stress Disorder Assessment

Because of the lifelong and persistent exposure to trauma that TNB people experience, scholars have noted the need to assess PTSD symptoms accurately. For instance, scholars have found that MHPs working with TNB clients selected events of discrimination that did not meet Criterion A of the PTSD diagnosis (such as witnessing violence; American Psychiatric Association, 2022) as the "traumatic event." These same MHPs were then found to identify a client's symptoms as related to internalized transprejudice instead of accurately identifying these as related to trauma. Considering these findings, Valentine et al. (2023) suggest five critical areas for MHPs to provide accurate and TNB-affirming trauma assessment: (a) use a collaborative approach, affirming each of the experiences of stress and trauma that TNB clients describe; (b) conduct a thorough assessment of both discrimination and trauma experiences, ensuring follow-up questions that help distinguish both; (c) use trauma-relatedness probes ("Did [symptom endorsed] get worse after [index traumatic event]?") to ensure one is identifying symptoms related to traumatic events accurately; (d) be mindful that when TNB people are vigilant about violence risk, this does not translate to being hypervigilant; and (e) educate clients so that they understand the risk of and healing from both experiences of discrimination and trauma can have similar journeys, but also may be distinct (Valentine et al., 2023, p. 392). Ultimately, these scholars recommend that treatment planning designed to address discrimination and trauma for TNB clients can use PTSD protocols for exploring stress related to discrimination, such as identifying the impacts on self-blame cognitive distortions and influence on self-esteem.

Using the Minority Stress Model to Assess Risk and Resilience

In addition to the importance of accurate and TNB-affirming PTSD diagnosis, MHPs can apply the Minority Stress Model (Meyer, 2015) to TNB communities (Hendricks & Testa, 2012) to guide assessment of risk and resilience. In the Minority Stress Model, there are two sources of stressors MHPs can explore: distal (emerging from society) and proximal (within the client, emerging from minoritizing societal influences). Distal stressors include gender-related discrimination, gender-related rejection, gender-related, victimization, and non-affirmation of gender identity each of which have an influence on TNB mental and physical health. Proximal stressors also impact TNB mental and physical health and include internalized transprejudice, negative expectations of societal maltreatment, and concealment of TNB gender identity. Within this model, community connectedness and pride are proposed as resilience factors that TNB clients experience as well.

Gender and Intersectional Microaggressions

Alongside the Minority Stress Model, researchers have suggested that assessment of gender and other intersectional microaggressions should be completed with TNB clients (Shipherd et al., 2019). These everyday slights and indignities related to TNB clients' experiences can include being misgendered, experiencing abusive language, being asked intrusive questions about one's gender journey (including hyper-focusing on one's sex assigned at birth and anatomy), seeing anti-TNB media, and being left out or pushed out of a group or community, amongst many other events (Anzani et al., 2021). Because there can be overlaps between discrimination and trauma experiences for TNB communities, assessment of both should be robust—including an assessment of gender microaggressions.

Using Socioecological Approaches

Because trauma experiences are framed by culture and society with impact on multiple levels, sociological frameworks can help MHPs with trauma assessment when working with TNB clients. As noted by dickey et al. (2017), the Centers for Disease Control and Prevention (CDC) encourages MHPs to consider how the levels within socioecological frameworks (individual, relationship, community, society) influence trauma experiences. These researchers suggest that MHPs further delineate these socioecological levels (intrapersonal, interpersonal, institutional, community, public policy, international levels) when assessing trauma experiences.

At the intrapersonal level, MHPs can explore experiences of internalized transprejudice and other negative cognitions and emotions driven by trauma. With the interpersonal level, MHPs can assess the types of interpersonal trauma and people with whom these were experienced across the lifespan. At the institutional level, they can ask questions elucidating microaggressions, discrimination, and traumatic experiences within society, such as difficulty accessing safe bathrooms and experiencing bias, prejudice, discrimination, and harassment in educational settings. When assessing the community level of trauma, MHPs can explore how the expressed and implied values, norms, and regulations have influenced TNB clients. At the public policy level, MHPs ensure they are assessing how the past, present, and future barriers or opportunities of public policies (e.g., local, state, regional, and national laws and policies) have shaped TNB client experiences of trauma. Finally, MHPs can explore how trauma may have been experienced by TNB clients at the international level of global affairs.

TREATMENT CONSIDERATIONS: USING TRAUMA-INFORMED APPROACHES

Trauma-informed care has been widely discussed in substance-abuse settings (e.g., Substance Abuse and Mental Health Services Administration, Trauma and Justice Strategic Initiative, 2014) and in K–12 settings (through the use of trauma-informed education; Thompson & Carello, 2022). The six principles of trauma-informed care include (a) safety; (b) trustworthiness and transparency; (c) peer support; (d) collaboration and mutuality; (e) empowerment, voice, and choice; and (f) cultural, historical, and gender issues (CDC, 2020). The Substance Abuse and Mental Health Services Administration described these principles as being applied not only to MHPs, but also to the organization where care is provided.

Applying these six principles (CDC, 2020) to trauma work with TNB clients, the first step of safety involves an assessment of physical and psychological safety. This safety includes the setting in which the MHP practices and safety within the counseling relationship. This safety can be addressed from the moment the TNB client contacts the MHP. To ensure this, MHPs can ask the following questions: What will the TNB client see on the MHPs website and intake materials that will intentionally set the expectation that this will be a safer environment for them? What will TNB clients experience during the first phone call and session with the MHP, and how will these experiences include an explicit attention to safety as the highest priority?

Throughout the client's experience in receiving mental health services, MHPs can attend to safety within the session through not only doing the trauma assessments discussed in the previous section, but also through reflecting at the end of the session on the client's experience of safety with the MHP to build modeling, expectations, and an experience of how safety can be experienced within an interpersonal relationship and within a health care setting. In the example of Rae, MHPs can start by acknowledging what might help them to feel safer in the session by providing Rae the ability to not answer certain questions, prioritize certain topics over others, and to discuss specific techniques and strategies to help them feel safer.

The second principle of trustworthiness and transparency (CDC, 2020) involves ensuring TNB clients have the opportunity to build and maintain trust with the MHP and can experience the counseling setting as one that is supportive. MHPs can cultivate this trusting relationship by building upon the safety explorations and regularly checking in on the client's experience through asking questions such as: "Trust is an important part of the counseling relationship— how are we doing building that trust together?" and "What needs do you have that would help us build a trusting therapeutic relationship with one another?" Trauma-informed care with trust involves transparency, so ensuring the MHP is also sharing the reasons why they may be asking questions, for instance, about a TNB client's social and medical transition or the content of conversations they are having or will have with collaborative care providers, is vitally important.

MHPs can also explore the third principle of trauma-informed care—peer support (CDC, 2020)—with TNB clients. Peer support is a form of mutual aid involving connecting TNB survivors of trauma with other TNB survivors of trauma and related appropriate resources for healing. From a trauma-informed approach, these survivors of trauma can provide other survivors an experience of hope and continued safety for their healing journeys. For TNB clients, these connections will only be able to be facilitated through MHPs collaborating and identifying these mutual TNB support networks that exist locally or online. MHPs can maintain these resources through regular connections with TNB community organizations and include these in resource materials shared within their offices.

The fourth trauma-informed care principle entails collaboration and mutuality (CDC, 2020). MHPs hold a significant amount of power in the helping relationship, as they are viewed as experts by clients. Therefore, identifying ways to share power and provide education to demystify therapeutic approaches, and show what the process of counseling and healing from trauma actually comprises, can be vital aspects of building on safety and trust in the therapeutic relationship. In many ways, this principle of collaboration and mutuality builds on the third principle of transparency, as the TNB client begins to understand that decision making can be collaborative and that they play a critical role in their own healing.

In the fifth principle of trauma-informed care, MHPs can explore TNB clients' experiences of empowerment, voice, and choice (CDC, 2020). Building upon collaboration and mutuality, MHPs find ways to amplify TNB client strengths and the resilience they have developed navigating trauma. In doing so, TNB clients can identify new boundaries for their interpersonal relationships and overall lives that help them not only navigate healing from trauma, but also help them move from resiliency to thriving. Through this principle, clients can explore self-advocacy skills they have and ones they may want to build to support their healing from trauma, so that they are empowered to connect with, value, and believe their voice that knows what they need to heal and the choices that come from connecting with that inner knowing.

Finally, the sixth principle of trauma-informed care is ensuring that cultural, historical, and gender issues (and their interlocking relationships; CDC, 2020) are explored throughout the counseling relationship. Using interventions that help TNB survivors of trauma reflect on their social identities beyond stereotypes and internalized oppression enables them to connect with their thoughts, feelings, needs, and other important aspects of their personhood. In doing so, MHPs can explore how intergenerational cultural, historical, and gender traumas have influenced their mental healing and what healing they need in order to support their own well-being.

CHAPTER SUMMARY

Given that trauma-informed care is a necessary component of affirmative practice, MHPs must stay informed about contemporary experiences of trauma at the various ecological levels that impact their TNB practice. Noting specific considerations for conceptualization and treatment that are affirmative of TNB individuals and communities will only improve clinical care. Concurrently, MHPs must center their advocacy to ensure that traumatic stress for TNB people is minimized and demand justice within economic, political, and social institutions and systems for TNB communities.

REFERENCES

Alizaga, N. M., Aguayo-Romero, R. A., & Glickman, C. P. (2022). Experiences of health care discrimination among transgender and gender nonconforming people of color: A latent class analysis. *Psychology of Sexual Orientation and Gender Diversity, 9*(2), 141–151. https://doi.org/10.1037/sgd0000479

American Psychiatric Association. (1994). *Diagnostic and statistical manual of mental disorders* (4th ed.). https://doi.org/10.1176/appi.books.9780890420614.dsm-iv

American Psychiatric Association. (2013). *Diagnostic and statistical manual of mental disorders* (5th ed.). https://doi.org/10.1176/appi.books.9780890425596

American Psychiatric Association. (2022). *Diagnostic and statistical manual of mental disorders* (5th ed., text rev.). https://doi.org/10.1176/appi.books.9780890425787

American Psychological Association. (n.d.). *Placing clinical practice guidelines in context*. https://www.apa.org/about/offices/directorates/guidelines/context

American Psychological Association. (2017). *Clinical practice guideline for the treatment of PTSD*. https://www.apa.org/ptsd-guideline

Anzani, A., Sacchi, S., & Prunas, A. (2021). Microaggressions towards lesbian and transgender women: Biased information gathering when working alongside gender and sexual minorities. *Journal of Clinical Psychology, 77*(9), 2027–2040. https://doi.org/10.1002/jclp.23140

Barbee, H., & Schrock, D. (2019). Un/gendering social selves: How nonbinary people navigate and experience a binarily gendered world. *Sociological Forum, 34*(3), 572–593. https://doi.org/10.1111/socf.12517

Barr, S. M., Snyder, K. E., Adelson, J. L., & Budge, S. L. (2021). Posttraumatic stress in the trans community: The roles of anti-transgender bias, non-affirmation, and internalized transphobia. *Psychology of Sexual Orientation and Gender Diversity, 9*(4), 410–421. https://doi.org/10.1037/sgd0000500

Bloemen, E. M., Rosen, T., LoFaso, V. M., Lasky, A., Church, S., Hall, P., Weber, T., & Clark, S. (2019). Lesbian, gay, bisexual, and transgender older adults' experiences with elder abuse and neglect. *Journal of the American Geriatrics Society, 67*(11), 2338–2345. https://doi.org/10.1111/jgs.16101

Brave Heart, M. Y. H. (1999). Oyate Ptayela: Rebuilding the Lakota Nation through addressing historical trauma among Lakota parents. *Journal of Human Behavior in the Social Environment, 2*(1–2), 109–126. https://doi.org/10.1300/J137v02n01_08

Briere, J., & Scott, C. (2014). *Principles of trauma therapy: A guide to symptoms, evaluation, and treatment* (2nd ed.). Sage Publications.

Bryant-Davis, T. (2010). Cultural considerations of trauma: Physical, mental and social correlates of intimate partner violence exposure. *Psychological Trauma: Theory, Research, Practice, and Policy, 2*(4), 263–265. https://doi.org/10.1037/a0022040

Bryant-Davis, T. (2019). The cultural context of trauma recovery: Considering the posttraumatic stress disorder practice guideline and intersectionality. *Psychotherapy, 56*(3), 400–408. https://doi.org/10.1037/pst0000241

Burnes, T. R., Dexter, M. D., Richmond, K., Singh, A. A., & Cherrington, A. (2016). The experiences of transgender survivors of trauma who undergo social and medical transition. *Traumatology, 22*(1), 75–84. https://doi.org/10.1037/trm0000064

Carter, R. T., & Pieterse, A. (2020). *Measuring the effects of racism: Guidelines for the assessment and treatment of race-based traumatic stress injury*. Columbia University Press.

Centers for Disease Control and Prevention. (2020). *Infographic: 6 guiding principles to a trauma-informed approach.* https://www.cdc.gov/orr/infographics/6_principles_trauma_info.htm

Chen, D., Berona, J., Chan, Y. M., Ehrensaft, D., Garofalo, R., Hidalgo, M. A., Rosenthal, S. M., Tishelman, A. C., & Olson-Kennedy, J. (2023). Psychosocial functioning in transgender youth after 2 years of hormones. *The New England Journal of Medicine, 388*(3), 240–250. https://doi.org/10.1056/NEJMoa2206297

Cicero, E. C., Reisner, S. L., Silva, S. G., Merwin, E. I., & Humphreys, J. C. (2019). Health care experiences of transgender adults. *Advances in Nursing Science, 42*(2), 123–138. https://doi.org/10.1097/ANS.0000000000000256

Ciprikis, K., Cassells, D., & Berrill, J. (2024). Transgender self-employment outcomes: Evidence from the USA. *Small Business Economics, 63*(3), 871–896. https://doi.org/10.1007/s11187-023-00845-4

Conlin, S. E., & Douglass, R. P. (2023). Feminist therapy with gender questioning adolescents: Clinical case example. *Women & Therapy, 46*(1), 58–75. https://doi.org/10.1080/02703149.2023.2189777

Courtois, C. A., & Ford, J. D. (2013). *Treatment of complex trauma: A sequenced, relationship-based approach*. The Guilford Press.

Cross, K., & O'Donnell, K. (2022). Introduction. In K. O'Donnell & K. Cross (Eds.), *Bearing witness: Intersectional perspectives on trauma theology* (pp. i–viii). SCM Press.

Dawson, L., & Kates, J. (2022). *Youth access to gender affirming care: The federal and state policy landscape*. KFF. https://www.kff.org/other/issue-brief/youth-access-to-gender-affirming-care-the-federal-and-state-policy-landscape/

DeGruy, J. (2017). *Post traumatic slave syndrome: America's legacy of enduring injury and healing*.

dickey, l. m., Singh, A. A., & Walinsky, D. (2017). Treatment of trauma and nonsuicidal self-injury in transgender adults. *Psychiatric Clinics of North America, 40*, 41–50. http://doi.org/10.1016/j.psc.2016.10.007

Estrellado, J. E. (2022). *A trauma recovery model for transgender, nonbinary, and gender expansive people of color* [Conference presentation]. Annual Convention of the American Psychological Association, Minneapolis, MN, United States.

Estrellado, J. E., & Balsam, K. F. (2023). Introduction to the special issue on feminist therapy with transgender, nonbinary, and gender expansive people. *Women & Therapy, 46*(1), 1–13. http://doi.org/10.1080/02703149.2023.2189774

Fabbre, V. D., & Gaveras, E. (2020). The manifestation of multilevel stigma in the lived experiences of transgender and gender nonconforming older adults. *American Journal of Orthopsychiatry, 90*(3), 350. http://doi.org/10/1037/ort0000440

Farvid, P., Vance, T. A., Klein, S. L., Nikiforova, Y., Rubin, L. R., & Lopez, F. G. (2021). The health and wellbeing of transgender and gender non-conforming people of colour in the United States: A systematic literature search and review. *Journal of Community & Applied Social Psychology, 31*(6), 703–731. https://doi.org/10.1002/casp.2555

Fielding, L. (2021). *Trans sex: Clinical approaches to trans sexualities and erotic embodiments*. Routledge.

Flores, A. R., Meyer, I., Langton, L. L., & Herman, J. L. (2021). Gender identity disparities in criminal victimization: National crime victimization survey, 2017–2018. *American Journal of Public Health, 111*(4), 726–729. http://doi.org/10.2105/AJPH.2020.306099

Foo, S. (2022). *What my bones know: A memoir of healing from complex trauma*. Ballantine Books.

Francis, A., Jasani, S., & Bachmann, G. (2018). Contraceptive challenges and the transgender individual. *Women's Midlife Health, 4*, 1–4. http://doi.org/10/1186/s40695-018-0042-1

Fuller, K. A., & Riggs, D. W. (2021). Intimate relationship strengths and challenges amongst a sample of transgender people living in the United States. *Sexual and Relationship Therapy, 36*(4), 399–412. https://doi.org/10.1080/14681994.2019.1679765

Gamio Cuervo, Á., Herrawi, F., Horne, S. G., & Wilkins-Yel, K. G. (2022). "I'm just so glad that I saved my life": A grounded theory analysis of transgender and nonbinary Latinx people navigating family rejection and intergenerational violence. *LGBTQ+ Family: An Interdisciplinary Journal, 18*(5), 403–428.

Gill-Peterson, J. (2018). *Histories of the transgender child*. University of Minnesota Press.

Gold, S. N. (2020). *Contextual trauma therapy: Overcoming traumatization and reaching full potential*. American Psychological Association. https://doi.org/10.1037/0000176-000

Gratton, F. V. (2019). *Supporting transgender autistic youth and adults: A guide for professionals and families*. Jessica Kingsley Publishers.

Grocott, L. R., Schlechter, T. E., Wilder, S. M., O'Hair, C. M., Gidycz, C. A., & Shorey, R. C. (2022). Social support as a buffer of the association between sexual assault and trauma symptoms among transgender and gender diverse individuals. *Journal of Interpersonal Violence, 38*(1–2), NP1738–NP1761. https://doi.org/10.1177/08862605221092069

Gunby, N., & Butler, C. (2022). What are the relationship experiences of in which one member identifies as transgender? A systematic review and meta-ethnography. *Journal of Family Therapy, 45*(2), 167–196. https://doi.org/10.1111/1467-6427.12409

Hart, B., & Shakespeare-Finch, J. (2022). Intersex lived experience: trauma and post-traumatic growth in narratives. *Psychology & Sexuality, 13*(4), 912–930.

Hendricks, M. L., & Testa, R. J. (2012). A conceptual framework for clinical work with transgender and gender nonconforming clients: An adaptation of the Minority Stress Model. *Professional Psychology: Research and Practice, 43*(5), 460–467. https://doi.org/10.1037/a0029597

Hereth, J., Pardee, D. J., & Reisner, S. L. (2020). Gender identity and sexual orientation development among young adult transgender men sexually active with cisgender men: 'I had completely ignored my sexuality . . . that's for a different time to figure out'. *Culture, Health & Sexuality, 22*(Suppl. 1), 31–47. http://doi.org/10.1080/13691058.2019.1636290

Herman, J. L. (1992). *Trauma and recovery: The aftermath of violence—From domestic abuse to political terror*. Basic Books.

Herman, J. L. (2015). *Trauma and recovery: The aftermath of violence—From domestic abuse to political terror* [eTextbook]. Basic Books. (Original work published 1992)

InterACT. (2021). *Annual report 2021*. https://interactadvocates.org/wp-content/uploads/2022/10/interACT_Annual_Report_2021.pdf

Keeley, S. (2022). Integrative family therapy with transgender, gender diverse, and non-binary (TGDNB) young people. *Australian and New Zealand Journal of Family Therapy, 43*(1), 151–162. https://doi.org/10/1002/anzf.1480

Khanna, N. (2021). Invisibility and trauma in the intersex community. In E. M. Lund, C. Burgess, & A. J. Johnson (Eds.), *Violence against LGBTQ+ persons: Research, practice, and advocacy* (pp. 185–194). https://doi.org/10.1007/978-3-030-52612-2_14

Knight, C. (2020). Trauma-informed supervision: Historical antecedents, current practice, and future directions. In C. Knight & L. D. Borders (Eds.), *Trauma-informed supervision: Core components and unique dynamics in varied practice contexts* (pp. 7–37). Routledge.

LaMartine, S., Nakamura, N., & García, J. J. (2023). "Even the officers are in on it:" Black transgender women's experiences of violence and victimization in Los Angeles. *Women & Therapy, 46*(2), 103–129. http://doi.org/10.1080/02703149.2023.2226012

Mangin, M. M. (2020). Transgender students in elementary schools: How supportive principals lead. *Educational Administration Quarterly, 56*(2), 255–288. https://doi.org/10.1177/0013161X19843579

McGrew, S. J., Caulfield, N. M., Boffa, J. W., Houtsma, C., Capron, D. W., Vujanovic, A. A., Franklin, C. L., & Raines, A. M. (2023). The role of distress intolerance in suicidality among military sexual trauma survivors. *Traumatology, 29*(2), 261–264. https://doi.org/10.1037/trm0000383

Menakem R. (2017). *My grandmother's hands: Racialized trauma and the pathway to mending our hearts and bodies*. Central Recovery Press.

Merrick, M. T., Ford, D. C., Ports, K. A., Guinn, A. S. (2018). Prevalence of adverse childhood experiences from the 2011–2014 behavioral risk factor surveillance system in 23 states. *Pediatrics, 172*(11), 1038–1044. http://doi.org/10.1001/jamapediatrics.2018.2537

Meyer, I. H. (2015). Resilience in the study of minority stress and health of sexual and gender minorities. *Psychology of Sexual Orientation and Gender Diversity, 2*(3), 209–213. https://doi.org/10.1037/sgd0000132

Mizock, L., & Lundquist, C. (2016). Missteps in psychotherapy with transgender clients: Promoting gender sensitivity in counseling and psychological practice. *Psychology of Sexual Orientation and Gender Diversity, 3*(2), 148–155. https://doi.org/10.1037/sgd0000177

Moran, M. (2022). Impact of culture, race, social determinants reflected throughout new DSM-5-TR. *Psychiatric News.* https://psychnews.psychiatryonline.org/doi/10.1176/appi.pn.2022.03.3.20

Morris, E. R., Lindley, L., & Galupo, M. P. (2020). "Better issues to focus on": Transgender microaggressions as ethical violations in therapy. *The Counseling Psychologist, 48*(6), 883–915. https://doi.org/10.1177/0011000020924391

National Center for Transgender Equality. (2022). *Remembrance report.* https://transequality.org/sites/default/files/docs/resources/TDOR%20Remembrance%20Report%20by%20NCTE_Nov%202022%20%281%29.pdf

Oswald, A. G., Avory, S., & Fine, M. (2022). Intersectional expansiveness borne at the neuroqueer nexus. *Psychology & Sexuality, 13*(5), 1122–1133. http://doi.org/10.1080/19419899.2021.1900347

Ouhmad, N., Deperrois, R., El Hage, W., & Combalbert, N. (2023). Cognitive distortions, anxiety, and depression in individuals suffering from PTSD. *International Journal of Mental Health, 53*(24), 336–352. http://doi.org/10.1080/00207411.2023.2219950

Perone, A. K. (2020). Protecting health care for transgender older adults amidst a backlash of US federal policies. *Journal of Gerontological Social Work, 63*(8), 743–752. https://doi.org/10.1080/01634372.2020.1808139

Ramos, N., & Marr, M. C. (2023). Traumatic stress and resilience among transgender and gender diverse youth. *Child and Adolescent Psychiatric Clinics, 32*(4), 667–682. https://doi.org/10.1016/j.chc.2023.04.001

Richmond, K. A., Burnes, T., & Carroll, K. (2012). Lost in trans-lation: Interpreting systems of trauma for transgender clients. *Traumatology, 18*(1), 45–57. http://doi/org/10.1177/1534765610396726

Richmond, K., Burnes, T. R., Singh, A. A., & Ferrara, M. (2017). Assessment and treatment of trauma with TGNC clients: A feminist approach. In A. Singh & l. m. dickey (Eds.), *Affirmative counseling and psychological practice with transgender and gender nonconforming clients* (pp. 191–212). American Psychological Association. https://doi.org/10.1037/14957-010

Romanelli, M., & Lindsey, M. A. (2020). Patterns of healthcare discrimination among transgender help-seekers. *American Journal of Preventive Medicine, 58*(4), e123–e131. https://doi.org/10.1016/j.amepre.2019.11.002

Rusow, J. A., Hidalgo, M. A., Calvetti, S., Quint, M., Wu, S., Bray, B. C., & Kipke, M. D. (2022). Health and service utilization among a sample of gender-diverse youth of color: The TRUTH study. *BMC Public Health, 22*(1), 1–13.

Shalka, T. R., & Leal, C. C. (2022). Sense of belonging for college students with PTSD: The role of safety, stigma, and campus climate. *Journal of American College Health, 70*(3), 698–705. https://doi.org/10.1080/07448481.2020.1762608

Sherman, A. D., Poteat, T. C., Budhathoki, C., Kelly, U., Clark, K. D., & Campbell, J. C. (2020). Association of depression and post-traumatic stress with polyvictimization and emotional transgender and gender diverse community connection among Black and Latinx transgender women. *LGBT Health, 7*(7), 358–366. https://doi.org/10.1089/lgbt.2019.0336

Shipherd, J. C., Berke, D., & Livingston, N. A. (2019). Trauma recovery in the transgender and gender diverse community: Extensions of the Minority Stress Model for treatment planning. *Cognitive and Behavioral Practice, 26*, 629–646. https://doi.org/10/1016/j.cbpra.2019.06.001

Spivey, L. A., & Edwards-Leeper, L. (2019). Future directions in affirmative psychological interventions with transgender children and adolescents. *Journal of Clinical Child & Adolescent Psychology, 48*(2), 343–356. https://doi.org/10.1080/15374416.2018.1534207

Staples, J. M., & Fuller, C. C. (2021). Adult sexual assault severity among transgender people of color: The impact of double marginalization. *Journal of Aggression, Maltreatment & Trauma, 30*(5), 694–706. http://doi.org/10.1080/10926771.2021.1894291

Substance Abuse and Mental Health Services Administration, Trauma and Justice Strategic Initiative. (2014). *SAMHSA's concept of trauma and guidance for a trauma-informed approach.* https://library.samhsa.gov/product/samhsas-concept-trauma-and-guidance-trauma-informed-approach/sma14-4884

Suyemoto, K. L., & Roemer, L. (2018). *Adapting mindfulness- and acceptance-based practices to address racism related stress among people of color* [Conference presentation]. Annual Convention of the American Psychological Association, San Francisco, CA, United States.

Tankersley, A. P., Grafsky, E. L., Dike, J., & Jones, R. T. (2021). Risk and resilience factors for mental health among transgender and gender nonconforming (TGNC) youth: A systematic review. *Clinical Child and Family Psychology Review, 24*, 183–206. https://doi.org/10.1007/s10567-021-00344-6

Taylor, J. (2020). *Biden calls anti-trans violence an 'epidemic that needs national leadership.'* NBC News. https://www.nbcnews.com/feature/nbc-out/biden-calls-anti-trans-violence-epidemic-needs-national-leadership-n1243932

Thompson, P., & Carello, J. (Eds.). (2022). *Trauma-informed pedagogies: A guide for responding to crisis and inequality in higher education.* Springer Publishing.

Tishelman, A., & Neumann-Mascis, A. (2018). Gender-related trauma. In C. Keo-Meier & D. Ehrensaft (Eds.), *The gender affirmative model: An interdisciplinary approach to supporting transgender and gender expansive children* (pp. 85–100). American Psychological Association. https://doi.org/10.1037/0000095-006

Valentine, S. E., Smith, A. M., Miller, K., Hadden, L., & Shipherd, J. C. (2023). Considerations and complexities of accurate PTSD assessment among transgender and gender diverse adults. *Psychological Assessment, 35*(5), 383–395. http://doi.org/10.1037/pas0001215

Viehl, C., Ginicola, M. M., Ellis, A., & Charette II, R. J. (2022). Understanding and responding to affectional and transgender prejudice and victimization. In L. L. Levers (Ed.), *Trauma counseling: Theories and interventions for managing trauma, stress, crisis, and disaster* (p. 283). https://doi.org/10.1891/9780826150851.0018

World Health Organization. (2019). *International statistical classification of diseases and related health problems* (11th ed.). https://icd.who.int/

Zongrone, A. D., Truong, N. L., & Clark, C. M. (2022). Transgender and nonbinary youths' experiences with gender-based and race-based school harassment. *Teachers College Record, 124*(8), 121–144. https://doi.org/10.1177/01614681221121531

13

TRANS AND NONBINARY SUICIDALITY AND SUICIDE RISK MANAGEMENT

JAYME PETA AND ASPEN THOMSON

Researchers have long identified significant mental health inequities for trans and nonbinary (TNB) communities, including higher rates of depression, anxiety, posttraumatic stress disorder, substance use, as well as suicidal thoughts and behaviors (STB; Grant et al., 2010; Tebbe & Budge, 2022). STB data captures have varied widely, with suicidal ideation lifetime prevalence ranging from 37–83% and suicide attempt lifetime prevalence ranging from 9.8–44% for TNB communities (McNeil et al., 2017; Reisner et al., 2016). In one of the largest nonclinical surveys of adult TNB people from the United States, 40% self-reported at least one previous suicide attempt, which is 9 times the rate of the general population (James et al., 2016). Of those, 7% reported attempting suicide in the past year, 12 times the rate of the general population (James et al., 2016). In this chapter, we describe risk and prevalence rates across the TNB lifespan, review considerations for crisis and safety planning, and describe advocacy strategies important for mental health providers (MHPs) who work with TNB communities across a wide spectrum of social identities and experiences of interlocking oppressions and privileges.

---

https://doi.org/10.1037/0000471-014
Affirmative Counseling and Psychological Practice With Trans and Nonbinary Clients, Second Edition, A. Singh and R. McCullough (Editors)
Copyright © 2026 by the American Psychological Association. All rights reserved.

PREVALENCE RATES OF SUICIDAL THOUGHTS AND BEHAVIORS IN TRANS AND NONBINARY COMMUNITIES

Mental health inequities related to STB are present throughout the lifespan for TNB people, and there are important considerations related to social identities and experiences of multiplicative oppression. For instance, the rates of suicidal ideation for TNB children and adolescents are twice as high as their cisgender peers (Becerra-Culqui et al., 2018; Thoma et al., 2019). TNB adolescents are also at substantially higher risk of not only suicide attempts, but also suicide attempts resulting in the need for medical treatment (Thoma et al., 2019). The self-reported prevalence of a previous suicide attempt for nonbinary adolescents specifically is 41.8% (Toomey et al., 2018). For binary transgender adolescents, rates are comparable, ranging from 30–50%, but are 2 to 4 times higher if they identify as lesbian, gay, bisexual, or queer (Thoma et al., 2019). In addition, several studies have found differences in TNB adolescent STB rates based on gender assigned at birth, but without controlling for access to gender-affirming care, which is highly relevant to consider with TNB STB and may vary based on gender, geographical location, and other factors (Becerra-Culqui et al., 2018; Toomey et al., 2018). It is also important to know that reported past-year suicide attempts decrease with age (James et al., 2016); however, these figures have a survivorship bias, and rates of past suicide attempts for TNB individuals are consistently at least five times higher than the general U.S. population.

TNB people of color (POCs) are reportedly at increased risk of suicide over their lifespan, with a 9% past-year suicide attempt prevalence reported by Latine or Black TNB adults and 10% for Native Americans and multiracial survey respondents, compared to the 7% average for TNB people (James et al., 2016). There are important considerations for TNB POCs related to the intersections of their racial and gender identities, which can influence STB (K. M. de Vries & Sojka, 2020; Vance et al., 2023). For instance, Millar and Brooks (2021) found that Latine and Black TNB people reported the most gender discrimination and victimization, while Asian TNB individuals reported the least, by a small margin. In addition, transfeminine POCs experience poorer physical and mental health internationally, including higher suicidality and reduced access to gender-affirming mental health counseling (Kota et al., 2023; Lett et al., 2022). In one of the few studies examining the intersection of TNB gender and race with adolescent participants, Park et al. (2022) found that multiracial TNB youth reported higher rates of depression and suicidal ideation compared to white and cisgender peers. See Chapter 2 for further discussion of the experiences of TNB communities of color.

Religiosity remains a relatively underexamined area of research regarding TNB suicidality. Research shows seemingly contradictory findings. Some researchers have found that religiosity contributes to suicide risk for TNB youth (Price-Feeney et al., 2021), but others have found religiosity to be a protective factor for TNB youth (Grossman et al., 2016). Rabasco & Andover (2023) added a possible explanation for the contradiction. They found that TNB adults who adhered to religious practices, and whose strong religious beliefs conflicted with their gender identity, experienced greater suicidal ideation severity. However, those who had resolved conflicts between their religious beliefs and gender identity had less severe suicidal ideation than the nonreligious participants. This suggests that religiosity may be a strong protective or risk factor, depending on whether TNB people participating in a religion have found ways to reconcile both aspects of their identities. Chapter 14 in this volume describes religion, spirituality, and faith among TNB people in more detail.

TNB veterans are between two and three times as likely to die by suicide as cisgender veterans, and over five times as likely as the general U.S. population (Boyer et al., 2021; Shaine et al., 2021). One possible reason for this is anti-TNB stigma in the military, including the former ban on TNB military service. Those discharged for reasons related to their TNB status are less likely to have received an honorable discharge, and veterans who were Black or Latine and assigned female at birth were more likely to be discharged explicitly due to being TNB (James et al., 2016).

TNB people with disabilities such as autism are at additional risk of suicidality as well, potentially due to greater barriers to accessing medical care and other interactions that are not yet fully understood (Kung, 2023; Strang et al., 2023; Strauss et al., 2021). A client's intersecting identities, cultural background, religion, and the narratives around mental health, suicide, and STB risk factors should be carefully considered, especially while so little research is available on subpopulations of TNB communities.

TRANS AND NONBINARY SUICIDALITY IN CONTEXT

Given the recent and dramatic rise in anti-TNB state legislation, anti-TNB narratives promoted by politicians on both sides of the aisle, and recent executive orders, we can reasonably anticipate rising rates of suicidality, depression, anxiety, and other mental health concerns in TNB communities (Du Bois et al., 2018; Pharr et al., 2022; Price et al., 2024; Restar et al., 2024). TNB youth are especially impacted, with over 93% living in states where anti-TNB legislation has been passed or proposed (Redfield et al., 2024). TNB minors in these states are significantly more likely to attempt suicide (Lee et al., 2024). Even minors living in states that have not proposed or passed anti-TNB legislation experience negative mental health impacts (Dhanani & Totton, 2023).

While there is little doubt that suicide among TNB communities is a crucial area of research and intervention—especially given the current political climate—there is also risk in adding to stigma by over-associating TNB people with suicide. Given the reemerging cultural narrative of depicting TNB people as mentally ill, sick, or perverse, it is important to balance the issue of suicide with the understanding that TNB people also experience a normal and healthy range of feelings regarding human gender identity and expression. Further, many of the arguments for improved access to gender-affirming care are based on the idea that without such care, TNB people will be at risk of suicide. This creates an expectation that TNB people must report extreme mental states and receive psychiatric s of gender dysphoria to be considered deserving of the medical care they need (Dewey & Gesbeck, 2015; MacKinnon, 2018). Together, this reinforces the historical pathologizing narrative that TNB people are "mentally ill" (Dewey & Gesbeck, 2015; Inch, 2016). Clinicians who are skilled at working with TNB clients and populations see TNB people as resilient and strong self-advocates for living authentically rather than solely focusing on suicidality as the center point of TNB lives or the key to obtain the services they need.

THEORETICAL MODELS FOR UNDERSTANDING TRANS AND NONBINARY SUICIDAL THOUGHTS AND BEHAVIORS

In this chapter we will focus on the Minority Stress Model and the interpersonal model to conceptualize TNB suicidality, as both models' utility has been supported for TNB adults (Testa et al., 2017) and youth (Austin et al., 2020; Sher et al., 2022).

Minority Stress Theory

Minority Stress Theory was developed by Meyer (1995) to explain mental and physical health disparities in gay men due to related societal stigma. This was later adapted as the *gender minority stress model* (GMSM) for TNB populations by Hendricks and Testa (2012) and Testa et al. (2015). The GMSM posits that TNB people in a cissexist society experience chronic psychological stress due to experiences such as victimization and anti-TNB discrimination, and that these experiences lead to negative perceptions of the self and others, thus contributing to poor mental health. Gender minority stress has been linked to poor overall mental health (J. M. A. de Vries et al., 2022; Kota et al., 2020). Having multiple marginalized identities, such as being a POC as well as being queer or trans, is known as *multiple minority stress* and compounds risk factors (Parra & Hastings, 2018). In a meta-analysis of 85 studies, Pellicane and Ciesla (2022) found that for TNB people, constructs of distal stress, concealment, expectations of rejection, and internalized stigma were associated with depression and suicidality.

Distal Stress (or external stress) refers to external sources of minority stress, including direct victimization by physical violence, sexual violence, harassment, and bullying, as well as institutional discrimination such as in employment, health care, and housing (Hendricks & Testa, 2012; Pellicane & Ciesla, 2022; Testa et al., 2015). Transfeminine POCs are particularly at risk of distal stressors such as sexual violence (Kota et al., 2023). To reduce the risk of these adverse experiences, TNB people may conceal their TNB status and refrain from disclosing their TNB identity or self-advocating in certain settings, although this is not always possible. This concealment can cause stress due to the dysphoria of suppressing one's identity, negative experiences such as misgendering that could result consequently, and isolation from potential community with other TNB people (Hendricks & Testa, 2012).

Whether a TNB individual is attempting to conceal their TNB status or not, they may experience anticipatory stress due to *expectations of rejection*. Expectations of rejection include hypervigilance toward signs of rejection, as well as the stressor of realistically anticipating rejection from others based on identity or appearance (Pellicane & Ciesla, 2022). Chronic heightened vigilance may be required to assess the risk versus reward of presenting as one's authentic gender expression at various times and places, and to attempt to mitigate the harm of distal stressors. This can lead to exhaustion, frequent fearfulness, and internalization (Rood et al., 2016). MHPs are encouraged to take a client-centered approach to developing treatment goals regarding concealment and anticipatory stress, and to avoid pathologizing thoughts and behaviors that appear harmful but may also be protective (Rood, Maroney, et al., 2017).

Internalized stigma refers to prejudices and negative attitudes from external sources being incorporated into a TNB person's self-image (Hendricks & Testa, 2012; Testa et al., 2015). For example, a trans woman may work to seem less threatening out of necessity for her own safety and internalize the idea that her presence is inherently threatening, or a nonbinary person may second-guess the authenticity of their own identity. Intersecting identities may increase severity of internalized stigma. For example, TNB individuals with autism may be at a higher risk for internalized stigma and, therefore, suicidality (Kung, 2023). TNB POCs may experience greater internalized sigma, but there is also evidence that they may be more prepared to be resilient to anti-trans messages

(Barr et al., 2022; Rood, Reisner, et al., 2017). Expectations of rejection and internalized stigma had the largest effect sizes in Pellicane and Ciesla's (2022) analysis, suggesting that TNB clients may benefit from an affirmative therapy approach to minimize STB, help reduce internalized stigma, and reduce suicide risk (e.g., Austin & Craig, 2015; Matsuno, 2019).

Interpersonal Theory of Suicide

The *Interpersonal-Psychological Theory of Suicide* (IPTS) proposes that the most dangerous STB come from prolonged thwarted belongingness and perceived burdensomeness without hope for remedy, and that access to means of completing suicide is distinct from desire to perform suicidal behaviors (Van Orden et al., 2010). Thwarted belongingness and perceived burdensomeness are separate but related constructs, and the IPTS considers each an internal factor that may be influenced by external factors such as the behaviors of others. *Thwarted belongingness* refers to social isolation, loneliness, the loss of a loved one, or a lack of social support. For example, a TNB person who has been rejected by their family or a TNB POC struggling to find friends who can relate to their circumstances may experience this. A TNB person who is a POC, lives with autism, has an undocumented status in the United States, or has other "multiple jeopardy" social identities or statuses may be especially vulnerable to experiencing thwarted belongingness as defined by the IPTS and expectations of rejection as defined by the GMSM. Research has suggested that TNB POCs are more likely to be forced out of a religious community than their white TNB counterparts (James et al., 2016), which can also lead to thwarted belongingness and perceived burdensomeness.

Perceived burdensomeness can include self-hatred or a self-image of "being so flawed as to be a liability on others" (Van Orden et al., 2010, p. 12). For TNB people, the experience of family stress or conflict at school or work as a result of their gender identity may be perceived as being a "burden" to others. The TNB individual may be caught between addressing their need for gender affirmation and perceiving themselves as causing problems, conflict, or even shame to those around them. TNB people, who are highly likely to have experienced rejection, and therefore thwarted belongingness, are also subject to potentially simultaneous perceived burdensomeness. They may still have social connections even if their need for belonging is completely thwarted (e.g., the professional bond with bigoted coworkers or the relational bond with rejecting family). Therefore, the sense of being a burden on others is possible even without direct social interactions. For example, a TNB person may feel they are shaming their family by simply existing in the same town, even if all contact has been cut off (Van Orden et al., 2010). When thwarted belongingness is combined with perceived burdensomeness, the result can be especially lethal.

Testa et al. (2017) show that experiences of minority stress, thwarted belongingness, and perceived burdensomeness are each highly correlated in TNB populations, and together they contribute to high risk for suicidality. This suggests that, for MHPs, attention to TNB clients' perceptions of themselves and their ability to belong, as well as their experiences of minority stress, will be key to understanding and predicting suicide risk. As TNB human rights become increasingly politicized, MHPs should be aware of the institutional discrimination TNB clients may face locally and nationally. Puckett et al. (2024) found that TNB people's perceptions of anti-TNB bias in their state correlated with greater minority stress for these TNB communities. In addition, TNB adults have greater psychological distress and higher rates of STB when they live in states with more discriminatory laws (Price et al., 2024).

Multiple studies have also supported the IPTS's explanatory power for STB in TNB youth (Grossman et al., 2016). Interpersonal microaggressions, such as misgendering, increase lifetime risk of suicide attempt (Austin et al., 2020; Sher et al., 2022). Inversely, correct name use reduces STB risk (Russell et al., 2018). TNB youth who feel isolated at school and neglected by family have higher short-term suicidality. Programs to reduce bullying and harassment increased social support, and knowing other TNB people was shown to reduce this risk of STB (Sher et al., 2022; Strauss et al., 2020). Family support is especially beneficial, as TNB children who are supported report developmentally appropriate levels of depression, commensurate to cisgender peers, and only mildly elevated anxiety (Olson et al., 2016). Therefore, MHP advocacy for familial, school, and community support for TNB youth, such as was outlined by Parker-Barnes et al. (2022) in their guidelines designed for LGBTQ+ clients of color, is crucial to client well-being. See Chapter 7 and Chapter 8 for further discussions on TNB children and adolescents.

PROTECTIVE FACTORS FROM INCREASED SUICIDAL THOUGHTS AND BEHAVIORS FOR TRANS AND NONBINARY CLIENTS

Researchers have identified a number of factors that have been shown to protect TNB people from increased STB risk. For example, Moody and Smith (2013) suggest that social support from friends and family was an important predictor of lower rates of suicidal behavior. In a further study on protective factors against suicide in TNB adults, Moody et al. (2015) confirmed these findings by demonstrating the importance of reasons for living, such as caring for existing children and wanting to be a positive role model. Both studies also emphasize the role of gender-affirming care in reducing risk. Access to and hope for the ability to access medical transition is highly protective in reducing STB risk in TNB clients (Coleman et al., 2022). When desired, obtaining gonadotropin releasing analogue (known colloquially as *puberty blockers*) is associated with reduced suicidality and improved mental health for TNB youth and continues to reduce STB into adulthood (Carmichael et al., 2021; Turban, King, et al., 2020). Multiple longitudinal studies on TNB youth and adults have found that access to gender-affirming hormones (GAH) reduces anxiety, depression, and suicidality (Aldridge et al., 2021; Allen et al., 2019; Chen et al., 2023). Inversely, when COVID-19 abruptly reduced access to gender-affirming health care, those who lost access experienced increased suicidal ideation (Jarrett et al., 2021).

While there is a strong consensus that access to various forms of medical transition improves TNB mental health and reduces suicidality, improvements are not necessarily linear. For instance, a TNB client (especially one who experiences multiple interlocking oppressions) may experience more minority stress immediately following disclosure of their TNB identity, or in the early stages of using GAH, but reduced STB risk long-term (Sher et al., 2022). The opposite of gender-affirming care, *conversion* or *"reparative" therapy*, is associated with worsened mental health, greater suicidal ideation, a higher lifetime risk of a suicide attempt (Turban, Beckwith, et al., 2020) and is strongly discouraged by the World Professional Association for Transgender Health's *Standards of Care* (Coleman et al., 2022).

Adolescent access to GAH is associated with further reduced rates of suicidal ideation compared to adult access, meaning that approaches emphasizing delaying use of GAH with a client that is age-appropriate to receive gender-affirming medical care may be deadly (Rafferty et al., 2018; Turban et al., 2022). Some medical providers may outright refuse care, falsely believing that gender-affirming medical care is relatively risky or untested (see Coleman et al., 2022). It is crucial for MHPs to consider the impact of being denied access to gender-affirming medical care for TNB youth and adults, especially in areas where access to this care is threatened by current political movements to restrict or ban it (Hughes et al., 2021).

CRISIS INTERVENTION

Despite the higher risk of suicidal ideation, suicide attempts, and completed suicides, gender-affirming, effective approaches to suicidal crisis intervention have been dramatically unresearched and rarely addressed in the literature

(Haas et al., 2010). The literature that exists has been focused on crisis intervention for LGBTQ+ youth. Yet, the literature reveals a deep need for suicide intervention that can specifically address the needs of suicidal TNB people. For example, Nemoto et al. (2005) found that 87% of TNB POCs in San Francisco had accessed crisis intervention services. In 2015 and 2016, 11% of those contacting the Crisis Text Line in the United States identified as TNB (Larsen et al., 2019). The isolation and stressors related to the COVID-19 pandemic seem to have intensified mental health crises for TNB individuals: In 2020, Trans Lifeline, a peer crisis line for TNB people, reported an 89% increase in calls related to suicidal crises since the beginning of the COVID-19 pandemic (Stabbe, 2020). More recently, Pisani et al. (2022) and Gould et al. (2021) found that 7.5% to 7.9% of callers accessing national U.S. crisis lines were TNB. These percentages are far higher than the estimated prevalence of TNB people in the United States (Goodman et al., 2019).

BARRIERS TO SUICIDE INTERVENTION

Further, stigma and barriers to mental health treatment for depression and suicidality have resulted in TNB individuals' reluctance to engage in treatment and premature discontinuation of treatment. MHPs are undertrained in TNB mental health overall, let alone crisis intervention with TNB communities, adding to the undertreatment of suicidality in TNB people and the reluctance of TNB people to obtain help during times of distress (Baguso et al., 2022; Snow et al., 2019). In a systemic literature review, Snow et al. (2019) found that past experiences of MHP incompetence, lack of nuance, and outright pathologization were major barriers for TNB individuals in accessing mental health treatment when needed. Shipherd et al. (2010) found that 40% of TNB individuals who avoided mental health services despite needing them did so due to past poor experiences or hearing of someone else's past poor experiences with mental health care. TNB people report refusal to obtain mental health help when experiencing distress due to fears of being misgendered, discriminated against, or forced into residential treatment with gender-based housing inappropriate for their identity (Hunt et al., 2020; Snow et al., 2019; Vermeir et al., 2018).

Due to having such negative experiences when seeking care, TNB people experiencing suicidality may not seek the treatment they need. Those who do obtain care report that concerns about treatment were justified; many experienced discrimination, victimization, and gender invalidation as part of their experience when getting treatment during a suicidal crisis (Vermeir et al., 2018). Studies on the experiences of TNB people seeking emergency mental health care have found that many had to educate their MHPs and—in emergency settings—are often required to do this with a lack of privacy from other patients (Mizock & Lundquist, 2016; Vermeir et al., 2018). The gender binary structure in inpatient settings can reinforce discrimination and victimization while causing increased distress for TNB patients (Walton & Baker, 2019). A number of studies have found that encountering transprejudice, inadequate treatment, mistreatment from peers, and undertrained or even hostile medical providers and MHPs have reduced the likelihood that TNB people would return to treatment during a crisis (Baguso et al., 2022; Mizock & Lundquist, 2016; Shipherd et al., 2010; Snow et al., 2019; Vermeir et al., 2018) and they are more likely to end inpatient treatment prematurely (Walton & Baker, 2019).

These experiences not only contribute to increased overall reluctance on the part of TNB people to seek help, but it stands to reason that they serve to increase the minority stress that drives suicidality in the first place. Indeed, research shows that TNB experiences of medical discrimination or negative encounters with law enforcement are associated with suicidality in TNB communities (interactions with medical and law enforcement systems are commonplace in suicide crisis intervention; Herman et al., 2014; Romanelli et al., 2018; Seelman et al., 2017).

NONDISCLOSURE OF SUICIDALITY

It is not unusual for those experiencing suicidality to exhibit reluctance about disclosing suicidal thinking (Calear & Batterham, 2019; Han et al., 2018; Mérelle et al., 2018). However, disclosure is a prerequisite to obtaining help with reducing suicidality and preventing suicide attempts (Fulginiti et al., 2016). The reluctance to seek help and disclose suicidality is compounded for TNB people due to the multiple barriers of expectations of inadequate and traumatizing treatment, poor past experiences (Reisner et al., 2015), and fears of discrimination or exploitation (Hunt et al., 2020). Meyer and colleagues (2015) found that only 23% of sexual minority individuals seek mental health or medical help during a suicidal crisis as compared to about 50% in a general community sample (Han et al., 2018; Luoma et al., 2002). While this study did not address specific TNB needs in psychiatric crisis, gender minorities—like sexual minorities—regularly report past negative experiences when seeking mental health care and may be less likely to seek help (Hunt et al., 2020; Shipherd et al., 2010; Snow et al., 2019).

In addition, greater levels of minority stress, especially internalized TNB stigma and expectations of rejection, are associated with higher levels of suicidality in adults (Bauer et al., 2015; Pellicane & Ciesla, 2022; Perez-Brumer et al., 2015; Testa et al., 2017). However, in a study of LGBTQ+ adolescents and young adults, minority stress was also connected to greater reluctance to access suicide services (Chang et al., 2022). Reisner et al. (2015) found that TNB adults had similar experiences where past discrimination, especially when experienced in health care settings, was associated with a much greater likelihood of avoiding or delaying care. This suggests a double jeopardy for TNB clients with STB. Those who are most likely to experience suicidality due to minority stress are least likely to reach out for assistance, and TNB clients with STB who do reach out for help may likely encounter further minority stress at the hands of crisis response services or MHPs. Chang et al. (2022) suggest that MHPs work with clients on reducing minority stress (particularly internalized transprejudice) which may raise the likelihood of disclosing suicidal intent.

There are two strategies MHPs can use to increase disclosure of suicidality in TNB individuals. First, ensuring that health care providers are TNB-competent is crucial. In a study on the use of LGBTQ+ crisis lines, TNB people in particular indicated they would not have used any crisis line that wasn't identified as one with MHPs specifically for LGBTQ+ clients—MHPs who likely were aware of TNB client needs (Goldbach et al., 2019). Clients who are already connected to clinics and MHPs known to be TNB friendly may be more likely to disclose. Thus, ensuring that clients are aware of TNB-affirming crisis support as well as using a TNB-affirming approach is key to increasing the likelihood of disclosure.

The second strategy is reducing internalized transprejudice as a suicide prevention measure. Not only is lower internalized transprejudice associated with lower suicidality, having less internalized stigma may also be associated with a higher likelihood of disclosure of suicidality (Chang et al., 2022; Perez-Brumer et al., 2015). Therefore, TNB-affirming approaches to reducing minority stress, especially with a focus on addressing internalized transprejudice and rejection expectation, are extremely important in reducing overall suicidality but also increasing the likelihood of disclosing suicidality. For a review of TNB-affirming approaches to reducing minority stress, see Austin & Craig (2015) and Matsuno (2019).

SUICIDE SAFETY PLANS FOR TRANS AND NONBINARY CLIENTS

Planning for potential increases in suicidal risk may also be key in both raising the likelihood of disclosure of suicidality and preventing suicide attempts in TNB clients. Suicide safety plans are crafted with the client to create easy-to-access guides to resources, coping strategies, and support should suicidal intent increase, given that when clients can manage moments of peak suicidal intent, the risk for suicide may diminish (Nuij et al., 2021; Stanley & Brown, 2012). Although there is wide variation in the recommendations regarding suicide treatment, suicide safety planning has been shown to be effective in reducing suicidal behaviors (Nuij et al., 2021; Stanley & Brown, 2012) and is recommended by the Suicide Prevention Resource Center (https://www.sprc.org/).

According to Stanley and Brown (2012), key elements of safety plans include (a) recognizing signs and triggers; (b) distracting, especially by connecting with social contacts; (c) contacting those who might be able to help resolve the crisis; (d) getting professional help; and (e) reducing lethal means. However, little research has been published on how to create culturally adapted suicide safety plans (i.e. suicide safety plans designed to meet the unique needs of those with minoritized identities), and no research has suggested clear adaptations to address the specific concerns of suicidal TNB clients.

The Cultural Theory and Model of Suicide (Chu et al., 2010) is the most prominent work on cultural adaptations of suicide safety planning to LGBTQ+ clients, as it is one of the first efforts to describe the integration of multiple cultural factors into an understanding of suicidality for LGBTQ+ people. The authors emphasize the need to understand the specific drivers of suicidality as they relate to gender, sexual orientation, race, and other aspects of identity. For example, they discuss the role of shame that may be a particular driver for some sexual and gender minority people in Black or Asian American families.

The Cultural Assessment for Risk of Suicide (CARS; Chu et al., 2013) was developed based on the Chu et al. (2010) model and is recommended as an approach to capture multiple forms of minority stress as they relate to suicide. However, be aware that questions relevant to TNB clients fall under the subheading "sexual minority stress." Alerting clients to this may be important. Chu and colleagues (2017) applied the CARS and suicidality model to a case example with an Asian American TNB veteran. This approach may be useful to review for an example of one application of a culturally adapted suicide prevention treatment for a TNB client. Similarly, Kauten et al. (2023) illustrate an approach to suicide safety planning with a TNB veteran by addressing minority stress factors. Both articles emphasize the need to determine the specific drivers for client suicidality, with a focus on how factors related to identity may be involved. However, neither approach fully outlines the specific needs that TNB clients may have related to suicidality.

Given that research suggests the importance of minority stress in driving suicidality and preventing disclosure of suicidality, any suicide crisis plan for TNB people must include mechanisms to rapidly reduce specific factors related to minority stress that may be driving suicidality for a TNB client, as well as increase resiliency to minority stress. Social support may be one of the most important protective factors against suicidality for TNB people who have experienced victimization and discrimination (Bariola et al., 2015; Bauer et al., 2015; dickey & Budge, 2020; Tebbe & Moradi, 2016; Testa et al., 2014; Trujillo et al., 2017). Therefore, an important treatment for TNB clients experiencing suicidality is to increase connection with other TNB individuals and supportive allies (dickey & Budge, 2020; Edwards et al., 2020). In times of acute suicidal crisis, connection with people who affirm the gender of the person in crisis is a central element in the suicide prevention plan (Kauten et al., 2023).

The Trans and Nonbinary Adapted Suicide Safety Plan

Considering the research on suicide safety planning with LGBTQ+ clients, we present an approach to suicide safety planning with TNB clients that focuses on the reduction of minority stress and increased connection with TNB community and allies. This approach has been applied to each step of Stanley and Brown's (2012) suicide safety plan.

In the first step, *recognizing signs and triggers*, a screener such as the CARS may be useful in identifying which factors could be triggering suicidal thinking and developing a case conceptualization of the drivers leading to the suicidal crisis (Jobes et al., 2018; Kauten et al., 2023). As discussed earlier, internalized stigma (Perez-Brumer et al., 2015; Testa et al., 2017), thwarted belongingness (including rejection and social isolation; Bauer et al., 2015; Chu et al., 2017; Testa et al., 2017), and expectations of rejection (Testa et al., 2017) are major drivers for suicidality in TNB people and may be helpful to examine with the client. Through the use of the CARS and careful inquiry about the thoughts, feelings, and events that led up to suicidal thinking or behavior, guided by the GMSM and IPTS models of suicide, MHPs can identify specific drivers and triggers for crisis. Identification of these can also contribute to treatment targets.

The second step, *distracting*, may be adapted for TNB clients by adding affirming aspects to distraction; this could include watching gender-affirming movies or doing affirming activities such as applying makeup or working out. This step may also be used to help boost social connection by distracting with affirming friends, attending an affirming event, going to a local LGBTQ+ center, or participating in online groups with other TNB people. It is important to discuss any activities with clients to ensure that gender dysphoria is not triggered.

The third step, *contacting helpful others*, can be crucial to connect clients to helpful others who are prepared to support the client who is feeling suicidal. However, adapting for TNB clients also means helping the client connect with community that shares the client's identity or identities, and with those who are especially able to help reduce minority stress for the client. For clients with multiple marginalized identities, this may mean prioritizing relationships with people who share some of their most salient identities, when possible. Collaboration with the client is key, as the most supportive friends and family in a crisis may share few identities. Thus, it is important to choose the support list carefully to ensure they can be affirming and are prepared to help the TNB client solve issues involving suicidality triggers. When internalized TNB stigma is a major driver, for example, those on the contact list may be given a list of ways to affirm the client. If the driver is rejection or isolation, those on the list might be selected for their ability to be in contact via phone, video, or in person to ensure a sense of connection and to help the client rebuild a sense of hope for belongingness.

The fourth step, *getting professional help*, should be planned with attention to addressing fears and concerns that clients may have about encountering harmful or nonaffirming professionals. In this step, minority stress may play a role in hindering the client's willingness to escalate their request for help due to fears of harmful encounters. Several crisis lines, such as Trans Lifeline (https://translifeline.org/), have recently been formed specifically for TNB callers. Trans Lifeline's website also offers links to other forms of community support. Given the history of violent and nonaffirming experiences with law enforcement for many TNB people, and especially TNB POCs, planning to avoid police involvement may be a key part of engagement with safety planning, which will be addressed in the following section.

Lastly, *reducing lethal means* is a standard practice in suicide prevention. As with any client, determining a TNB client's plan is essential in suicide prevention. Blosnich et al. (2021) found that TNB veterans were more likely to use firearms or self-poisoning than cisgender veterans in completed suicides. In a national sample, however, TNB people were more likely to have used hanging or poisoning than their cisgender counterparts (Patten et al., 2022). As with all clients, it is important to inquire carefully about the means and availability of those methods. However, with TNB clients, it is important to set aside assumptions about the stereotypes regarding gender and means. That is, while it is commonly assumed that men are more likely to use a gun, the MHP should inquire widely about means for all gendered presentations.

MAXIMIZING DISCLOSURE OF SUICIDALITY WITH THE TRANS AND NONBINARY CLIENT

In addition to a culturally adapted safety plan, we also recommend an approach that maximizes the likelihood that the TNB client will disclose suicidality and be willing to make use of the plan. Two important principles that may ease reluctance of TNB people to engage with suicide safety plans are those of collaboration and transparency. These principles may be helpful to encourage clients to share their concerns about a safety plan and provide affirmation that the MHP will address concerns that may arise if intervention must be escalated in a suicidal crisis.

Collaboration ensures that the client is afforded autonomy in the development of any plan and may be particularly important with TNB clients who have reasons to hold concerns about nonaffirmation, discrimination, and victimization when encountering crisis and inpatient services. An excellent approach with a focus on collaboration and transparency was developed by Jobes (2016) and Jobes et al. (2018): *The Collaborative Assessment and Management of Suicidality*. Although it was not designed specifically for TNB clients, this approach fully involves the client in the planning and allows TNB clients to make key decisions for themselves. The power to make important decisions about one's medical care is often removed for TNB people who have been subject to paternalistic gatekeeping or nonaffirming care from medical systems (Shuster, 2019). Thus, highly collaborative and transparent care is a key recommendation in a 2021 scoping review of literature regarding ethical and culturally competent TNB medical care (Sundus et al., 2021).

Similarly, transparency helps ensure that TNB clients are aware of the possibilities and limitations of the MHP within the plan, further allowing TNB clients to make choices that help them avoid nonaffirming care and increase coping and resiliency in the case where avoiding such care is not possible. For example, the MHP might inform the client what scenarios may trigger a call to mobile crisis services so that the client is aware of how to avoid this escalation. They may also plan together for how a client can respond in the face of a less affirming MHP. In an example of transparency of limitations, the client should be made aware that the MHP may be able to suggest inpatient facilities that are known to be more TNB friendly, but cannot be guaranteed that the client will go to one of those facilities. This way, the MHP and client can plan together for when the client is unable to make choices or is forced to encounter less than optimal care.

"CONCERN POINTS" IN WORKING WITH TRANS AND NONBINARY CLIENTS EXPERIENCING SUICIDAL THOUGHTS AND BEHAVIORS

Using the approach of collaboration and transparency with TNB clients experiencing STB, we suggest MHPs identify and address what we term *concern points*. These are the feared scenarios that interfere with the client's ability to disclose suicidality or follow the plan, especially for those with a high risk of needing crisis stabilization or hospitalization. For example, clients who are fearful of returning to a nonaffirming inpatient placement may be reluctant to contact an MHP when suicidal ideation is increasing. In these cases, addressing these areas before a rise in suicidal ideation may be important. Based on surveys of negative experiences reported by TNB clients, concern points to be aware of include: encountering non-affirming MHPs in crisis systems; encountering police or law enforcement; being outed to MHPs, peers, or family; victimization by staff or peers in crisis treatment; being denied future gender-affirming medical procedures based on their mental health; and not being given a choice about housing when housing is assigned by gender (James et al., 2015; Mizock & Fleming, 2011; Mizock & Lundquist, 2016; Rosentel et al., 2021; Shipherd et al., 2010; Smith et al., 2019).

Special concern should be noted related to police involvement in suicide crises. A 2014 report of the Williams Institute showed that 61% of TNB people who have attempted suicide in their life reported being harassed by the police and 57% reported that police treated them with disrespect (Herman et al., 2014). TNB clients of color are more likely to have experienced police violence and harassment, as well as increased negative experiences when attempting to engage in mental health services (Nemoto et al., 2005; Rosentel et al., 2021; Sutter & Perrin, 2016). As a result, concerns about engaging police must be discussed and alternative plans made if possible.

Advocacy

Once concern points are identified, MHPs can take steps to advocate for clients or help them advocate for themselves. Some areas that should be considered for all TNB people include identifying key affirming resources before they are needed. For example, the MHP and client can investigate and choose crisis hotlines that are LGBTQ+ friendly or, if not TNB-affirming, do not involve the police. Trans Lifeline offers resources about community crisis care (https://translifeline.org/resource/community-based-crisis-support/hotlines-that-avoid-police/). Many urban areas in the United States offer crisis intervention MHPs who are available to respond on site to an individual having a crisis. These mobile crisis units allow clients to avoid involvement with law enforcement and can help client's avoid trips to the local emergency department. By identifying these local services, clients who need immediate assessment can make use of these services rather than calling the police or emergency services.

In addition, MHPs can advocate on behalf of clients by speaking to local mobile crisis units to ensure they are aware of the needs of TNB clients and can advocate for training. Choosing hospitals and crisis units carefully can reassure clients about possible outcomes of disclosing suicidality. Calling potential placement sites to learn about policies regarding gendered housing, gender-affirming medications and belongings, and staff training on names and pronoun use with TNB clients can help allay fears about inpatient experiences.

Planning for Resiliency and Concern Points

MHPs can also help clients build resiliency and plan for unwanted experiences if they cannot be avoided. Together, MHPs and clients can decide the best strategies for responding to misgendering on the part of peers on an inpatient unit or ensuring that emergency contacts do not include family members to whom they are not "out." Clients can plan with the MHP to have prescriptions for gender-affirming hormones on hand should they need to present them in an inpatient or hospital setting. It may also be beneficial to reassure clients regarding their choices. For example, clients that choose to conceal their TNB identity as part of engaging in emergency services may worry that MHPs will then see the identity as unimportant; TNB clients may also fear that disclosing suicidality could delay gaining access to hormone treatment. MHP validation and reassurance can help clients release fears that they will be seen as less authentic in their identity as a result of their choices while in crisis (Friley & Venetis, 2022).

Other forms of preparation involving the principle of transparency can also help address concerns. Clients should know how to avoid escalation of a crisis response to an unwanted outcome. For example, voluntarily contacting MHPs before a suicidal crisis escalates may help prevent further action from being taken, whereas missing appointments or refusing to engage with services may result in a call to mobile crisis services. Additionally, MHPs can acknowledge and educate the client about the possibility of negative encounters. Honesty about the possibility of experiencing misgendering or negative experiences from peers while in an inpatient setting may open opportunities to prepare for such events and to reassure the client that MHPs have no illusions about the experiences of mental health care for TNB people in crisis.

After the Suicidal Crisis

Lastly, taking time after a suicidal crisis to review the safety plan and the experiences of the TNB client may both help refine the plan and provide an opportunity to process and address minority stress experiences that arose. Negative experiences of lack of gender affirmation, discrimination, victimization, misgendering, or negative interactions with peers can be discussed through the approach of TNB-affirming treatment to help the client address negative thoughts and feelings that arose, as well as shore up resiliency factors. For example, helping clients identify thoughts of shame and internalized stigma related to the negative events or reframing the negative events as ignorance and cultural stigma rather than due to the client's identity may help clients prevent further distress related to these experiences. Clients may also benefit from increased contact with affirming others who can reassure the client that their negative experiences are not due to the client's identity. In this way, the likelihood of client disclosure during future suicidal crises may be increased during a suicidal crisis.

Despite the higher rates of suicide among TNB adults, few approaches to addressing suicidal crises with these communities have been investigated. Considering the negative experiences many TNB people have had with MHPs, hospital systems, law enforcement systems, and medical systems, combined with internalized stigma related to identity, it stands to reason that willingness to disclose suicidality and engage with a suicide plan is diminished for TNB people. However, with TNB-affirming psychotherapy to reduce internalized stigma, combined with a collaborative and transparent approach to planning for suicide crisis and increasing resilience factors, many clients may find themselves more willing to disclose and engage.

SUMMARY

In summary, TNB communities have higher rates of suicide attempts, as well as rates of nonsuicidal self-injury. Research regarding TNB suicide point strongly to the impact of minority stress, loss of belongingness, and perceived burdensomeness as possible factors in these higher rates. Despite these documented higher rates of suicidality and distress, there is very little research on crisis intervention for TNB people who are experiencing suicidal risk. Unfortunately, when TNB people seek help for suicidality, they are highly likely to experience minority stressors, which can further contribute to heightened suicidal risk. As a result, TNB people may be less likely to disclose suicidality. We described a culturally adapted approach to suicide crisis intervention with TNB clients. This approach emphasizes a collaborative, transparent approach that enhances client autonomy. Key aspects include reducing minority stress, increasing social connections and resiliency, identifying obstacles to making use of a safety plan, and addressing those obstacles in ways that address minority stress–related fears and concerns.

REFERENCES

Aldridge, Z., Patel, S., Guo, B., Nixon, E., Pierre Bouman, W., Witcomb, G. L., & Arcelus, J. (2021). Long-term effect of gender-affirming hormone treatment on depression and anxiety symptoms in transgender people: A prospective cohort study. *Andrology, 9*(6), 1808–1816. https://doi.org/10.1111/andr.12884

Allen, L. R., Watson, L. B., Egan, A. M., & Moser, C. N. (2019). Well-being and suicidality among transgender youth after gender-affirming hormones. *Clinical Practice in Pediatric Psychology, 7*(3), 302–311. https://doi.org/10.1037/cpp0000288

Austin, A., & Craig, S. L. (2015). Transgender affirmative cognitive behavioral therapy: Clinical considerations and applications. *Professional Psychology: Research and Practice, 46*(1), 21–29. https://doi.org/10.1037/a0038642

Austin, A., Craig, S. L., D'Souza, S., & McInroy, L. B. (2020). Suicidality among transgender youth: Elucidating the role of interpersonal risk factors. *Journal of Interpersonal Violence, 37*(5–6), NP2696–NP2718. https://doi.org/10.1177/0886260520915554

Baguso, G. N., Aguilar, K., Sicro, S., Mañacop, M., Quintana, J., & Wilson, E. C. (2022). "Lost trust in the system": System barriers to publicly available mental health and substance use services for transgender women in San Francisco. *BMC Health Services Research, 22*(1), 930. https://doi.org/10.1186/s12913-022-08315-5

Bariola, E., Lyons, A., Leonard, W., Pitts, M., Badcock, P., & Couch, M. (2015). Demographic and psychosocial factors associated with psychological distress and resilience among transgender individuals. *American Journal of Public Health, 105*(10), 2108–2116. https://doi.org/10.2105/AJPH.2015.302763

Barr, S. M., Snyder, K. E., Adelson, J. L., & Budge, S. L. (2022). Posttraumatic stress in the trans community: The roles of anti-transgender bias, non-affirmation, and internalized transphobia. *Psychology of Sexual Orientation and Gender Diversity, 9*(4), 410–421. https://doi.org/10.1037/sgd0000500

Bauer, G. R., Scheim, A. I., Pyne, J., Travers, R., & Hammond, R. (2015). Intervenable factors associated with suicide risk in transgender persons: A respondent driven sampling study in Ontario, Canada. *BMC Public Health, 15*(1), 525. https://doi.org/10.1186/s12889-015-1867-2

Becerra-Culqui, T. A., Liu, Y., Nash, R., Cromwell, L., Flanders, W. D., Getahun, D., Giammattei, S. V., Hunkeler, E. M., Lash, T. L., Millman, A., Quinn, V. P., Robinson, B., Roblin, D., Sandberg, D. E., Silverberg, M. J., Tangpricha, V., & Goodman, M. (2018). Mental health of transgender and gender nonconforming youth compared with their peers. *Pediatrics, 141*(5), e20173845. https://doi.org/10.1542/peds.2017-3845

Blosnich, J. R., Boyer, T. L., Brown, G. R., Kauth, M. R., & Shipherd, J. C. (2021). Differences in methods of suicide death among transgender and nontransgender patients in the Veterans Health Administration, 1999–2016. *Medical Care, 59*, S31–S35. https://doi.org/10.1097/MLR.0000000000001384

Boyer, T. L., Youk, A. O., Haas, A. P., Brown, G. R., Shipherd, J. C., Kauth, M. R., Jasuja, G. K., & Blosnich, J. R. (2021). Suicide, homicide, and all-cause mortality among transgender and cisgender patients in the Veterans Health Administration. *LGBT Health, 8*(3), 173–180. https://doi.org/10.1089/lgbt.2020.0235

Calear, A. L., & Batterham, P. J. (2019). Suicidal ideation disclosure: Patterns, correlates and outcome. *Psychiatry Research, 278*, 1–6. https://doi.org/10.1016/j.psychres.2019.05.024

Carmichael, P., Butler, G., Masic, U., Cole, T. J., De Stavola, B. L., Davidson, S., Skageberg, E. M., Khadr, S., & Viner, R. M. (2021). Short-term outcomes of pubertal suppression in a selected cohort of 12 to 15 year old young people with persistent gender dysphoria in the UK. *PLOS One, 16*(2), e0243894. https://doi.org/10.1101/2020.12.01.20241653

Chang, C. J., Kellerman, J., Feinstein, B. A., Selby, E. A., & Goldbach, J. T. (2022). Greater minority stress is associated with lower intentions to disclose suicidal thoughts among LGBTQ+ youth. *Archives of Suicide Research, 26*(2), 626–640. https://doi.org/10.1080/13811118.2020.1818656

Chen, D., Berona, J., Chan, Y.-M., Ehrensaft, D., Garofalo, R., Hidalgo, M. A., Rosenthal, S. M., Tishelman, A. C., & Olson-Kennedy, J. (2023). Psychosocial functioning in transgender youth after 2 years of hormones. *The New England Journal of Medicine, 388*(3), 240–250. https://doi.org/10.1056/NEJMoa2206297

Chu, J., Floyd, R., Diep, H., Pardo, S., Goldblum, P., & Bongar, B. (2013). A tool for the culturally competent assessment of suicide: The Cultural Assessment of Risk for Suicide (CARS) measure. *Psychological Assessment, 25*(2), 424–434. https://doi.org/10.1037/a0031264

Chu, J., Goldblum, P., Floyd, R., & Bongar, B. (2010). The cultural theory and model of suicide. *Applied & Preventive Psychology, 14*(1–4), 25–40. https://doi.org/10.1016/j.appsy.2011.11.001

Chu, J., Hoeflein, B. T. R., Goldblum, P., Bongar, B., Heyne, G. M., Gadinsky, N., & Skinta, M. D. (2017). Innovations in the practice of culturally competent suicide risk management. *Practice Innovations, 2*(2), 66–79. https://doi.org/10.1037/pri0000044

Coleman, E., Radix, A. E., Bouman, W. P., Brown, G. R., de Vries, A. L. C., Deutsch, M. B., Ettner, R., Fraser, L., Goodman, M., Green, J., Hancock, A. B., Johnson, T. W., Karasic, D. H., Knudson, G. A., Leibowitz, S. F., Meyer-Bahlburg, H. F. L., Monstrey, S. J., Motmans, J., Nahata, L., . . . Arcelus, J. (2022). Standards of care for the health of transgender and gender diverse people, version 8. *International Journal of Transgender Health, 23*(Suppl. 1), S1–S259. https://doi.org/10.1080/26895269.2022.2100644

de Vries, J. M. A., Downes, C., Sharek, D., Doyle, L., Murphy, R., Begley, T., McCann, E., Sheerin, F., Smyth, S., & Higgins, A. (2022). An exploration of mental distress in transgender people in Ireland with reference to minority stress and dissonance theory. *International Journal of Transgender Health, 24*(4), 469–486. https://doi.org/10.1080/26895269.2022.2105772

de Vries, K. M., & Sojka, C. J. (2020). Transitioning gender, transitioning race: Transgender people and multiracial positionality. *International Journal of Transgender Health, 23*(1–2), 97–107. https://doi.org/10.1080/26895269.2020.1838388

Dewey, J. M., & Gesbeck, M. M. (2015). (Dys) functional diagnosing: Mental health diagnosis, medicalization, and the making of transgender patients. *Humanity & Society, 41*(1), 37–72. https://doi.org/10.1177/0160597615604651

Dhanani, L. Y., & Totton, R. R. (2023). Have you heard the news? The effects of exposure to news about recent transgender legislation on transgender youth and young adults. *Sexuality Research & Social Policy, 20*(4), 1345–1359. https://doi.org/10.1007/s13178-023-00810-6

dickey, l. m., & Budge, S. L. (2020). Suicide and the transgender experience: A public health crisis. *American Psychologist, 75*(3), 380–390. https://doi.org/10.1037/amp0000619

Du Bois, S. N., Yoder, W., Guy, A. A., Manser, K., & Ramos, S. (2018). Examining associations between state-level transgender policies and transgender health. *Transgender Health, 3*(1), 220–224. https://doi.org/10.1089/trgh.2018.0031

Edwards, L. L., Torres Bernal, A., Hanley, S. M., & Martin, S. (2020). Resilience factors and suicide risk for a sample of transgender clients. *Family Process, 59*(3), 1209–1224. https://doi.org/10.1111/famp.12479

Friley, L. B., & Venetis, M. K. (2022). Decision-making criteria when contemplating disclosure of transgender identity to medical providers. *Health Communication, 37*(8), 1031–1040. https://doi.org/10.1080/10410236.2021.1885774

Fulginiti, A., Pahwa, R., Frey, L. M., Rice, E., & Brekke, J. S. (2016). What factors influence the decision to share suicidal thoughts? A multilevel social network analysis of disclosure among individuals with serious mental illness. *Suicide & Life-Threatening Behavior, 46*(4), 398–412. https://doi.org/10.1111/sltb.12224

Goldbach, J. T., Rhoades, H., Green, D., Fulginiti, A., & Marshal, M. P. (2019). Is there a need for LGBT-specific suicide crisis services? *Crisis, 40*(3), 203–208. https://doi.org/10.1027/0227-5910/a000542

Goodman, M., Adams, N., Corneil, T., Kreukels, B., Motmans, J., & Coleman, E. (2019). Size and distribution of transgender and gender nonconforming populations: A narrative review. *Endocrinology and Metabolism Clinics of North America, 48*(2), 303–321. https://doi.org/10.1016/j.ecl.2019.01.001

Gould, M. S., Chowdhury, S., Lake, A. M., Galfalvy, H., Kleinman, M., Kuchuk, M., & McKeon, R. (2021). National Suicide Prevention Lifeline crisis chat interventions: Evaluation of chatters' perceptions of effectiveness. *Suicide and Life-Threatening Behavior, 51*(6), 1126–1137. https://doi.org/10.1111/sltb.12795

Grant, J. M., Mottet, L., Tanis, J., Herman, J. L., Harrison, J., & Keisling, M. (2010). *National transgender discrimination survey report on health and health care.* National Center for Transgender Equality and the National Gay and Lesbian Task Force. https://cancer-network.org/wp-content/uploads/2017/02/National_Transgender_Discrimination_Survey_Report_on_health_and_health_care.pdf

Grossman, A. H., Park, J. Y., & Russell, S. T. (2016). Transgender youth and suicidal behaviors: Applying the interpersonal psychological theory of suicide. *Journal of Gay & Lesbian Mental Health, 20*(4), 329–349. https://doi.org/10.1080/19359705.2016.1207581

Haas, A. P., Eliason, M., Mays, V. M., Mathy, R. M., Cochran, S. D., D'Augelli, A. R., Silverman, M. M., Fisher, P. W., Hughes, T., Rosario, M., Russell, S. T., Malley, E., Reed, R., Litts, D. A., Haller, E., Sell, R. L., Remafedi, G., Bradford, J., Beautrais, A., L., . . . Clayton, P. J. (2010). Suicide and suicide risk in lesbian, gay, bisexual, and transgender populations: Review and recommendations. *Journal of Homosexuality, 58*(1), 10–51. https://doi.org/10.1080/00918369.2011.534038

Han, J., Batterham, P. J., Calear, A. L., & Randall, R. (2018). Factors influencing professional help-seeking for suicidality: A systematic review. *Crisis, 39*(3), 175–196. https://doi.org/10.1027/0227-5910/a000485

Hendricks, M. L., & Testa, R. J. (2012). A conceptual framework for clinical work with transgender and gender nonconforming clients: An adaptation of the minority stress model. *Professional Psychology: Research and Practice, 43*(5), 460–467. https://doi.org/10.1037/a0029597

Herman, J. L., Haas, A. P., & Rodgers, P. L. (2014). *Suicide attempts among transgender and gender non-conforming adults.* UCLA: The Williams Institute. https://escholarship.org/uc/item/8xg8061f

Hughes, L. D., Kidd, K. M., Gamarel, K. E., Operario, D., & Dowshen, N. (2021). "These laws will be devastating": Provider perspectives on legislation banning gender-affirming care for transgender adolescents. *The Journal of Adolescent Health, 69*(6), 976–982. https://doi.org/10.1016/j.jadohealth.2021.08.020

Hunt, Q. A., Morrow, Q. J., & McGuire, J. K. (2020). Experiences of suicide in transgender youth: A qualitative, community-based study. *Archives of Suicide Research, 24*(Suppl. 2), S340–S355. https://doi.org/10.1080/13811118.2019.1610677

Inch, E. (2016). Changing minds: The psycho-pathologization of trans people. *International Journal of Mental Health, 45*(3), 193–204. https://doi.org/10.1080/00207411.2016.1204822

James, S. E., Brown, C., & Wilson, I. (2015). *2015 US transgender survey: Report on the experiences of Black respondents*. National Center for Transgender Equality. https://transequality.org/sites/default/files/docs/usts/USTSBlackRespondentsReport-Nov17.pdf

James, S. E., Herman, J. L., Rankin, S., Keisling, M., Mottet, L., & Anafi, M. (2016). *The report of the 2015 U.S. transgender survey*. National Center for Transgender Equality. https://transequality.org/sites/default/files/docs/usts/USTS-Full-Report-Dec17.pdf

Jarrett, B. A., Peitzmeier, S. M., Restar, A., Adamson, T., Howell, S., Baral, S., & Beckham, S. W. (2021). Gender-affirming care, mental health, and economic stability in the time of COVID-19: A multi-national, cross-sectional study of transgender and nonbinary people. *PLOS One, 16*(7), e0254215. https://doi.org/10.1371/journal.pone.0254215

Jobes, D. A. (2016). *Managing suicidal risk: A collaborative approach* (2nd ed.). Guilford Press.

Jobes, D. A., Gregorian, M. J., & Colborn, V. A. (2018). A stepped care approach to clinical suicide prevention. *Psychological Services, 15*(3), 243–250. https://doi.org/10.1037/ser0000229

Kauten, R. L., Carter, S. P., Stivers, M., Novak, L. A., Baer, M. M., LaCroix, J. M., Grant, N. E., Sickmann, B., Goldston, D. B., Soumoff, A., & Ghahramanlou-Holloway, M. (2023). Post-admission cognitive therapy for a transgender service member with a recent suicidal crisis: A case study of gender-affirming care. *Cognitive and Behavioral Practice, 30*(2), 273–286. https://doi.org/10.1016/j.cbpra.2021.10.007

Kota, K. K., Luo, Q., Beer, L., Dasgupta, S., & McCree, D. H. (2023). Stigma, discrimination, and mental health outcomes among transgender women with diagnosed HIV infection in the United States, 2015-2018. *Public Health Reports, 138*(5), 771–781. https://doi.org/10.1177/00333549221123583

Kota, K. K., Salazar, L. F., Culbreth, R. E., Crosby, R. A., & Jones, J. (2020). Psychosocial mediators of perceived stigma and suicidal ideation among transgender women. *BMC Public Health, 20*(1), 125. Advance online publication. https://doi.org/10.1186/s12889-020-8177-z

Kung, K. T. F. (2024). Autistic traits, gender minority stress, and mental health in transgender and non-binary adults. *Journal of Autism and Developmental Disorders, 54*(4), 1389–1397. https://doi.org/10.1007/s10803-022-05875-7

Larsen, M. E., Torok, M., Huckvale, K., Reda, B., Berrouiguet, S., & Christensen, H. (2019). Geospatial suicide clusters and emergency responses: An analysis of text messages to a crisis service. *2019 41st Annual International Conference of the IEEE

Engineering in Medicine and Biology Society (EMBC), 6109–6112. https://doi.org/10.1109/EMBC.2019.8856909

Lee, W. Y., Hobbs, J. N., Hobaica, S., DeChants, J. P., Price, M. N., & Nath, R. (2024). State-level anti-transgender laws increase past-year suicide attempts among transgender and non-binary young people in the USA. *Nature Human Behaviour, 8*(11), 2096–2106. https://doi.org/10.1038/s41562-024-01979-5

Lett, E., Abrams, M. P., Gold, A., Fullerton, F.-A., & Everhart, A. (2022). Ethnoracial inequities in access to gender-affirming mental health care and psychological distress among transgender adults. *Social Psychiatry and Psychiatric Epidemiology, 57*(5), 963–971. https://doi.org/10.1007/s00127-022-02246-6

Luoma, J. B., Martin, C. E., & Pearson, J. L. (2002). Contact with mental health and primary care providers before suicide: A review of the evidence. *The American Journal of Psychiatry, 159*(6), 909–916. https://doi.org/10.1176/appi.ajp.159.6.909

MacKinnon, K. R. (2018). Pathologising trans people: Exploring the roles of patients and medical personnel. *Theory in Action, 11*(4), 74–96. https://doi.org/10.3798/tia.1937-0237.1826

Matsuno, E. (2019). Nonbinary-affirming psychological interventions. *Cognitive and Behavioral Practice, 26*(4), 617-628. https://doi.org/10.1016/j.cbpra.2018.09.003

McNeil, J., Ellis, S. J., & Eccles, F. J. R. (2017). Suicide in trans populations: A systematic review of prevalence and correlates. *Psychology of Sexual Orientation and Gender Diversity, 4*(3), 341–353. https://doi.org/10.1037/sgd0000235

Mérelle, S., Foppen, E., Gilissen, R., Mokkenstorm, J., Cluitmans, R., & Van Ballegooijen, W. (2018). Characteristics associated with non-disclosure of suicidal ideation in adults. *International Journal of Environmental Research and Public Health, 15*(5), 943. https://doi.org/10.3390/ijerph15050943

Meyer, I. H. (1995). Minority stress and mental health in gay men. *Journal of Health and Social Behavior, 36*(1), 38–56. https://doi.org/10.2307/2137286

Meyer, I. H., Teylan, M., & Schwartz, S. (2015). The role of help-seeking in preventing suicide attempts among lesbians, gay men, and bisexuals. *Suicide and Life-Threatening Behavior, 45*(1), 25–36. https://doi.org/10.1111/sltb.12104

Millar, K., & Brooks, C. V. (2021). Double jeopardy: Minority stress and the influence of transgender identity and race/ethnicity. *International Journal of Transgender Health, 23*(1-2), 133–148. https://doi.org/10.1080/26895269.2021.1890660

Mizock, L., & Fleming, M. Z. (2011). Transgender and gender variant populations with mental illness: Implications for clinical care. *Professional Psychology: Research and Practice, 42*(2), 208–213. https://doi.org/10.1037/a0022522

Mizock, L., & Lundquist, C. (2016). Missteps in psychotherapy with transgender clients: Promoting gender sensitivity in counseling and psychological practice. *Psychology of Sexual Orientation and Gender Diversity, 3*(2), 148–155. https://doi.org/10.1037/sgd0000177

Moody, C., Fuks, N., Peláez, S., & Smith, N. G. (2015). "Without this, I would for sure already be dead": A qualitative inquiry regarding suicide protective factors among trans adults. *Psychology of Sexual Orientation and Gender Diversity, 2*(3), 266–280. https://doi.org/10.1037/sgd0000130

Moody, C., & Smith, N. G. (2013). Suicide protective factors among trans adults. *Archives of Sexual Behavior, 42*(5), 739–752. https://doi.org/10.1007/s10508-013-0099-8

Nemoto, T., Operario, D., & Keatley, J. (2005). Health and social services for male-to-female transgender persons of color in San Francisco. *International Journal of Transgenderism, 8*(2–3), 5–19. https://doi.org/10.1300/J485v08n02_02

Nuij, C., van Ballegooijen, W., de Beurs, D., Juniar, D., Erlangsen, A., Portzky, G., O'Connor, R. C., Smit, J. H., Kerkhof, A., & Riper, H. (2021). Safety planning-type interventions for suicide prevention: Meta-analysis. *The British Journal of Psychiatry, 219*(2), 419–426. https://doi.org/10.1192/bjp.2021.50

Olson, K. R., Durwood, L., DeMeules, M., & McLaughlin, K. A. (2016). Mental health of transgender children who are supported in their identities. *Pediatrics, 137*(3), e20153223. https://doi.org/10.1542/peds.2015-3223

Park, I. Y., Speer, R., Whitfield, D. L., Kattari, L., Walls, E. N., & Christensen, C. (2022). Predictors of bullying, depression, and suicide attempts among youth: The intersection of race/ethnicity by gender identity. *Children and Youth Services Review, 139*, 106536. https://doi.org/10.1016/j.childyouth.2022.106536

Parker-Barnes, L., McKillip, N., & Powell, C. (2022). Systemic advocacy for BIPOC LGBTQIA + clients and their families. *The Family Journal, 30*(3), 479–486. https://doi.org/10.1177/10664807221090947

Parra, L. A., & Hastings, P. D. (2018). Integrating the neurobiology of minority stress with an intersectionality framework for LGBTQ-Latinx populations. *New Directions for Child and Adolescent Development, 2018*(161), 91–108. https://doi.org/10.1002/cad.20244

Patten, M., Carmichael, H., Moore, A., & Velopulos, C. (2022). Circumstances of suicide among lesbian, gay, bisexual and transgender individuals. *The Journal of Surgical Research, 270*, 522–529. https://doi.org/10.1016/j.jss.2021.08.029

Pellicane, M. J., & Ciesla, J. A. (2022). Associations between minority stress, depression, and suicidal ideation and attempts in transgender and gender diverse (TGD) individuals: Systematic review and meta-analysis. *Clinical Psychology Review, 91*, 102113. https://doi.org/10.1016/j.cpr.2021.102113

Perez-Brumer, A., Hatzenbuehler, M. L., Oldenburg, C. E., & Bockting, W. (2015). Individual- and structural-level risk factors for suicide attempts among transgender adults. *Behavioral Medicine, 41*(3), 164–171. Advance online publication. https://doi.org/10.1080/08964289.2015.1028322

Pharr, J. R., Chien, L. C., Gakh, M., Flatt, J., Kittle, K., & Terry, E. (2022). Serial mediation analysis of the association of familiarity with transgender sports bans and suicidality among sexual and gender minority adults in the United States. *International Journal of Environmental Research and Public Health, 19*(17), 10641. https://doi.org/10.3390/ijerph191710641

Pisani, A. R., Murrie, D. C., Silverman, M., Turner, K. (2022). Prevention-oriented risk formulation. In M. Pompili (Ed.), *Suicide risk assessment and prevention* (pp. 120–138). https://safesideprevention.com/media/documents/External/Pisani-et-al-2022-risk-formulation-chapter-PROOF.pdf

Price, M. A., Hollinsaid, N. L., McKetta, S., Mellen, E. J., & Rakhilin, M. (2024). Structural transphobia is associated with psychological distress and suicidality in a large national sample of transgender adults. *Social Psychiatry and Psychiatric Epidemiology, 59*(2), 285–294. https://doi.org/10.1007/s00127-023-02482-4

Price-Feeney, M., Green, A. E., & Dorison, S. H. (2021). Suicidality among youth who are questioning, unsure of, or exploring their sexual identity. *Journal of Sex Research, 58*(5), 581–588. https://doi.org/10.1080/00224499.2020.1832184

Puckett, J. A., Huit, T. Z., Hope, D. A., Mocarski, R., Lash, B. R., Walker, T., Holt, N., Ralston, A., Miles, M., Capannola, A., Tipton, C., Juster, R.-P., & DuBois, L. Z. (2024). Transgender and gender-diverse people's experiences of minority stress, mental health, and resilience in relation to perceptions of sociopolitical contexts. *Transgender Health*, *9*(1), 14–23. https://doi.org/10.1089/trgh.2022.0047

Rabasco, A., & Andover, M. (2023). The relationship between religious practices and beliefs and suicidal thoughts and behaviors among transgender and gender diverse adults. *Psychology of Religion and Spirituality*, *15*(1), 25–31. https://doi.org/10.1037/rel0000453

Rafferty, J., AAP Committee on Psychosocial Aspects of Child and Family Health, AAP Committee on Adolescence, & AAP Section on Lesbian, Gay, Bisexual, and Transgender Health and Wellness. (2018). Ensuring comprehensive care and support for transgender and gender-diverse children and adolescents. *Pediatrics*, *142*(4), e20182162. https://doi.org/10.1542/peds.2018-2162

Redfield, E., Conron, K. J., & Mallory, C. (2024). *The impact of 2024 anti-transgender legislation on youth.* Williams Institute. https://williamsinstitute.law.ucla.edu/publications/2024-anti-trans-legislation/

Reisner, S. L., Poteat, T., Keatley, J., Cabral, M., Mothopeng, T., Dunham, E., Holland, C. E., Max, R., & Baral, S. D. (2016). Global health burden and needs of transgender populations: A review. *Lancet*, *388*(10042), 412–436. https://doi.org/10.1016/S0140-6736(16)00684-X

Reisner, S. L., Vetters, R., Leclerc, M., Zaslow, S., Wolfrum, S., Shumer, D., & Mimiaga, M. J. (2015). Mental health of transgender youth in care at an adolescent urban community health center: A matched retrospective cohort study. *Journal of Adolescent Health*, *56*(3), 274–279. https://doi.org/10.1016/j.jadohealth.2014.10.264

Restar, A., Layland, E. K., Hughes, L., Dusic, E., Lucas, R., Bambilla, A. J. K., Martin, A., Shook, A., Karrington, B., Schwarz, D., Shimkin, G., Grandberry, V., Xanadu, X., Streed, C. G., Jr., Operario, D., Gamarel, K. E., & Kershaw, T. (2024). Antitrans policy environment and depression and anxiety symptoms in transgender and nonbinary adults. *JAMA Network Open*, *7*(8), e2431306. Advance online publication. https://doi.org/10.1001/jamanetworkopen.2024.31306

Romanelli, M., Lu, W., & Lindsey, M. A. (2018). Examining mechanisms and moderators of the relationship between discriminatory health care encounters and attempted suicide among U.S. transgender help-seekers. *Administration and Policy in Mental Health and Mental Health Services Research*, *45*(6), 831–849. https://doi.org/10.1007/s10488-018-0868-8

Rood, B. A., Maroney, M. R., Puckett, J. A., Berman, A. K., Reisner, S. L., & Pantalone, D. W. (2017). Identity concealment in transgender adults: A qualitative assessment of minority stress and gender affirmation. *American Journal of Orthopsychiatry*, *87*(6), 704–713. https://doi.org/10.1037/ort0000303

Rood, B. A., Reisner, S. L., Puckett, J. A., Surace, F. I., Berman, A. K., & Pantalone, D. W. (2017). Internalized transphobia: Exploring perceptions of social messages in transgender and gender-nonconforming adults. *International Journal of Transgenderism*, *18*(4), 411–426. https://doi.org/10.1080/15532739.2017.1329048

Rood, B. A., Reisner, S. L., Surace, F. I., Puckett, J. A., Maroney, M. R., & Pantalone, D. W. (2016). Expecting rejection: Understanding the minority stress experiences of transgender and gender-nonconforming individuals. *Transgender Health*, *1*(1), 151–164. https://doi.org/10.1089/trgh.2016.0012

Rosentel, K., López-Martínez, I., Crosby, R. A., Salazar, L. F., & Hill, B. J. (2021). Black transgender women and the school-to-prison pipeline: Exploring the relationship between anti-trans experiences in school and adverse criminal-legal system outcomes. *Sexuality Research & Social Policy, 18*(3), 481–494. https://doi.org/10.1007/s13178-020-00473-7

Russell, S. T., Pollitt, A. M., Li, G., & Grossman, A. H. (2018). Chosen name use is linked to reduced depressive symptoms, suicidal ideation, and suicidal behavior among transgender youth. *The Journal of Adolescent Health, 63*(4), 503–505. https://doi.org/10.1016/j.jadohealth.2018.02.003

Seelman, K. L., Colón-Diaz, M. J. P., LeCroix, R. H., Xavier-Brier, M., & Kattari, L. (2017). Transgender noninclusive healthcare and delaying care because of fear: Connections to general health and mental health among transgender adults. *Transgender Health, 2*(1), 17–28. https://doi.org/10.1089/trgh.2016.0024

Shaine, M. J. D., Cor, D. N., Campbell, A. J., & McAlister, A. L. (2021). Mental health care experiences of trans service members and veterans: A mixed-methods study. *Journal of Counseling and Development, 99*(3), 273–288. https://doi.org/10.1002/jcad.12374

Sher, E., Hedrick, M., Paliotta, M., Dawson, L. J., Issa, N., & Gelman, D. (2022). Learn to affirm: Suicidality reduction in gender and sexual minority youth through interpersonal and systemic change. *Psychiatric Annals, 52*(8), 328–332. https://doi.org/10.3928/00485713-20220718-02

Shipherd, J. C., Green, K. E., & Abramovitz, S. (2010). Transgender clients: Identifying and minimizing barriers to mental health treatment. *Journal of Gay & Lesbian Mental Health, 14*(2), 94–108. https://doi.org/10.1080/19359701003622875

Shuster, S. M. (2019). Performing informed consent in transgender medicine. *Social Science & Medicine, 226*, 190–197. https://doi.org/10.1016/j.socscimed.2019.02.053

Smith, W. B., Goldhammer, H., & Keuroghlian, A. S. (2019). Affirming gender identity of patients with serious mental illness. *Psychiatric Services, 70*(1), 65–67. https://doi.org/10.1176/appi.ps.201800232

Snow, A., Cerel, J., Loeffler, D. N., & Flaherty, C. (2019). Barriers to mental health care for transgender and gender-nonconforming adults: A systematic literature review. *Health & Social Work, 44*(3), 149–155. https://doi.org/10.1093/hsw/hlz016

Stabbe, O. (2020, June 12). *Trans Lifeline's data during a pandemic*. Trans Lifeline. https://translifeline.org/trans-lifelines-data-during-a-pandemic/

Stanley, B., & Brown, G. K. (2012). Safety planning intervention: A brief intervention to mitigate suicide risk. *Cognitive and Behavioral Practice, 19*(2), 256–264. https://doi.org/10.1016/j.cbpra.2011.01.001

Strang, J. F., Anthony, L. G., Song, A., Lai, M.-C., Knauss, M., Sadikova, E., Graham, E., Zaks, Z., Wimms, H., Willing, L., Call, D., Mancilla, M., Shakin, S., Vilain, E., Kim, D.-Y., Maisashvili, T., Khawaja, A., & Kenworthy, L. (2023). In addition to stigma: Cognitive and autism-related predictors of mental health in transgender adolescents. *Journal of Clinical Child and Adolescent Psychology, 52*(2), 212–229. https://doi.org/10.1080/15374416.2021.1916940

Strauss, P., Cook, A., Watson, V., Winter, S., Whitehouse, A., Albrecht, N., Wright Toussaint, D., & Lin, A. (2021). Mental health difficulties among trans and gender diverse young people with an autism spectrum disorder (ASD): Findings from Trans

Pathways. *Journal of Psychiatric Research, 137*, 360–367. https://doi.org/10.1016/j.jpsychires.2021.03.005

Strauss, P., Cook, A., Winter, S., Watson, V., Wright Toussaint, D., & Lin, A. (2020). Associations between negative life experiences and the mental health of trans and gender diverse young people in Australia: Findings from Trans Pathways. *Psychological Medicine, 50*(5), 808–817. https://doi.org/10.1017/S0033291719000643

Sundus, A., Shahzad, S., & Younas, A. (2021). Ethical and culturally competent care of transgender patients: A scoping review. *Nursing Ethics, 28*(6), 1041–1060. https://doi.org/10.1177/0969733020988307

Sutter, M., & Perrin, P. B. (2016). Discrimination, mental health, and suicidal ideation among LGBTQ people of color. *Journal of Counseling Psychology, 63*(1), 98–105. https://doi.org/10.1037/cou0000126

Tebbe, E. A., & Budge, S. L. (2022). Factors that drive mental health disparities and promote well-being in transgender and nonbinary people. *Nature Reviews Psychology, 1*(12), 694–707. https://doi.org/10.1038/s44159-022-00109-0

Tebbe, E. A., & Moradi, B. (2016). Suicide risk in trans populations: An application of minority stress theory. *Journal of Counseling Psychology, 63*(5), 520–533. https://doi.org/10.1037/cou0000152

Testa, R. J., Habarth, J., Peta, J., Balsam, K., & Bockting, W. (2015). Development of the gender minority stress and resilience measure. *Psychology of Sexual Orientation and Gender Diversity, 2*(1), 65–77. https://doi.org/10.1037/sgd0000081

Testa, R. J., Jimenez, C. L., & Rankin, S. (2014). Risk and resilience during transgender identity development: The effects of awareness and engagement with other transgender people on affect. *Journal of Gay & Lesbian Mental Health, 18*(1), 31–46. https://doi.org/10.1080/19359705.2013.805177

Testa, R. J., Michaels, M. S., Bliss, W., Rogers, M. L., Balsam, K. F., & Joiner, T. (2017). Suicidal ideation in transgender people: Gender minority stress and interpersonal theory factors. *Journal of Abnormal Psychology, 126*(1), 125–136. https://doi.org/10.1037/abn0000234

Thoma, B. C., Salk, R. H., Choukas-Bradley, S., Goldstein, T. R., Levine, M. D., & Marshal, M. P. (2019). Suicidality disparities between transgender and cisgender adolescents. *Pediatrics, 144*(5), e20191183. https://doi.org/10.1542/peds.2019-1183

Toomey, R. B., Syvertsen, A. K., & Shramko, M. (2018). Transgender adolescent suicide behavior. *Pediatrics, 142*(4), e20174218. https://doi.org/10.1542/peds.2017-4218

Trujillo, M. A., Perrin, P. B., Sutter, M., Tabaac, A., & Benotsch, E. G. (2017). The buffering role of social support on the associations among discrimination, mental health, and suicidality in a transgender sample. *International Journal of Transgenderism, 18*(1), 39–52. https://doi.org/10.1080/15532739.2016.1247405

Turban, J. L., Beckwith, N., Reisner, S. L., & Keuroghlian, A. S. (2020). Association between recalled exposure to gender identity conversion efforts and psychological distress and suicide attempts among transgender adults. *JAMA Psychiatry, 77*(1), 68–76. https://doi.org/10.1001/jamapsychiatry.2019.2285

Turban, J. L., King, D., Carswell, J. M., & Keuroghlian, A. S. (2020). Pubertal suppression for transgender youth and risk of suicidal ideation. *Pediatrics, 145*(2), e20191725. https://doi.org/10.1542/peds.2019-1725

Turban, J. L., King, D., Kobe, J., Reisner, S. L., & Keuroghlian, A. S. (2022). Access to gender-affirming hormones during adolescence and mental health outcomes among transgender adults. *PLOS One, 17*(1), e0261039. Advance online publication. https://doi.org/10.1371/journal.pone.0261039

Vance, M. M., Wade, J. M., Brandy, M., Jr., & Webster, A. R. (2023). Contextualizing Black women's mental health in the twenty-first century: Gendered racism and suicide-related behavior. *Journal of Racial and Ethnic Health Disparities, 10*(1), 83–92. https://doi.org/10.1007/s40615-021-01198-y

Van Orden, K. A., Witte, T. K., Cukrowicz, K. C., Braithwaite, S. R., Selby, E. A., & Joiner, T. E., Jr. (2010). The interpersonal theory of suicide. *Psychological Review, 117*(2), 575–600. https://doi.org/10.1037/a0018697

Vermeir, E., Jackson, L. A., & Marshall, E. G. (2018). Barriers to primary and emergency healthcare for trans adults. *Culture, Health & Sexuality, 20*(2), 232–246. https://doi.org/10.1080/13691058.2017.1338757

Walton, H. M., & Baker, S. L. (2019). Treating transgender individuals in inpatient and residential mental health settings. *Cognitive and Behavioral Practice, 26*(4), 592–602. https://doi.org/10.1016/j.cbpra.2017.09.006

14

TRANS AND NONBINARY EXPERIENCES OF RELIGION, SPIRITUALITY, AND FAITH

RUBEN HOPWOOD AND JACK BRUNO

Religion, spirituality, faith, beliefs, and practices may play a central role in the daily lives of many trans and nonbinary (TNB) people (Porter et al., 2013). Just as there is no homogeneous experience, identity, or self-expression among TNB people, there is no homogeneous religion, faith, beliefs, or spiritual practices of TNB people (Levy & Lo, 2013). There are many factors that influence the expression and effects of religion, spirituality, and faith in TNB people's lives. Personal, social, and clinical language and attitudes about gender identity diversity as well as religious and spiritual beliefs and biases can maximize and incorporate or can minimize, pathologize, and harm TNB people (Kapitan & Kapitan, 2023). Antireligious and antispiritual ideologies can interfere with TNB people's ability to maintain support systems, access health care, and achieve well-being (Zinnbauer, 2013).

In this chapter, we discuss ways religious or spiritual beliefs may be integrated into the worldviews of TNB clients. We outline some general effects of religious and spiritual beliefs and practices on mental health and well-being. We conclude the chapter with two case studies and recommended strategies

---

The authors acknowledge the work of Tarryn Witten for her coauthorship of the 2015 version of this chapter and her tireless work to research and publish on trans and nonbinary aging and spirituality.

https://doi.org/10.1037/0000471-015
Affirmative Counseling and Psychological Practice With Trans and Nonbinary Clients, Second Edition, A. Singh and R. McCullough (Editors)
Copyright © 2026 by the American Psychological Association. All rights reserved.

mental health providers (MHPs) can use to explore the nuance and complexity of TNB people's involvement in faith communities.[1] We strive to be inclusive of varied systems of spirituality, faith, and cultural differences, while acknowledging that exhaustive coverage of the experiences of TNB people within all possible religious and spiritual systems and cultures is simply not possible in one chapter.

DEFINITIONS AND FUNCTIONS

Religion and spirituality are common concepts that remain poorly defined as separate constructs. Yet, there are overlaps and basic elements that are identifiable that we will use within the chapter. Generally, *spirituality* has to do with the search for whatever is sacred; *religiousness* or *religion* has to do with rituals, institutionally sanctioned behavior or actions, and beliefs; *faith* can refer to both spirituality and religion; and *sacred* has to do with whatever is considered *divine*, that which is outside human experience or understanding (i.e., existential) or larger than the self, fundamentally meaningful, or of primary concern to a person (Harris et al., 2018; Madrigal-Borloz, 2023).

Religion, spiritual practices, and faith communities teach worldviews that help people create or they provide meaning and purpose for everyday life events, both mundane and extraordinary. Faith communities teach values and morality to both inform and confirm one's actions in and interpretations of life. Religious involvement, or religiousness, may include specific behaviors, beliefs, rituals, objects, symbols, expressions, and thoughts; it draws upon or invites the presence of ancestors, cultural memories, and practices that help people stay connected to their histories and learn models for resilience in the face of suffering (Ai et al., 2013; Etengoff & Rodriguez, 2022; Rosenberg, 2017). Religious and spiritual practices and beliefs may contribute to positive mental health and resilience by providing a framework for people to order and make sense of their lives or by giving a sense of support and security through a higher power outside themselves to help manage challenges in life (McFadden et al., 2013; Rosenberg, 2017; Singh & McKleroy, 2011). Religion and spirituality may also play a central role in cultural identity and continuity, ancestral memory, heritage, values, and tribal sovereignty (Ai et al., 2013; Irwin, 1997; Kidwell et al., 2002; Rosenberg, 2017).

---

[1] The case examples in this chapter have been modified to disguise the clients' identities and protect their confidentiality.

EXPERIENCES AND IMPACT OF RELIGION AND SPIRITUALITY

The effects of religion, spirituality, and faith communities on TNB people occur across the lifespan regardless of gender identity or age (Porter et al., 2013). It is beneficial for MHPs to include questions about influences of these practices, beliefs, and communities as part of routine assessments for treatment. Involvement in religious and spiritual communities and practices may provide protective factors against suicidal thoughts or attempts and other negative outcomes in the general population (Gearing & Alonzo, 2018). There is also evidence that these protective factors from involvement in religious and spiritual communities and faith traditions may not be present for many TNB people (Rabasco & Andover, 2021). Self-concepts, worldviews, meaning, and purpose learned from religious, spiritual, and faith communities can be fraught with challenges (M. Campbell et al., 2019), including negative effects and religious or spiritual harm as a result of being singled out for rejection and discrimination based on gender identities that run counter to dominant cultural expectations (Okrey Anderson & McGuire, 2021). Nonetheless, some TNB people may stay in faith communities and may develop a distinction between religious and spiritual institutions, as well as personal practices and beliefs (Beagan & Hattie, 2015). MHPs should hold space for how clients may resonate with or differ from dominant definitions of religion, spiritualty, and systems of meaning making.

Positive Effects

Research indicates that participation in supportive religious and spiritual practices and communities may reduce stress, enhance coping, and improve meaningful integration of significant events in TNB people's lives (bautista et al., 2014; Golub et al., 2010; Singh & McKleroy, 2011). Participation may contribute to positive identity formation (Vieten et al., 2013) and inform end-of-life processes (Porter et al., 2013). Further, religious and spiritual involvement is linked to improved overall health and well-being; reduction of depressive symptoms, suicidal thinking, and anxiety; and increased longevity (Harris et al., 2018). These data suggest that one of the main benefits of participation in religious and spiritual communities may be improved coping and resilience in the face of challenges in life. As with any practice of cultural humility, MHPs should seek an awareness of their own experiences and biases regarding potential effects and protective factors from religion or spirituality while centering clients' understanding and experiences.

Negative Effects

Contrary to the positive benefits, for many TNB people, spirituality and religion may instead contribute to negative outcomes arising from religious and spiritual antiqueer and antitrans prejudice (McFadden et al., 2013; Porter et al., 2013). For TNB individuals who are marginalized within their faith traditions, these communities may cause more harm than good. This can be due to faith-based conversion practices (T. W. Jones et al., 2022), removing spiritual and sometimes tangible support, rejection, and condemnation of the person due to their gender variance from norms (Ginicola, Filmore, & Stokes, 2017). It is important for MHPs to engage TNB people in topics regarding religion or spirituality from a trauma informed lens. Research identifies higher risk of nonsuicidal self-injury or other risk-taking behaviors correlated with higher levels of religiosity (e.g., prayer, attending services, reading sacred texts, meditation) in TNB individuals who are in communities that stigmatize their identities (Golub et al., 2010; Longo et al., 2012).

Rejection from religious and spiritual communities combined with chronic experiences of discrimination and trauma are strongly correlated with high rates of mental health issues, substance abuse, and alarmingly high rates of attempted suicide among TNB people (James et al., 2016; Rabasco & Andover, 2021), higher rates of sexual risk-taking behaviors (Golub et al., 2010), and increased suicidality in TNB older adults (Witten, 2014). Rejections and existential wounds can take many forms, including loss of access to significant life and death rituals (Etengoff & Rodriguez, 2022) and denial of marriage ceremonies, last rights, and access to spiritual counseling (Witten, 2014). Some spiritual rejection and harm affect the TNB community vicariously when they witness other members of the TNB community having their identities and lives erased by families and religious communities who returned the deceased to a sex assigned at birth during funerals, memorials, or other postdeath rituals (Rothaus, 2014).

Negative experiences with religious and spiritual communities can significantly affect TNB people's mental health and well-being, directly and indirectly. Beagan and Hattie (2015) found the emotional and psychological harm to some queer and trans people from organized religion were extensive and often resulted in disconnection from one's body. Another study found positive correlations between levels of antiqueer and antitrans religious bias and beliefs in communities of upbringing, parents, and families—and found an increased frequency and severity of suicidal thoughts or behaviors and withdrawal from families of origin (Gibbs & Goldbach, 2015). Contrary to that study, in a more recent study, TNB individuals who held personal religious beliefs that reject their gender identity had significantly more severe suicidal thinking, but no more suicide attempts than TNB individuals who held religious beliefs that were accepting of their gender identity (Rabasco & Andover, 2021). Still, other studies found protective factors from religious practices and beliefs correlated to reduced prevalence and severity of suicidal thoughts and behaviors (Boppana & Gross, 2019; Grossman et al., 2016). Yüksel and colleagues (2017), as well as Bauer and colleagues (2015), found no relationship between religious and spiritual beliefs or practices and suicidal thinking or behaviors among TNB people. The data remain mixed and unclear due to limitations in scope of participants and different study methods. The connections between rejecting religious and spiritual beliefs and suicidality need to be explored more to fully understand the risk factors religion and spiritual beliefs and practices create for increased suicidal thoughts and attempts for TNB individuals.

Colonialism Effects

The interplay of identities and marginalization within TNB communities may show up as tensions between individuals and the impact of religion and spirituality. This tension may be particularly visible through the effects of powerful religion-based social systems that influence education, health care, and public opinion (e.g., media). Social and cultural factors from modern Western influence and ideologies, combined with continued damage from historic colonizing actions, continue to overlap and intertwine with religious and spiritual beliefs, practices, and institutions. This contributes to an unspoken centering of White and Western culture, people, and monotheistic faiths (e.g., belief there is only one god) as normative and superior. This is particularly troublesome for anyone with intersecting marginalized identities who experience ongoing misunderstanding and pathologizing by westernized White MHPs due to limitations and bias in clinicians' cultural knowledge and sensitivity (Curling et al., 2020; Rosmarin et al., 2021). As discussed later in the chapter, MHPs should consider their own relationship with colonial dynamics and the history of their field of practice related to religious and spiritual systems historically decentered or suppressed under colonialization as they engage with clients. A greater awareness may be gained by examining origins of measures used to evaluate people, exploring definitions of wellness or health, questioning who is included and excluded in research, and advocating for equitable organizational practices and policies of support around wellness sovereignty.

Literature on the impact of religious and spiritual systems on TNB people in general and characteristics and practices of involvement in religion and spirituality have primarily focused on White TNB people, youth and young adults, and those of middle and upper classes, leaving TNB people of color, older adults, and economically disadvantaged people largely misunderstood. One exception is the Trans Metlife Survey of TNB elders' religious and spiritual connections (Porter et al., 2013). The study found that more than half (56%) of the elders reported being affiliated with Christianity or some other nonspecific faith tradition that was affirming of queer and trans people, and less than a third (26%) reported no affiliation with any religion. Nonetheless, the participants were primarily White and middle to upper class, leaving a continued gap in the data. Without representation from racially, ethnically, and economically marginalized TNB populations, there are significant deficits to more fully understanding the benefits and risks of involvement in religion and spirituality for the estimated 1.3 million TNB people in the United States (Herman et al., 2022).

Studies suggest TNB people of color and those outside of Jewish and Christian religious paradigms find strength and resilience in faith traditions and negotiate gender identities differently than White TNB people (bautista et al., 2014; Sharzer et al., 2020). For instance, many practitioners of Indigenous spiritual beliefs contend that there is no division between the mundane and the sacred, and that ceremonial life is a time set aside to recognize the spiritually connected nature of the world (Kidwell et al., 2002). One study found that Two-Spirit, *Indigiqueer* (meaning queer and trans Indigenous people), and cisgender heterosexual Indigenous people showed no difference in how much importance they place on spirituality (Balsam et al., 2004). *Two-Spirit* is an identity term used by some Indigenous people to describe their sexual orientation or gender identity as existing outside of or apart from binary Western colonial body-based sexual and gender concepts, while simultaneously centering their experiences and knowledge of self as Indigenous people and members of specific tribes, bands, or other communities. The leadership responsibilities given to Two-Spirit community members in ceremonies are intrinsically tied to the spiritual health and wholeness of that individual and the community at large in a reciprocal act of resilience and spiritual well-being. In this way, Indigenous spiritualities are integrated, essential, and salient aspects of holistic community life that include Two-Spirit people as necessary for ritual and spiritual life to be complete.

The detrimental influence of religious institutions and beliefs is most visible globally in the ongoing effects of colonialism, assimilation, and the attempted genocide of whole populations that have reshaped the religious, spiritual, and faith traditions of Indigenous peoples. Colonialism left enduring conflicted relationships between communities and their members who both serve important spiritual roles within their cultures and traditions (e.g., Two-Spirit, Hijra, third sex) and reject imposed Western conceptualizations of a rigid gender binary. This conflict leaves the community spiritually wounded and challenged to reclaim a holistic spiritual and communal life.

Body Image Impact

All spiritualities and faith traditions do not lead people toward personal understanding and wholeness in the same way or at all, especially when dealing with the physical body, sexual and gender expressions, and beliefs. When exploring embodiment goals, gender euphoria, and dysphoria with TNB clients, the MHP does well to create space to discuss spiritual components of body, embodiment, expression, and emotional content that may accompany, shift, and change along the client's journey. Faith traditions have varied understandings of the physical body, whether there is a spiritual aspect of a person (e.g., "soul"), what people do with and to their bodies, and what happens to people after death. Traditions vary in conceptualizations of gender in relation to physical form (body), function and role of gender in society, and who or what has authority over a person's body. Disagreements exist across faith traditions around what constitutes self-knowledge and how one discerns what is the "real" or "true" self when it is considered contrary to the physical body (Sharzer et al., 2020). There are also diverging views on how to respond to TNB people and gender-affirming treatments. Responses range from prohibiting variance from an assigned gender to permission to express one's gender separate from the physical form, with a few that oblige TNB people to undergo gender-affirming surgeries (e.g., Islamic law in Iran) to uphold the belief systems, or possibly risk death (Sharzer et al., 2020).

Many Western religious traditions are rooted in beliefs that sex and gender as assigned at birth are fixed, binary constructs, that are divinely appointed (Appleton, 2011; Levy & Lo, 2013). These binary conceptualizations of sex and gender are typically used to shape language, laws, customs, privileges, and economies; influence social structures; and shape public discourse and freedoms—despite the reality that science cannot prove or falsify a causal relationship between gender identity and chromosomal sex (M. Campbell et al., 2019; Parkinson, 2023). Through the interplay of religious-based sociopolitical power and beliefs about an immutable binary nature of assigned sex and gender (Parkinson, 2023), dominant religious systems use political power to enforce their values and views across a culture (Miller et al., 2022) without regard to the beliefs, values, and sometimes lives of others. Within these beliefs and social structures, acknowledgement or support of TNB people is limited (Parkinson, 2023). MHPs can counter the impact of negating and dismissive public narratives about TNB people by working to acknowledge and address internalized narratives of self, creating space for discussing systems of marginalization and the material impacts of religious structure's interweaving with sociopolitical domains.

Existential Loss and Rejection

For TNB individuals and their families, denial of access to spiritual and religious care and rituals for various stages of life may represent a significant or ambiguous loss of being irrevocably cut off from personal meaning, communal identity, and belonging, extending beyond the ordinary losses expected in life to losses in an afterlife as well (Harris et al., 2018). MHPs can explore losses and their meaning in a way that respects the client's beliefs and needs. Offering compassionate support can empower individuals to connect to communities in ways that may lead toward healing or addressing existential wounds. MHPs, however, need to respectfully attend to client's needs around potential existential losses of one's soul or spirit; these are losses beyond human existence that cannot be recaptured or repaired.

Spiritual and existential rejection and losses may engender negative self-images, or loss of families who perceive the person as dead despite being tangibly alive (Norwood, 2013). MHPs are called on to support clients in their grief around experiences of acute and enduring losses by taking seriously the loss of these spaces, people, communities, and relationships. Religious and spiritual rejection may also lead to increased suicidal thoughts and attempts and may inculcate the idea that TNB people are of little or no inherent worth and value to something or someone sacred or beyond them (Harris et al., 2018; T. W. Jones et al., 2022; Okrey Anderson & McGuire, 2021). Other TNB individuals may restrict their own access to needed care or return to externally imposed expectations and demands on their identities and self-expression for safety or to gain access to spiritual and religious traditions that are important to them. Examples of this in the literature include TNB Muslim women who continue to present as men within or isolated from Islamic communities and religious activities (Etengoff & Rodriguez, 2022).

Over time, many people in Western societies, meaning Europe, parts of the Americas, and those cultures heavily influenced by Western European culture and colonization, have rejected the enforced value systems of dominant religious institutions and theistic spirituality (e.g., belief in a god or gods) as a hindrance to personal experiences and freedom of self-knowledge and expression (Curling et al., 2020). Nonetheless, TNB people may still identify with a broad spectrum of religious and spiritual beliefs and practices and may engage in various ways with a binary conceptualization of sex and gender found in many religious, spiritual, and faith traditions, such as conforming to a binary self-expression, living in celibacy, fulfilling religious obligations to have children before affirming a TNB gender identity, and living stealth or dual lives. It is important that the MHP openly reinforce the importance of client self-determination and honor their choices without judgement or undue pressure to choose a particular action.

In the next section we will offer short descriptions of a selection of religious and spiritual communities, beliefs, and faith traditions largely found in the United States. A full discussion of each religious and spiritual community and its particularities is beyond the scope of this chapter. The following descriptions provide a broad foundation and examples to illustrate the importance of considering the relationships of TNB people to religious or spiritual traditions of their own and of the dominant society in which they live. Exploring and addressing the impact of religious and spiritual beliefs and practices are a significant aspect of providing effective and relevant mental health services to TNB people and their significant others.

RELIGIOUS AND SPIRITUAL TRADITIONS

This section describes an historic and crude categorization of many rich and varied religious and spiritual traditions into two groups: "Eastern" and "Western." This division is rooted in Western scholarship and colonialism which often oversimplifies and obscures the complexities between and within religious groups and spiritual practices. References to *Western* and *Eastern* traditions highlight this reductionist framework that centers on a European (e.g., Western) perspective and bias toward traditions and practices historically found outside their context.

"Western" religions historically refer to traditions which originated in the Ancient Middle East: Judaism, Christianity, and Islam, and are today practiced in large numbers by people primarily associated with Western culture and values. "Eastern" religious traditions, as they are conceived of today, originated across the Asian continent. These include myriad cultures, traditions, and practices described in the 17th and 18th centuries by Western missionaries, merchants, and intellectuals, most of whom had never visited parts of the Far East (Ristuccia, 2013). These descriptions were built upon misinterpretations of earlier Roman or Latin Western explorers from the 13th and 14th centuries. These explorers conflated groups, defining and often disconnecting practices from populations and context. This historic anthropological lens oversimplified and obscured nuances and details to construct conceptualizations of unified and widespread religions using a Western Christian rubric as the comparison and grouping myriad practices into monolithic traditions that we continue today to combine under the blunt, two-dimensional categories of Hinduism, Buddhism, Daoism, Jainism, Shinto, etc. (Ristuccia, 2013). Traditions and practices that the Westerners did not perceive to have enough elements to qualify as a religion (e.g., organized rituals, hierarchy, asceticism, sacred texts, liturgical cycles) or practices they found confusing or offensive were depicted as immoral, magical, and demonic—as were the people who practiced those traditional rites and rituals (Ristuccia, 2013). These traditions, practices, and people were then dismissed as meaningless or suppressed as harmful. This legacy creates ongoing challenges and barriers to providing effective and relevant care for TNB and other people. MHPs may overlook and fail to inquire about, acknowledge, and respect religious and spiritual practices and belief traditions that do not fit into dominant cultural definitions and expectations. This section offers some terminology and context of this reductionist framework, offering a necessarily limited set of examples to broaden the context within which MHPs may examine and reduce their biases that may overlook the presence and importance of religious and spiritual practices and beliefs in TNB people's lives.

Abrahamic and Monotheistic Traditions

Within the United States, the largest and most visible religious groups (e.g., Judaism, Christianity, and Islam) have broadly tended to endorse binary concepts of sex and gender as divinely created (Lipka & Tevington, 2022; Parker et al., 2022). The literature indicates that evangelical Protestants, Catholics, and other religious groups tend to have more negative attitudes toward TNB people than Jewish and nonreligious individuals (M. Campbell et al., 2019; Cragun & Sumerau, 2015). TNB people cannot entirely, if at all, escape the negative effects and marginalization from this set of beliefs due to the predominance of structurally powerful religious systems and communities that shape and influence public policies, cultural narratives, discourse, and comprise large proportions of the population (i.e., 60% of Americans and 75% of Protestant Christians polled in the United States in 2022 believe that gender is determined by sex assigned at birth; Lipka & Tevington, 2022; Parker et al., 2022).

The Western religious traditions TNB people are affiliated with have a profound impact on their overall well-being. TNB people who are members of religious traditions that affirm their gender show increased ability to cope and decreased stress and mental health problems (Levy & Lo, 2013). However, there are significantly higher rates of psychological distress and poor mental health in TNB people who are members of more evangelical Protestant and conservative Christian religious traditions who are strongly correlated with the most rejecting messages toward TNB people (M. Campbell et al., 2019; Hopwood, 2022; Lipka & Tevington, 2022). It is important for MHPs to explore TNB clients' traditions, practices, and choices to remain in or distance from these traditions using an open attitude of humility and nonjudgemental curiosity. This approach can enable greater understanding of the TNB client and of how their choices regarding religious or spiritual practices may affect their meaning, purpose, community, and resilience. Some TNB people choose to remain in their religious and spiritual communities, despite rejecting messages, because the loss of their faith community may be experienced as even more spiritually harmful and emotionally painful. Others find ways to incorporate and interpret or recontextualize religious and spiritual beliefs in a more affirming or ambivalent way (Etengoff & Rodriguez, 2022). Some choose to leave faith communities and may find alternative religious or spiritual groups and practices that do not reject TNB people, such as Unitarian Universalism (Unitarian Universalist Association, n.d.) and Earth-based faith traditions and spirituality (Appleton, 2011; Kaldera, 2009; Smith & Horne, 2007).

Traditions of Indigenous, Earth-Based, Eastern, and Asian Regions

The following section is a brief introduction to some selected traditions and their role in the lives of many TNB individuals and communities. There are myriad religious and spiritual practices from so-called Eastern, Indigenous, and earth-based traditions, and many are important to numerous TNB people (3% of the U.S. population by self-report; Public Religion Research Institute, 2021). The range of diversity in spiritualities originating in Eastern and Asian geographic regions is not reducible to references such as "Eastern religions" or "Asian religions." As noted earlier, the pattern of grouping peoples into categories such as "the East" or "Asia" is a product of colonial essentialist generalizations and stereotypes that disclose the disinterest in fully understanding or preserving traditions outside Western belief systems (Blakemore, 2019; Kim, 2018). We use references to East and West as geographic placeholders and not as categorizations of people or traditions. Additionally, broad groupings of Indigenous and earth-based traditions do not inherently imply any particular geographic region, and such traditions may originate from many cultures and continents. Colonialism negatively affected religious and spiritual traditions of Indigenous people and, by default, the experiences of TNB people from myriad cultures across most of the globe.

Western colonizing actions exacted great costs from Indigenous communities across the American continent and disrupted, suppressed, or destroyed many spiritual traditions and practices. Colonialism in Asia, like in the Americas, separated people from their traditions, language, and heritage (Venkatraman & Yam, 2022) and brought and left a wake of violence, conflict, and genocide. It negatively affected many communities and their religious and spiritual practices, yet it had very minimal impact on China or Japan in particular (Haselby, 2019). In the East, colonialism broke down historic religious fluidity and the sharing of sacred spaces, festivals, and spiritual traditions by forcing clear distinctions between people like Muslims and Hindus. The process of forced divisions focused on differences between people, creating significant separations between India and Pakistan in particular (i.e., the 1952 Partition) and transforming what once were open and shared spiritual festivals and temples that welcomed women and TNB people into places of enforced normative gender roles, sex segregation, and religious animosity toward the "other" (Khalid, 2021).

Buddhism

Traditions from Southeast Asia, such as those within Buddhism, may offer opportunities for acceptance of TNB people within their myriad communities. Some Buddhist groups have stories of magical sex changes within their sacred texts (Mahayana) or reincarnation in another sex (Jain). This is more complex than this simplistic and brief comment can address, and many stories of sex change are influenced by Western thinking and based on an overarching belief that it is a punishment to be reborn a woman and that a person who is a third sex (i.e., identity based on gender identity and spirituality, not on sexual identity) is incapable of understanding dharma, or religious and moral law governing human conduct (Appleton, 2011; Natural History Museum, 2020). Despite this apparent negative view of "changing sex," at least toward femaleness, there may be more acceptance of TNB people within the U.S. Buddhist groups serving queer and trans communities (Sanghas).[2] To be supportive and responsive to client needs, the MHP needs to learn about the Sangha that a TNB person participates in to understand how they may be accepted, rejected, limited, or supported to express their gender and their community's beliefs regarding gender and gender-affirming medical interventions or changes to their bodies.

---

[2]See Queer Sangha at https://www.youtube.com/playlist?list=PL2aY7M6Jqybdvn2sd6 RXuSFpZbEgkGI_4 and LGBTQIA2S+Sangha at https://www.insightmeditationcenter. org/lgbtqueer-sangha/

Hinduism

Hinduism arises from India in South Asia. Prior to the influences of westernization, Hinduism historically accepted the existence of a third sex, integrating queer, trans, and third sex people into the Indian society and spiritual practices with specific roles in many religious rituals (Wilhelm, 2010). Within the wide spectrum of beliefs and practices of Hinduism, there are pockets of tolerance for people of a third sex; however, responses to marginalized sexual and gender identities may still be rejecting. Some Hindu communities express prejudice and violence toward queer and trans people (Wilhelm, 2010).[3] Some TNB people, however, find acceptance and personal meaning based in a variety of the Hindu forms of God and sacred narratives that represent a blending of male and female sexes (Shiva, Siva or Durga, and Ardhanarisvara), three genders (male, female, and a fluid blending of genders: Sri Arjuna, Brihannala), deities who cross-dress (Sri Bhagavati-devi), and other representations of the Hindu concept of a third sex (Wilhelm, 2010). As of 2014, one TNB group in India known as Hijra (i.e., taking on neither male or female gender, not transitioning to a binary sex, fluidity of gender and possession of the spirit of all genders) has full legal recognition and may participate in some historic cultural spiritual rituals and rites that are slowly being restored in some communities (Khaleeli, 2014; Laxman, 2022; Sapna, 2017).[4]

American Indian and Alaskan Native Spiritual Traditions, Indigenous Transgender, Indigiqueer, and Two-Spirit Individuals

Notably, due to colonial projects of attempted physical and cultural assimilation and genocide, adherents of various forms of Christianity have actively sought to eliminate Indigenous religious and spiritual traditions and Indigenous people on the American continent over the centuries. This shows up in part in the way in which religion, religious belief, and participation in a religious or faith community are operationalized in research that often continues to reflect colonial or Western theories of knowledge. For instance, a 2020 study of the religious landscape of the United States reported that 60% of American Indian and Alaskan Native people identify as Christians, while 28% are religiously unaffiliated (R. P. Jones et al., 2021). This obscures the presence of Indigenous spirituality, lifeways, and ceremonial involvement in addition to any Christian practices. While more culturally informed data is needed, initial findings from a nuanced study of two tribes suggest that, rather than passive recipients of colonial religious conversion, Indigenous individuals and communities actively

---

[3] See http://www.galva108.org for a further description of Vaishnava and Hindu views on a third gender from the Gay & Lesbian Vaishnava Association.
[4] For more information, see Khaleeli (2014), Laxman (2022), and Sapna (2017).

engage with Christian beliefs alongside tribally based spirituality and lifeways (P. N. Jones, 2005), as well as relatively more recent spiritual and religious movements such as the Native American Church (Garroutte et al., 2014). Individual Indigenous people may hold any number of religious or spiritual beliefs, and it is incumbent on MHPs to ask in more open-ended ways about religious or spiritual traditions and practices of any Indigenous and Indigiqueer people they may work with (P. N. Jones, 2005).

Although it is impossible to address all Indigenous spiritual beliefs as monolithic, many communities' belief systems include important spiritual and ceremonial roles for those who live outside of the Western colonial framework of a sex and gender binary. Many of the 225 Indigenous languages spoken across the North American continent include words for these community members and describe their positions within their community. These positions in Indigenous societies often include caretaking roles, occupational specialties, diplomatic and mediation responsibilities, and specific roles in keeping community spiritual and medicinal knowledge (Driskill et al., 2011; Gilley, 2006; Lang, 1998; Tafoya, 1997). When settler colonialism sought to eliminate or subjugate Indigenous communities, they often targeted these individuals specifically for their gendered presentation and choice of partners, which were framed as sinful within colonial Christian worldviews (Davies-Cole & Robinson, 2022; Gilley, 2006). As missionaries representing a number of Christian denominations strove to convert Indigenous communities, tribal beliefs regarding gendered life outside of a strict binary were particularly troublesome to these "civilizing" efforts, and the colonizing religious drive to exterminate "problematic" Indigenous conceptualizations of gender added fuel to genocidal processes.

It is within this context that the term Two-Spirit was coined in 1990 by Indigenous activists at the American Indian Gay and Lesbian Conference (Lang, 2016). Some tribal groups, families, and individuals had been able to maintain knowledge of their communities' Two-Spirit members who had lived in ways that were not represented in Western binaries and could hold space for those roles in their communities' spiritual life. For others, that knowledge has proven harder to access due to the history of genocidal oppression and supplanting tribal and community knowledge with colonial religions. Two-Spirit, TNB, and Indigiqueer or Indigenous people often found, and continue to find, their tribal knowledge replaced with antiqueer and anti-TNB bias in their home communities, as well as racism and settler colonialism in predominantly non-Indigenous queer and trans spaces. The creation of the term Two-Spirit was crucial in forming an identity label for Indigenous people with a variety of sexual orientations and gender presentations. With Two-Spirit as an Indigenous identity label, community members can align themselves politically, culturally, and spiritually with their Indigenous communities (Smithers, 2022). Individuals may also utilize a tribally specific term to describe themselves instead of or alongside Two-Spirit, Indigiqueer, or queer and trans.

RECLAIMING RELIGIOSITY AND SPIRITUALITY FOR TRANS AND NONBINARY CLIENTS

Negative self-image, ambiguous loss from experiences of religious and spiritual rejection, and loss of connection to faith communities, with the Divine, or something sacred, may lead to hopelessness and increase depression and suicidal thoughts in TNB populations (Okrey Anderson & McGuire, 2021; Rabasco & Andover, 2021). Joining an affirming religious or spiritual community—or developing affirming beliefs and spiritual practices—may reduce the harmful effects of spiritual rejection (Levy & Lo, 2013). Awareness of the self as a spiritual being may develop or increase for some as they wrestle with essentialist spiritual arguments about the role of the body in self-understanding, and TNB clients may shift away from conceptualizing the physical form as the totality of their being (Sharzer et al., 2020). Some TNB people may equate their life course and coming out experiences to spiritual discernment and integration of their bodies and spirits. Other TNB people may use the experiences of religious or spiritual prejudice to either develop their own individual spiritual and religious beliefs that may help them integrate their gender with their faith (Levy & Lo, 2013) or to find hope for the future and cope with negative life events (Singh & McKleroy, 2011). For TNB people with additional marginalized identities, engagement in their community's cultural religious and spiritual practices, such as services, ceremonies, and rituals, may also contribute to a greater sense of cultural belonging and holistic well-being (Ansloos et al., 2021; Limb & Hodge, 2008).

Case Studies

This section provides two brief case studies of the ways an MHP might encounter and work with a client's religion or spirituality in treatment. The individuals' names and situations are composites of several individuals and are modified to protect identities while retaining the key elements of presenting concerns and approaches to care.

Carolyn

Carolyn is a Caribbean American TNB woman in her 50s and uses she/her/hers pronouns. Carolyn came to counseling seeking support around her gender affirmation process and help to manage distress and navigate self-advocacy, specifically with her religious community. Carolyn was in a very conservative Christian community that was deeply meaningful to her, yet it rejected her relationship with a man because community members viewed it as "homosexual" in nature due to Carolyn's birth-assigned sex as male, despite her history of gender-affirming medical treatment. Members rejected her gender identity on the basis of their belief in "God's mandated and immutable" creation of sex and gender as binary and unchangeable. Despite these rejections, the religious community welcomed her to attend services and included her in the community as a participant only, without the ability to join in religious leadership.

This experience of rejection was painful for Carolyn. A primary focus of treatment was understanding and supporting her need to stay actively connected to this community and to build additional coping skills to reduce emotional and spiritual harm. The connection to her faith community continued to provide strength and empowerment in ways that were at times difficult for the MHP to understand. Carolyn's resilience was based in her personal belief that she was being faithful to the only "true" religion. Her beliefs were primary to her well-being. The clinician honored Carolyn's religious and spiritual beliefs and practices and sought to understand her faith and community involvement more fully. With greater understanding of its role in her life, the MHP was able to support Carolyn's continued involvement with her faith community. This collaborative treatment was effective in helping Carolyn manage the stressors in her gender affirmation process.

Previous providers supported Carolyn's gender while rejecting her religious beliefs and disparaging her faith community. They overlooked or dismissed the existential significance of her beliefs and involvement in this community. Several discouraged Carolyn's involvement in her faith community and pressured her to leave her faith entirely. This rejection of her faith community by her health care team paralleled her faith community's rejection of her gender and her health care providers and caused Carolyn significant distress and destabilization. In previous treatment, Carolyn felt trapped in an impossible choice between her religious beliefs and faith community or herself and her health care. Her mental health declined (clinical depression, suicidality) and her physical health deteriorated (two heart attacks).

Finding a clinician who was sensitive and accepting of her faith and spirituality enabled Carolyn to engage in gender-affirming mental health treatment and aided in her physical health improvement and stabilization. A spiritually affirming approach included her religious practices as valuable coping tools and invited her beliefs into meaningful dialogue. With no need to defend her religious beliefs and practices against her MHP's views, Carolyn was able to improve her sense of self-worth and self-advocate for changes within her personal and religious life that allowed her to feel more accepted and affirmed as a trans woman. These changes enabled significant improvements in her relationships and her overall quality of life.

Raul

Raul is a first-generation immigrant from the Dominican Republic in their early 20s and uses they/them/theirs pronouns. They came to counseling in an integrated community health clinic for support to transition. Raul talked about experiences they had interpreted as spiritual directives to express a "transgender identity." Raul described unusual physiological sensations outside their control, loss of consciousness, black-out periods, as well as thoughts and behaviors that Raul reported as distressing and foreign to their self-concept. The MHP felt the experiences needed further evaluation. It was unclear whether gender dysphoria was present, or if Raul's spirituality was illusory or detrimental. The MHP decided that uncertainty about the causes of their experiences combined with the ego-dystonic aspects of Raul's interpretations required exploration from a spiritually sensitive and gender-affirming approach that included sensitivity to possible neurological concerns.

Raul was reluctant to continue the assessment when the MHP asked them to wait to begin gender-affirming hormone treatment while the care team gained insight into any neurological or other health needs. Raul had future-oriented hopefulness based on their spiritual interpretation of these events and agreed. Despite the ego-dystonic gender aspects of the interpretations, Raul expressed commitment to following what they felt was a spiritual calling to change their life in relation to gender.

The MHP worked to balance assessment of possible risks and centering respectful attention to understanding the role of Raul's religious and spiritual beliefs in decision making. Through nonjudgmental exploration to increase understanding of religious beliefs and practices in Raul's faith tradition and culture, the MHP demonstrated respect for Raul's beliefs. This supportive approach enabled the MHP to gain insight into how a TNB identity fits within Raul's spiritual framework and developing identity. The collaborative therapeutic work enabled the MHP to build trust and support Raul in coordinating medical assessments of possible underlying concerns. Increased understanding of the spiritual experiences enabled the MHP to explore possible reinterpretations that were culturally attuned and more aligned with Raul's self-concept (e.g., ego-syntonic). Raul was able to better clarify their sense of gender identity, how their identity fit into their belief system and culture, and receive support to access appropriate gender-affirming care while developing alternate ways to describe their spiritual experiences that could reduce pathologization by other Western providers while remaining culturally accurate.

INTEGRATING RELIGION AND SPIRITUALITY INTO COUNSELING WITH TRANS AND NONBINARY CLIENTS

Skilled and affirmative care includes competency in issues of spiritual and religious diversity, as well as sexual and gender identity diversity, that goes beyond familiarity with one's own identities, beliefs, and practices. Many people seeking counseling prefer an MHP who has spiritual values and integrates the client's religious and spiritual concerns into therapy (Ginicola, Furth, & Smith, 2017). Mental health treatment can be ineffective, even detrimental, when it ignores or disparages a client's religious and spiritual beliefs and practices (Plante, 2024). However, there is little to no training for MHPs in how to integrate religion and spirituality into their clinical practice (Plante, 2024; Vieten et al., 2013). MHPs should seek training and supervision in spiritually informed or integrated therapy; they should learn to recognize any limitations in their knowledge and refer or seek supervision when appropriate (American Counseling Association, 2010; Vieten et al., 2013).

Clinical Assessment Practices

Providing care within an accepted standard of counseling practice remains imperative, while also making room to include a client's spirituality; this could look like inviting in and using spiritually meaningful language, metaphors, prayers, rituals, or imagery when helpful to the client. Understanding the role of religion and spirituality in a client's life and its role in treatment planning begins with the initial evaluation for services. A comprehensive evaluation includes inquiring about religious and spiritual upbringing and current beliefs and practices (American Psychological Association, 2015; Plante, 2024). Assessing risk factors, strengths, coping skills, and resilience is informed by understanding the effects in a TNB person's life from chronic and acute experiences of acceptance, rejection, and condemnation (Hendricks & Testa, 2012). Especially when working with TNB people who may have a damaged sense of hope and self-image based on religious or spiritual discrimination, it is imperative to understand where a person derives meaning, purpose, and hope in life

(Hendricks & Testa, 2012) and how this has changed over time. Routinely asking for details, such as religious and spiritual upbringing, experiences, conflicts, beliefs, and practices aids in risk assessments and enables clients to bring their whole selves into the process with less fear (Rodriguez & Follins, 2012).

Understanding the worldview and values of clients without judging them is crucial to providing relevant, respectful, and appropriate interventions (Vieten et al., 2013). Not all methods of inquiry and exploration of a client's beliefs and practices are equivalent or even helpful. Sensitive and respectful inquiries require acknowledging the conundrum that "psychological evaluation has the potential to clarify the paths, destinations, and integrity of the sacred, but it also has the potential to insult, pathologize, and oppress" (Zinnbauer, 2013, p. 86). Exploration of religion and spirituality needs to include a balanced approach. Clinicians need information to assess needs and to build an informed understanding of whether an individual's beliefs and practices may be contributing to well-being, may be detrimental, or in very rare instances, might be indicators of obsessive-compulsive characteristics or psychotic disorders (Vieten et al., 2013; Zinnbauer, 2013). MHPs who have taken the time to understand the role of religion and spirituality in the client's life are more equipped to support TNB individuals as they explore the person's own expectations and those of their religious and spiritual communities, families, and society to know how these affect choices about making any changes in their lives (Levy & Lo, 2013).

Treatment

Religious and spiritually based practices are used commonly in many mental health and other self-improvement settings (e.g., yoga, mindfulness, meditation). It is less common, however, for MHPs to be aware of the spiritual origins of these practices or to be aware of their own religious and spiritual biases (Vieten et al., 2013). Knowledge of the sources of these practices is important to better enable using interventions that align with a client's culture, practices, or beliefs (Plante, 2024; Vieten et al., 2013). Effective treatment that also mitigates harm is possible when clinicians know where practices come from and how to incorporate them sensitively into the religious beliefs and spirituality of the client (Karpen, 2018). For example, knowledge of meditative or centering and healing practices from various traditions allows clinicians and clients to explore, modify, or avoid practices that would cause spiritual problems. This individualized treatment capitalizes on the client's strengths, sense of agency, and desire to improve well-being without making assumptions or overlooking crucial information (Zinnbauer, 2013).

Plante (2024) describes common spiritual and religious practices and values that can be used effectively in therapy. These include

- meditation and prayer (e.g., quieting the mind, focusing attention);
- meaning, purpose, calling in life (e.g., life direction, decision-making);
- acceptance of self and others (e.g., empathy, compassion);
- being part of something larger and greater than oneself (e.g., connection to community, history, traditions, culture);
- forgiveness, gratitude, love, kindness, compassion, volunteerism, and charity (e.g., social connections, purpose, value);
- rituals and community events (e.g., honoring important moments and stages in life);
- social justice models (e.g., teachers, prophets, exemplars) of thinking and behavior from spiritual and religious traditions; and
- bibliotherapy (e.g., reading materials for insight and knowledge).

Mental Health Provider Self-Awareness

Knowledge of self is essential to gaining knowledge of others (Karpen, 2018). It is important for MHPs to engage in active self-examination, supervision, continuing education, and training to develop appropriate and sensitive ways to address and incorporate religious and spiritual concerns in clinical practice with TNB people (Plante, 2024; Vieten et al., 2013). The MHP's knowledge of their own beliefs and practices aids in identifying and actively interrupting their biases and stereotypes around religion or spirituality (Plante, 2024). Unexamined attitudes about religion and spirituality may appear as skewed clinical assessments and poorly informed or biased conclusions about clients' situations and needs. For example, conclusions that someone for whom religion and spirituality are formative and meaningful is misguided, delusional, gullible, or rigid, or someone who does not hold religion and spirituality as important is immoral and unethical (Plante, 2024; Vieten et al., 2013).

In addition to self-awareness, an MHP's understanding of systemic and interpersonal factors that may interfere with exploration of religion and spirituality in TNB people's lives is also crucial. For example, some Indigenous clients may be guarded or selective in sharing specifics of spiritual practices and beliefs with providers from dominant social groups due to the complexities and harmful effects of anti-Indigenous bias in the larger culture. Hesitancy on the part of some Indigenous clients may be due to the effect of historical trauma on their communities and corresponding mistrust of medical and MHPs. Additional inhibitions to disclose some information may include cultural norms of restricting information shared outside specific groups of community members (i.e.

those initiated, members of certain clans, or those holding specific identities). Other concerns regarding the legality of traditional medicines used in ceremonies, such as peyote, and customs related to the seasonal appropriateness of discussing spiritual matters also affect how and whether information may be disclosed (Hodge & Limb, 2010a).

MHPs need to mitigate routine inquiry practices that may feel intrusive with respect of client boundaries during clinical assessments and treatment. To do this, MHPs can proactively express and respect the right of any client to refuse to disclose or discuss anything they feel uncomfortable talking about without implying judgement or obligation to disclose information. Rather than insisting on disclosure of specific details, the MHP might explore ways Indigenous clients benefit from engaging in ceremony, ritual, or spiritual life broadly. Hodge and Limb (2010b) suggest considering the use of spiritual histories or *lifemaps* to invite Indigenous clients to share elements of their spiritual selves with practitioners. These two approaches were rated highly for cultural consistency amongst a group of predominantly Native American social workers. Hodge & Limb (2010a) also note the importance of skills in clinical encounters, such as acknowledging and honoring cultural boundaries regarding disclosure, allowing more time for engagement and assessment phases of treatment, employing awareness and sensitivity to historical spiritual oppression, emphasizing trust building, and providing transparency into why spiritual information is being collected and how it will be used, documented, or shared.

STRATEGIES TO INTEGRATE TRANS AND NONBINARY CLIENT SPIRITUALITY INTO PSYCHOLOGICAL PRACTICE

There are eight essential strategies MHPs can use to learn about the role of religion, spiritual practices, and traditions in the lives of TNB clients. First, MHPs can gather information from a broad biological, social, cultural, and spiritual approach to improve care, diagnosis, and treatment planning regardless of the presenting problem (Plante, 2024). How a clinician conceptualizes gender, religion, and spirituality affects approaches to gathering and interpreting information from a person which may be helpful or harmful (Kapitan & Kapitan, 2023; Zinnbauer, 2013). Openness to learn about and respect clients' backgrounds, cultural systems of value, beliefs, and spiritual practices to integrate these into treatment in culturally relevant and sensitive ways can be helpful for the TNB client (Vieten et al., 2013). Understanding the client as accurately as possible necessitates reflecting back, clarifying, and verifying concepts and meanings shared by both client and clinician.

Second, MHPs can explore how TNB clients may use religion and spirituality to avoid, mask, or justify other psychological or medical problems (e.g., displacement of conflict onto the body through self-punishment, subjection to emotional or physical harm, denial of medical conditions such as anorexia, psychosis, or stress reactions; Zinnbauer, 2013). It is within the legal and ethical responsibilities of clinical practice to evaluate and report instances of suspected abuse or neglect that may be couched within the belief structure or practices of a particular religious group (e.g., refusal to access medical care for a dependent who is critically ill; the use of corporal punishment or significant physical and emotional harm—as legally defined—against another person.). Third, it is important to resist assumptions that clients are disinterested in exploring and integrating religious or spiritual concerns and practices into treatment. Routinely assess religious and spiritual histories, past experiences, current beliefs, and past or current spiritual practices of all kinds (e.g., yoga, Tai Chi, Tarot, vision quests, Sweats, mandalas, labyrinth walking, meditation beads, etc.).

Fourth, it is crucial to explore the roles spiritual practices have in a person's formation, coping, and current life situations (C. L. Campbell & Catlett, 2019; Plante, 2024; Vieten et al., 2013) and remain open to listening for spiritual practices or religious beliefs and interests that may appear in the routine conversations of therapy, and to explore those things and their meaning. Fifth, MHPs can facilitate unbiased collaborative and respectful exploration of possible or desired changes in practices and beliefs to improve functioning, mental health, and well-being with TNB clients (Plante, 2024; Vieten et al., 2013). Sixth, MHP self-reflection is vital. Acknowledge the limits of your own knowledge and exercise humility. Seek actively to learn more about your own traditions and about traditions of which you are not a part. Check in with clients often and identify when your personal beliefs and implicit biases or assumptions about religion and spirituality are interfering with your ability to provide respectful and unbiased clinical treatment.

Seventh, avoid imposing personal beliefs or spiritual interpretations onto clients. Engage in collaborative work on religious and spiritual issues or concerns outside your scope of training and knowledge, including collaborating with religious leaders in the client's tradition. Refer clients to another provider for treatment when appropriate (Etengoff & Rodriguez, 2022; Merino et al., 2018; Plante, 2024). Finally, use best practices of intersectional, positive-growth, and strengths-based approaches to explore religious and spiritual practices and beliefs. Actively seek regular supervision, peer and expert consultation, and continuing education to support spiritually integrated treatment skills (Plante, 2024; Snodgrass, 2019; Vieten et al., 2013).

CHAPTER SUMMARY

In this chapter we highlighted a variety of important issues for members of the TNB community, their significant others, friends, family, and supporters, as well as those in the religious and spiritual communities with which they are affiliated. There is a need for additional research to understand the role and impact of religion and spirituality in the lives of TNB people. There is an urgent need to incorporate TNB people's religious and spiritual beliefs and practices into the therapeutic work they are engaged in right now to increase relevance and holistic support of this community. It is important that MHPs recognize and explore the effects of religion and spirituality in the lives of TNB people and normalize their involvement or their desire to be involved in religious or spiritual communities and practices.

REFERENCES

Ai, A. L., Bjorck, J. P., Appel, H. B., & Huang, B. (2013). Asian American spirituality and religion: Inherent diversity, uniqueness, and long-lasting psychological influences. In K. I. Pargament, J. J. Exline, & J. W. Jones (Eds.), *APA handbook of psychology, religion, and spirituality: Vol. 1. Context, theory, and research* (pp. 581–598). American Psychological Association. https://doi.org/10.1037/14045-032

American Counseling Association. (2010). Competencies for counseling with transgender clients. *Journal of LGBT Issues in Counseling, 4*(3–4), 135–159. https://doi.org/10.1080/15538605.2010.524839

American Psychological Association. (2015). Guidelines for psychological practice with transgender and gender nonconforming people. *American Psychologist, 70*(9), 832–864. https://doi.org/10.1037/a0039906

Ansloos, J., Zantingh, D., Ward, K., McCormick, S., & Bloom Siriwattakanon, C. (2021). Radical care and decolonial futures: Conversations on identity, health, and spirituality with Indigenous Queer, trans, and two-spirit youth. *International Journal of Child, Youth & Family Studies, 12*(3–4), 74–103. https://doi.org/10.18357/ijcyfs123-4202120340

Appleton, N. (2011). In the footsteps of the Buddha? Women and the bodhisattva path in Theravada Buddhism. *Journal of Feminist Studies in Religion, 27*(1), 33–51. https://doi.org/10.2979/jfemistudreli.27.1.33

Balsam, K. F., Huang, B., Fieland, K. C., Simoni, J. M., & Walters, K. L. (2004). Culture, trauma, and wellness: A comparison of heterosexual and lesbian, gay, bisexual, and Two-Spirit Native Americans. *Cultural Diversity & Ethnic Minority Psychology, 10*(3), 287–301. https://doi.org/10.1037/1099-9809.10.3.287

Bauer, G. R., Scheim, A. I., Pyne, J., Travers, R., & Hammond, R. (2015). Intervenable factors associated with suicide risk in transgender persons: A respondent driven sampling study in Ontario, Canada. *BMC Public Health, 15*(1), 525. Advance online publication. https://doi.org/10.1186/s12889-015-1867-2

bautista, d., Mountain, Q., & Reynolds, H. M. (2014). Religion and spirituality. In L. Erickson-Schroth (Ed.), *Trans bodies, trans selves: A resource for the transgender community* (pp. 62–79). Oxford University Press.

Beagan, B. L., & Hattie, B. (2015). Religion, spirituality, and LGBTQ identity integration. *Journal of LGBT Issues in Counseling, 9*(2), 92–117. https://doi.org/10.1080/15538605.2015.1029204

Blakemore, E. (2019). *What is colonialism? The history of colonialism is one of brutal subjugation of Indigenous peoples*. National Geographic. https://www.nationalgeographic.com/culture/article/colonialism

Boppana, S., & Gross, A. M. (2019). The impact of religiosity on the psychological well-being of LGBT Christians. *Journal of Gay & Lesbian Mental Health, 23*(4), 412–426. https://doi.org/10.1080/19359705.2019.1645072

Campbell, C. L., & Catlett, L. (2019). Silent illumination: A case study exploring the spiritual needs of a transgender-identified elder receiving hospice care. *Journal of Hospice and Palliative Nursing, 21*(6), 467–474. https://doi.org/10.1097/NJH.0000000000000596

Campbell, M., Hinton, J. D. X., & Anderson, J. R. (2019). A systematic review of the relationship between religion and attitudes toward transgender and gender-variant people. *International Journal of Transgenderism, 20*(1), 21–38. https://doi.org/10.1080/15532739.2018.1545149

Cragun, R. T., & Sumerau, J. E. (2015). The last bastion of sexual and gender prejudice? Sexualities, race, gender, religiosity, and spirituality in the examination of prejudice toward sexual and gender minorities. *Journal of Sex Research, 52*(7), 821–834. https://doi.org/10.1080/00224499.2014.925534

Curling, D., Barnes, C., & Forbes, J. R. (2020). Religion, spirituality, and counseling psychology. In M. Olufunmilayo Adekson (Ed.), *Handbook of counseling and counselor education* (pp. 153–167). Routledge. https://doi.org/10.4324/9781351164207

Davies-Cole, M. E., & Robinson, M. (2022). Berdache to Two-Spirit and beyond. In M. Walter, T. Kukutai, A. A. Gonzales, & R. Henry (Eds.), *The Oxford handbook of Indigenous sociology* (pp. 450–463). Oxford University Press. https://doi.org/10.1093/oxfordhb/9780197528778.013.27

Driskill, Q.-L., Finley, C., Gilley, B. J., & Morgensen, S. L. (Eds.). (2011). *Queer indigenous studies: Critical interventions in theory, politics, and literature*. University of Arizona Press. https://uapress.arizona.edu/book/queer-indigenous-studies

Etengoff, C., & Rodriguez, E. M. (2022). "At its core, Islam is about standing with the oppressed": Exploring transgender Muslims' religious resilience. *Psychology of Religion and Spirituality, 14*(4), 480–492. https://doi.org/10.1037/rel0000325

Garroutte, E. M., Beals, J., Anderson, H. O., Henderson, J. A., Nez-Henderson, P., Thomas, J., Croy, C., Manson, S. M., & the AI-SUPERPFP Team. (2014). Religiospiritual participation in two American Indian populations. *Journal for the Scientific Study of Religion, 53*(1), 17–37. https://doi.org/10.1111/jssr.12084

Gearing, R. E., & Alonzo, D. (2018). Religion and suicide: New findings. *Journal of Religion and Health, 57*(6), 2478–2499. https://doi.org/10.1007/s10943-018-0629-8

Gibbs, J. J., & Goldbach, J. (2015). Religious conflict, sexual identity, and suicidal behaviors among LGBT young adults. *Archives of Suicide Research, 19*(4), 472–488. https://doi.org/10.1080/13811118.2015.1004476

Gilley, B. (2006). *Becoming Two-Spirit: Gay identity and social acceptance in Indian country*. University of Nebraska Press.

Ginicola, M. M., Filmore, J. M., & Stokes, M. (2017). Working with LGBTQI+ clients who have experienced religious and spiritual abuse using a trauma-informed approach. In M. M. Ginicola, C. Smith, & J. M. Filmore (Eds.), *Affirmative counseling with LGBTQI+ people* (pp. 329–342). American Counseling Association. https://doi.org/10.1002/9781119375517.ch24

Ginicola, M. M., Furth, B. H., & Smith, C. (2017). The role of religion and spirituality in counseling the LGBTQI+ client. In M. M. Ginicola, C. Smith, & J. M. Filmore (Eds.), *Affirmative counseling with LGBTQI+ people* (pp. 297–312). American Counseling Association. https://doi.org/10.1002/9781119375517.ch22

Golub, S. A., Walker, J. J., Longmire-Avital, B., Bimbi, D. S., & Parsons, J. T. (2010). The role of religiosity, social support, and stress-related growth in protecting against HIV risk among transgender women. *Journal of Health Psychology, 15*(8), 1135–1144. https://doi.org/10.1177/1359105310364169

Grossman, A. H., Park, J. Y., & Russell, S. T. (2016). Transgender youth and suicidal behaviors: Applying the interpersonal psychological theory of suicide. *Journal of Gay & Lesbian Mental Health, 20*(4), 329–349. https://doi.org/10.1080/19359705.2016.1207581

Harris, K. A., Howell, D. S., & Spurgeon, D. W. (2018). Faith concepts in psychology: Three 30-year definitional content analyses. *Psychology of Religion and Spirituality, 10*(1), 1–29. https://doi.org/10.1037/rel0000134

Haselby, S. (2019, May 29). *Europeans came to Asia not as conquerors but as customers.* Aeon. https://aeon.co/essays/europeans-came-to-asia-not-as-conquerors-but-as-customers

Hendricks, M. L., & Testa, R. J. (2012). A conceptual framework for clinical work with transgender and gender nonconforming clients: An adaptation of the Minority Stress Model. *Professional Psychology: Research and Practice, 43*(5), 460–467. https://doi.org/10.1037/a0029597

Herman, J. L., Flores, A. R., & O'Neill, K. K. (2022). *How many adults and youth identify as transgender in the United States?* [Data Set]. Williams Institute, UCLA School of Law. https://williamsinstitute.law.ucla.edu/publications/trans-adults-united-states/

Hodge, D. R., & Limb, G. E. (2010a). Conducting spiritual assessments with Native Americans: Enhancing cultural competency in social work practice courses. *Journal of Social Work Education, 46*(2), 265–284. https://doi.org/10.5175/JSWE.2010.200800084

Hodge, D. R., & Limb, G. E. (2010b). A Native American perspective on spiritual assessment: The strengths and limitations of a complementary set of assessment tools. *Health & Social Work, 35*(2), 121–131. https://doi.org/10.1093/hsw/35.2.121

Hopwood, R. A. (2022). Approaching intersections of spirituality, religion, and nontraditional gender identities in psychotherapy. In S. J. Sandage & B. D. Strawn (Eds.), *Spiritual diversity in psychotherapy: Engaging the sacred in clinical practice* (pp. 223–248). American Psychological Association. https://doi.org/10.1037/0000276-010

Irwin, L. (1997). Freedom, law, and prophecy: A brief history of Native American religious resistance. *American Indian Quarterly, 21*(1), 35–55. https://doi.org/10.2307/1185587

James, S. E., Herman, J. L., Rankin, S., Keisling, M., Mottet, L., & Anafi, M. (2016). *The report of the 2015 U.S. Transgender Survey.* National Center for Transgender Equality. http://www.transequality.org/sites/default/files/docs/USTS-Full-Report-FINAL.PDF

Jones, P. N. (2005). The American Indian Church and its sacramental use of peyote: A review for professionals in the mental-health arena. *Mental Health, Religion & Culture, 8*(4), 277–290. https://doi.org/10.1080/13674670412331304348

Jones, R. P., Jackson, N., Orcés, D., & Huff, I. (2021). *The 2020 PRRI census of American religion* [Research survey report]. Public Religion Research Institute. https://www.prri.org/wp-content/uploads/2021/07/PRRI-Jul-2021-Religion.pdf

Jones, T. W., Power, J., & Jones, T. M. (2022). Religious trauma and moral injury from LGBTQA+ conversion practices. *Social Science & Medicine, 305*, 115040. https://doi.org/10.1016/j.socscimed.2022.115040

Kaldera, R. (2009). *Hermaphrodeities: The transgender spirituality workbook*. Asphodel Press.

Kapitan, A., & Kapitan, L. (2023). Language is power: Anti-oppressive, conscious language in art therapy practice. *International Journal of Art Therapy*, 1–9. https://doi.org/10.1080/17454832.2022.2112721

Karpen, S. C. (2018). The social psychology of biased self-assessment. *American Journal of Pharmaceutical Education, 82*(5), 6299. https://doi.org/10.5688/ajpe6299

Khaleeli, H. (2014, April 16). Hijra: India's third gender claims its place in law. *The Guardian*. http://www.theguardian.com/society/2014/apr/16/india-third-gender-claims-place-in-law

Khalid, H. (2021, Apr. 13). *How colonialism eroded Pakistan's history of religious fluidity*. Al Jazeera. https://www.aljazeera.com/features/2021/4/13/how-colonialism-eroded-pakistans-history-of-religious-fluidity

Khatri, S. (2017). Hijras: The 21st century untouchables. *Washington University Global Studies Law Review, 16*(2), 387–410.

Kidwell, C. S., Noley, H., & Tinker, G. E. (2002). *A Native American theology*. Orbis Books.

Kim, D. W. (Ed.). (2018). *Colonial transformation and Asian religions in modern history*. Cambridge Scholars Publishing.

Lang, S. (1998). *Men as women, women as men: Changing gender in Native American cultures* (J. L. Vantine, Trans.). University of Texas Press.

Lang, S. (2016). Native American men-women, lesbians, Two-Spirits: Contemporary and historical perspectives. *Journal of Lesbian Studies, 20*(3–4), 299–323. https://doi.org/10.1080/10894160.2016.1148966

Laxman, S. (2022, November 25). *Two-Spirit and Hijra: The common stories uniting us*. Indiaspora. https://www.indiaspora.org/features/two-spirit-and-hijra-the-common-stories-uniting-us

Levy, D. L., & Lo, J. R. (2013). Transgender, transsexual, and gender queer individuals with a Christian upbringing: The process of resolving conflict between gender identity and faith. *Journal of Religion & Spirituality in Social Work, 32*(1), 60–83. https://doi.org/10.1080/15426432.2013.749079

Limb, G. E., & Hodge, D. R. (2008). Developing spiritual competency with Native Americans: Promoting wellness through balance and harmony. *Families in Society, 89*(4), 615–622. https://doi.org/10.1606/1044-3894.3816

Lipka, M., & Tevington, P. (2022). *Attitudes about transgender issues vary widely among Christians, religious 'nones' in U.S.* Pew Research Center. https://www.pewresearch.org/short-reads/2022/07/07/attitudes-about-transgender-issues-vary-widely-among-christians-religious-nones-in-u-s/

Longo, J., Walls, N. E., & Wisneski, H. (2012). Religion and religiosity: Protective or harmful factors for sexual minority youth? *Mental Health, Religion & Culture, 16*(3), 273–290. https://doi.org/10.1080/13674676.2012.659240

Madrigal-Borloz, V. (2023, June 21). *Freedom of religion or belief not incompatible with equality for LGBT persons: UN expert* [Press release: Special procedures]. United Nations Human Rights Office of the High Commissioner. https://www.ohchr.org/en/press-releases/2023/06/freedom-religion-or-belief-not-incompatible-equality-lgbt-persons-un-expert

McFadden, S. H., Frankowski, S., Flick, H., & Witten, T. M. (2013). Resilience and multiple stigmatized identities: Lessons from transgender persons' reflections on aging. In J. D. Sinnott (Ed.), *Positive psychology* (pp. 247–267). Springer. https://doi.org/10.1007/978-1-4614-7282-7_16

Merino, Y., Adams, L., & Hall, W. J. (2018). Implicit bias and mental health professionals: Priorities and directions for research. *Psychiatric Services, 69*(6), 723–725. https://doi.org/10.1176/appi.ps.201700294

Miller, K. K., Park, M., & Peterson, J. (2022, February). Colonization and the health of lesbian, gay, bisexual, transgender, queer/questioning and intersex (LGBTQI) populations: A narrative review of three case studies. *Pediatrics, 149*(1 Meeting Abstracts February 2022), 585.

Natural History Museum. (2020). *Beyond gender: Indigenous perspectives, Mapuche*. https://nhm.org/stories/beyond-gender-indigenous-perspectives-mapuche

Norwood, K. (2013). Grieving gender: Trans-identities, transition, and ambiguous loss. *Communication Monographs, 80*(1), 24–45. https://doi.org/10.1080/03637751.2012.739705

Okrey Anderson, S., & McGuire, J. K. (2021). "I feel like God doesn't like me": Faith and ambiguous loss among transgender youth. *Family Relations, 70*(2), 390–401. https://doi.org/10.1111/fare.12536

Parker, K., Horowitz, J. M., & Brown, A. (2022). *Americans' complex views on gender identity and transgender issues*. Pew Research Center. https://www.pewresearch.org/social-trends/2022/06/28/americans-complex-views-on-gender-identity-and-transgender-issues/

Parkinson, P. (2023). Gender identity discrimination and religious freedom. *The Journal of Law and Religion, 38*(1), 10–37. https://doi.org/10.1017/jlr.2022.45

Plante, T. G. (2024). *Spiritually informed therapy: Wisdom and evidence based strategies that work*. Cognella Academic Publishing.

Porter, K. E., Ronneberg, C. R., & Witten, T. M. (2013). Religious affiliation and successful aging among transgender older adults: Findings from the Trans MetLife Survey. *Journal of Religion, Spirituality and Aging, 25*(2), 112–138. https://doi.org/10.1080/15528030.2012.739988

Rabasco, A., & Andover, M. (2021). The relationship between religious practices and beliefs and suicidal thoughts and behaviors among transgender and gender diverse adults. *Psychology of Religion and Spirituality, 15*(1), 25–31. https://doi.org/10.1037/rel0000453

Ristuccia, N. J. (2013). Eastern religions and the West: The making of an image. *History of Religions, 53*(2), 170–204. https://doi.org/10.1086/673185

Rodriguez, E. M., & Follins, L. D. (2012). Did God make me this way? Expanding psychological research on queer religiosity and spirituality to include intersex and transgender individuals. *Psychology and Sexuality, 3*(3), 214–225. https://doi.org/10.1080/19419899.2012.700023

Rosenberg, R. (2017). The importance of Jewish ritual in the secular, postmodern world of *Transparent. Jewish Film & New Media, 5*(1), 75–101. https://doi.org/10.13110/jewifilmnewmedi.5.1.0075

Rosmarin, D. H., Pargament, K. I., & Koenig, H. G. (2021). Spirituality and mental health: Challenges and opportunities. *The Lancet Psychiatry, 8*(2), 92–93. https://doi.org/10.1016/S2215-0366(20)30048-1

Rothaus, S. (2014, November 21). *Transgender woman dies suddenly, presented at funeral in open casket as a man.* Miami Herald. http://www.miamiherald.com/news/local/community/gay-south-florida/article4055600.html

Sharzer, L. A., Jones, D. A., Alipour, M., & Pacha, K. J. (2020). Religious attitudes toward gender-confirming surgery. In L. S. Schechter (Ed.), *Gender confirmation surgery: Principles and techniques for an emerging field* (pp. 237–257). Springer Nature. https://doi.org/10.1007/978-3-030-29093-1_23

Singh, A. A., & McKleroy, V. S. (2011). "Just getting out of bed is a revolutionary act": The resilience of transgender people of color who have survived traumatic life events. *Traumatology, 17*(2), 34–44. https://doi.org/10.1177/1534765610369261

Smith, B., & Home, S. (2007). Gay, lesbian, bisexual and transgendered (GLBT) experiences with Earth-spirited faith. *Journal of Homosexuality, 52*(3–4), 235–248. https://doi.org/10.1300/J082v52n03_11

Smithers, G. D. (2022). *Reclaiming Two-Spirits: Sexuality, spiritual renewal & sovereignty in Native America.* Beacon.

Snodgrass, J. L. (2019). The future of spiritually integrated psychotherapy in the AAPC tradition. *The Journal of Pastoral Care & Counseling, 73*(3), 153–156. https://doi.org/10.1177/1542305019867867

Tafoya, T. (1997). Native gay and lesbian issues: The Two-Spirited. In B. Greene (Ed.), *Ethnic and cultural diversity among lesbians and gay men* (pp. 1–10). Sage.

Unitarian Universalist Association. (n.d.). *Lesbian, gay, bisexual, transgender, and queer justice.* https://www.uua.org/lgbtq

Venkatraman, S., & Yam, K. (2022, September 13). *Across generations, South and Southeast Asians reflect on colonialism's impact on identity.* NBC News. https://www.nbcnews.com/news/asian-america/generations-south-southeast-asians-reflect-colonialisms-impact-identit-rcna47092

Vieten, C., Scammell, S., Pilato, R., Ammondson, I., Pargament, K. I., & Lukoff, D. (2013). Spiritual and religious competencies for psychologists. *Psychology of Religion and Spirituality, 5*(3), 129–144. https://doi.org/10.1037/a0032699

Wilhelm, A. D. (2010). *Tritiya-Prakriti: People of the third sex: Understanding homosexuality, transgender identity, and intersex conditions through Hinduism.* Xlibris.

Witten, T. M. (2014). It's not all darkness: Robustness, resilience, and successful transgender aging. *LGBT Health, 1*(1), 24–33. https://doi.org/10.1089/lgbt.2013.0017

Yüksel, Ş., Aslantaş Ertekin, B., Öztürk, M., Bikmaz, P. S., & Oğlağu, Z. (2017). A clinically neglected topic: Risk of suicide in transgender individuals. *Nöro Psikiyatri Arşivi, 54*(1), 28–32. https://doi.org/10.5152/npa.2016.10075

Zinnbauer, B. J. (2013). Models of healthy and unhealthy religion and spirituality. In K. I. Pargament, A. Mahoney, & E. P. Shafranske (Eds.), *APA handbook of psychology, religion, and spirituality: Vol. 2. An applied psychology of religion and spirituality* (pp. 71–89). American Psychological Association. https://doi.org/10.1037/14046-004

15

TRANS AND NONBINARY PARTICIPATION IN PHYSICAL ACTIVITIES, COMPETITIVE SPORTS, AND PHYSICAL EDUCATION CLASSES

JOHN GLEAVES, MATT ENGLAR-CARLSON, AND MAX USMAN

For many, the success of collegiate swimmer Lia Thomas, an openly trans woman, in the spring of 2022 drew their attention to trans and nonbinary (TNB) people taking part in competitive sports, organized exercise spaces, and physical education classes.[1] Thomas's success coincided with two other factors that helped generate significant media attention. First, the International Olympic Committee, the highest governing body in international sport, had just implemented significant reforms to its policies governing TNB athletes that afforded greater freedoms to each sport to set their own TNB eligibility policies. Second, a growing number of legislative efforts, both in the United States and around the world, had turned TNB participation into "a politicized issue," according to trans athlete Chris Mosier (Block, 2022).[2] Unfortunately, instead of heralding Thomas's success as the culmination of many historical

---

[1] What we will collectively refer to as physical activities unless otherwise noted.

[2] At the time of this chapter's publication, the Trump Administration signed an executive order designed to prevent transgender athletes from participating in girls' or women's sports in the United States. Though not the focus of this chapter, that action illustrates the sociopolitical nature of trans and nonbinary participation in physical activities, competitive sports, and physical education classes. Actions like this are significant and highlight the need for mental health professionals to advocate for their trans and nonbinary clients, but more importantly, to engage in public advocacy to combat falsehoods about this topic.

https://doi.org/10.1037/0000471-016
Affirmative Counseling and Psychological Practice With Trans and Nonbinary Clients, Second Edition, A. Singh and R. McCullough (Editors)
Copyright © 2026 by the American Psychological Association. All rights reserved.

efforts to protect sport and physical activity as a human right *and* encourage TNB participation in physical activities, some far-right groups planned and fueled contentious and politically divisive conversations and legislation that amplified inaccuracies about TNB communities in sports using anti-TNB tropes (e.g., that TNB athletes won because of "unfair advantages" and TNB athlete participation would result in a lack of "safety" for cisgender women). The focus on TNB people in competitive sport across the media spectrum, thus, fell upon entrenched political lines, dominating discussion, while the health focus on physical activity was minimized and TNB human rights to participate in sports was intentionally erased (Barnes, 2023).

As we have seen recently, this politicization has intensified—shaping conversations about TNB participation in physical education classes, as well as TNB access to grassroots sports participation and elite sport competitions. Most of this rhetoric has focused on removing TNB access to physical activities, with lesser efforts seeking to protect TNB people's rights to participate. While trans athlete Renée Richards was under scrutiny in the 1970s for her participation in professional tennis, discussions over TNB rights to physical activity was not part of a "political culture war," according to Jason Pierceson, a political science professor at the University of Illinois Springfield, in an interview with National Public Radio (Kurtzleben, 2021). For instance, it was not until the 2010s that a series of bills designed to regulate TNB access to bathrooms and locker rooms was followed by efforts to regulate TNB participation in sports and physical activities based on designated sex at birth (ibid).

The success of several higher profile TNB athletes drew increased media attention which resulted in wider public awareness, although there was often misinformation from the media about their participation and the far right seized on this increased media attention, using it to magnify the anti-TNB tropes noted earlier (Thorpe et al., 2023). A survey of the politicization of TNB sport found that "the issue of [TNB] inclusion in sport (a subset of legislative efforts against [TNB] people) has escalated a form of symbolic politics which is as much about partisan contestation as it is about addressing a perceived problem" (Harris et al., 2023, p. 757). At the same time, several countries and states in the United States have made efforts to protect TNB rights in physical activity and sports. However, the politicization of TNB sports has made the climate for TNB participation inconsistent across geographic locations, resulting in some neighboring states and school districts having conflicting positions on the issue.

This divisive political climate has also negatively affected TNB participation in physical activities. For example, many TNB persons report the politicized landscape has increased their avoidance of participating in physical activity due to fear of discrimination, harassment, and concern for their safety (Pérez-Samaniego et al., 2019), even when TNB persons have laws protecting their participation rights. Moreover, frequent revisions to international and national sporting policies by sporting organizations between 2015 and 2023 have made TNB participation rights precarious with new policies sometimes taking effect weeks or days before contests, leaving TNB athletes fearing whether they can continue participating (Ivy, 2023). Mental health providers (MHPs) should be aware of the negative effects this politicized environment have on TNB client's perceptions and experience of physical activity.

In this chapter, we draw attention to important questions regarding TNB participation in physical activities and present what is currently known on the topic. This is a rapidly changing field influenced by science and politics. In this way, we hope to separate the needs, challenges, and issues of TNB people from some of the public discourse over physiological fairness, designated sex categories, and locker room access. Many of the answers to our questions are partial. There simply is not room to go in depth on facets of the topic. At other times, partial answers are due to limited TNB-affirmative scholarship, focusing specifically on physical activities. Moreover, the chapter mostly focuses on topics beyond the inclusion of TNB athletes in elite competitions because even though elite sport often dominates the headlines, those issues relate to a small percentage of TNB people and a small percentage of people overall engaging in physical activities (Ivy, 2021; Gleaves & Lehrbach, 2016). Instead, the chapter's focus on recreational sport, exercise gyms, group fitness settings, and physical education classes reflects the overwhelming evidence discussed throughout this chapter supporting the health benefits of physical activity as well as the need for assisting clients in creating exercise habits that have biopsychosocial benefits. For some, that might include elite sport, but for most it does not. In that spirit, this chapter includes discussion about the experiences and needs of TNB people in the many areas of meaningful physical activity spaces. As such, the chapter takes an affirmative approach to TNB participation in physical activities across age ranges and ability levels.

GENDER AS PART OF SPORT AND PHYSICAL ACTIVITY

Historically, sport and physical activity has reinforced society's notions about femininity and masculinity. This is particularly true when examining the influence of Anglo-European culture on the development of modern sport culture. Historian Allan Guttmann (1994) documents how modern sport not only takes shape in the 18th century, but also reflects much of British culture's hegemonic feminine and masculine norms of this time. Gender roles were strictly defined and enforced, with men being expected to embody strength, courage, and physical prowess, while women were relegated to the domestic sphere and viewed as physically and emotionally fragile. Sport and physical activity (or the lack thereof) provided spaces for developing and demonstrating these attributes. The limited opportunities available for women to participate in sports and physical activities reflected the dominant view that sport was essentially a masculine preserve, making women's participation in sports deemed inappropriate. Boys and men were encouraged to participate in sport as training to develop traditional "masculine" traits required for military service, political office, or leadership. Failure to sufficiently display masculine qualities in sporting spaces threatened men's status (Harrow, 2016).

While women fought for greater opportunities to participate in sports in the late 19th and early 20th centuries, White, patriarchal gender stereotypes and expectations continued to be reinforced through sports. "Women's" sports were often limited to activities that were seen as more "feminine," such as gymnastics, figure skating, and synchronized swimming, while "men's" sports were focused on more "masculine" activities, such as football, boxing, and weightlifting (Cahn, 2015). Athletes were often prevented from violating these norms through formal policies, and those who tried faced discouragement or social sanctions. This gender reinforcement continued well into the 20th century, with enforced, strict gender segregation and limiting opportunities for women to compete and excel in sports (Schultz, 2014).

In the 21st century, there is an effort to dismantle these narrow notions of masculinity and femininity. Sports and physical activity reside within a contextual space, thus societal biases and deeply held notions about gender are reflected in sporting realms. These tacit biases shape people's attitudes and experiences in sport, from participants to coaches, referees, spectators, and even the authorities who operate gyms, recreational sporting leagues, and youth community sports. The greater contextual biases about gender—and sexuality—in different sport settings impacts engagement and participation. For example, sport has shown greater tolerance towards lesbian women, while gay men still face negative consequences if they openly acknowledge their sexuality during their sporting careers (Schultz, 2018). Such residual biases continue to shape norms and attitudes within contemporary sport culture, whether it relates to weightlifting at a local community center or competing in the Olympic Games (Barnes, 2023).

Societal biases around race are also pervasive and intersect with gender. World athletics has attempted to regulate women's bodies since women began participating in elite sports (Pieper, 2016). Scholars have noted that historic associations of White, hegemonic femininity foster the conditions under which women of color are more scrutinized (Cooky & Dworkin, 2013; Pieper, 2014). Instead of being celebrated, the historic triumphs of Black female athletes, such as Millie McDaniel, Willye White, and Wilma Rudolph often reinforced stereotypes of Black women being less feminine than White women (Pieper, 2016). For women of color, mainly from the Global South, racism has played a prominent role as they have endured more gender verification testing, such as being investigated for high levels of naturally occurring testosterone (Karkazis & Jordan-Young, 2020).

When considering the experiences of TNB persons in sport and physical activity, such historical biases about gender act in complex ways. One person may have experienced sport in a negative way while being identified in their gender assigned at birth, while another person may have had positive experiences. For example, a TNB person assigned female at birth may have enjoyed how sports permitted them to move their body, get dirty, or display traditionally "masculine" traits not allowed in other areas of their life, where social expectations required more "feminine" gender performances; TNB persons assigned male at birth may have found the expectations for traditionally "masculine" displays of aggression or competitiveness in sport off-putting and received social censure for disliking such activities. On the other hand, the very reason that one person had negative views or positive views may change after socially or medically transitioning (Elling & d'Escury, 2017; Elling-Machartzki, 2017). A person assigned female at birth may have been stigmatized for their "boyish" behavior only to find that sports provide them a space to publicly display an expression of their masculinity that feels meaningful to them.

While the nuances of gendered experiences are discussed in the chapter, the important point is to understand that "traditional" notions of masculine and feminine behavior often shape sporting spaces encountered by TNB persons. Some TNB people may enjoy physical activity or consider sports as places they flourish and others may not. These experiences may relate both to participation in physical activities as a TNB person, but also to their past experiences participating in physical activities as their gender assigned at birth. Thus, it is important to consider physical activities in a gender-affirming context, while keeping in mind the historical ways that sport, physical education, and physical activity have defined and reinforced traditional gendered narratives. For MHPs working with TNB persons, the key takeaway is that there are often much deeper layers beyond just participating in physical activities and sports. TNB people often must confront their own ingrained biases about gender and sport, while at the same time navigating the ingrained biases of others who share the sporting or physical activity arena. Further, many TNB people have to manage transphobic, homophobic, and racist social contexts while negotiating gender dysphoria, all while enduring the onslaught of anti-TNB legislation that attacks the rights, bodies, and existence of TNB people (Williams et al., 2023).

THE IMPORTANCE OF PHYSICAL ACTIVITIES FOR TRANS AND NONBINARY PERSONS

Physical activity is vital for health and well-being across the lifespan of all people, including TNB communities. Regular exercise offers various benefits such as improved physical and mental health, better cognitive performance, increased social skills, and the establishment of healthy habits (Singh et al., 2012). The benefits of regular exercise may be especially pronounced for TNB adults as it can mitigate health disparities overrepresented in TNB adults (James et al., 2016). For example, Streed et al. (2021) found that TNB adults experience cardiovascular health disparities likely caused by the experience of significant social stressors such as experiences of discrimination or harassment and possible side effects from the use of gender-affirming hormone therapy. Physical activity helps maintain a healthy weight, reduces the risk of heart disease, diabetes, and cancer, and improves cardiovascular health, blood pressure, and cholesterol levels (Katzmarzyk et al., 2019). Moreover, Mücke et al. (2018) showed in a systematic review that physical activity reduces the cardiovascular impact of social stressors associated with TNB cardiovascular health disparities. Thus, for TNB persons, the benefits of physical activity may be more pronounced if they were experiencing elevated social stressors (Reisner et al., 2015). Additionally, the World Professional Association for Transgender Health noted this kind of physiopsychosocial approach to health care has notably favorable outcomes when treating TNB populations in their *Standards of Care for the Health of Transgender and Gender Diverse People* (Coleman et al., 2022). The examination of the lives of TNB people through a social lens provides a better picture of what health looks like for them.

For TNB youth and adolescents, physical activity can reduce many of the noted physical and mental health disparities (Veale et al., 2017; Williams et al., 2023). Exercise boosts mood and cognitive function in youth by improving attention span and academic performance (Hillman et al., 2008). Group activities and sports help youth in developing social and communication skills, leadership, and teamwork (Eime et al., 2013), though failure to prevent discrimination and harassment of TNB youth in physical activity spaces may reduce these benefits. It is important to not only prevent TNB discrimination in sports, but to also actively reach out and include TNB youth in sports and group activities—especially because many narratives around TNB participation in sports focus on TNB discrimination (Taha-Thomure et al., 2022). Additionally, the perception of sports and athletics is that there are little to no inclusive and comfortable environments for TNB people (Jones et al., 2017).

Finally, engaging in physical activity at a young age is also linked to greater enjoyment of exercise and a commitment to staying active throughout adulthood, while maintaining lifelong healthy habits (Carson et al., 2016). Such benefits are vital as TNB youth have reduced engagement in physical activity when compared to peer groups and closing the physical activity gap between TNB youth and their peer groups can promote better health outcomes earlier in life (Bishop et al., 2020; Jones et al., 2018). However, Bishop et al. (2020) recommends that for TNB youth, physical activity behaviors should be adjusted based on gender identity and gender identity subgroups. A challenge in creating new spaces for TNB people to engage in physical activity can be the underlying disparity felt by TNB people who want to engage in team-based activities. Sports and physical activity are often key to the social development of young people. When TNB people are unable to participate in sports and physical activity because of environmental or social barriers, their social development can become altered. This altering of social development can be a threat to the ongoing mental health of young TNB people. See Chapters 9 and 10 for further discussion of TNB children and adolescents.

Regarding mental health disparities, Haas et al. (2014) noted TNB adults showed higher rates of depression, anxiety, and suicidality reported compared to cisgender adults. However, physical activity is a natural mood booster that reduces stress, anxiety, and depression and improves cognitive function, memory, and self-esteem. Exercise also increases energy levels, productivity, focus, and concentration; improves sleep quality; and reduces the risk of falls and injuries. Engaging in regular exercise can help adults lead longer, healthier lives with a better quality of life, so it is crucial for TNB older adults (55 and older) as it offers numerous benefits that address the TNB physical and mental health disparities (Zelle & Arms, 2015).

Trans and Nonbinary Embodiment and Physical Activity

Physical activities play an important role in connecting people's sense of self to their physical body. Indeed, the human body serves as the core of our lived experiences and sense of self. The phenomenological body of work by Maurice Merleau-Ponty (2004) remains especially helpful on this point. Merleau-Ponty explains the body is not merely an object one possesses, or a tool one uses, but rather an integral part of one's subjective experience. Through our lived body, we actively engage with our surroundings, making sense of the world through embodied actions, sensations, and perceptions. The role of physical activity is especially pronounced when it comes to developing the link between self, the lived body, and experiences of gender. Works by Iris Marion Young have suggested that physical activities not only allow people to experience their gendered body's capacities, but also provide performative platforms where people display these capacities in public settings, shaped by dominant gendered discourses and structures (Young, 1980, 2002). Such experiences play into what Gleaves (2017) has called "meaningful narratives," which allow people to both define and identify with themselves and others through shared physical activity. Meaningful narratives combine the inward subjective sense of self and the outward performance of self through embodied physical performances. An example of this could be a TNB athlete who identifies as male playing in a sport where their physical prowess is not only praised by their teammates, but also becomes part of the athlete's own identity because they are recognized by peers as a physically strong man.

This complex interplay between embodied subjectivity and the management of gendered bodies becomes even more salient within the TNB community (Torres et al., 2022). The significance of adopting an embodied approach when considering the TNB experience lies in the ongoing process of how individuals come to understand and identify with their own gender, which is shaped by their lived experiences and interactions with their bodies starting at birth (Fausto-Sterling, 2021). Moon (2019) has explored how the embodied experience shapes the affective interpellation of TNB identity and "being" their identity. This connection between one's body and identity is particularly pronounced in TNB youth, as their bodily development not only influences how they interact with the outside world, but also shapes their interpretations of internal signals forming their awareness of their own bodies (Langer, 2019). Several researchers, such as Durwood et al. (2017) and Olson et al. (2016), have stressed the importance of delving into the bodily experiences of TNB people, with a focus on the phenomenological perspective rather than solely on emotional or biological aspects. Their findings indicate that changes related to affirming a body that aligns with one's felt gender identity can have profound positive psychological effects and help to counteract internalized stigma.

Thus, physical activities provide additional benefits for TNB persons since such activities provide a wide array of embodied experiences. For example, Elling-Machartzki (2017) concluded that "the body-self narratives also indicated that [physical activity and sport] had been important enabling and empowering activities at different times in the lives of transgender people" (p. 256). In particular, Elling-Machartzki (2017) noted that TNB people often identified physical activities as a source of coping strategy in the pretransition phase as well as supporting body-subject awareness, gender recognition, and pride in their body-self.

COMMON EXPERIENCES AND UNIQUE CHALLENGES

TNB people report some common experiences in physical activity, but there are also significant differences that are important to recognize. One common experience is that TNB people describe facing barriers and challenges in accessing physical activity spaces, especially while transitioning (Jones et al., 2017). The same is true with TNB youth and adolescent participation (Storr et al., 2022). This can include feeling uncomfortable or unsafe in gender-segregated facilities, experiencing discrimination or harassment, being required to wear uniforms or athletic wear that may signify gender, or feeling like they do not belong in traditional gendered sports and activities (Hargie et al., 2017; Jones et al., 2017). So even when a TNB person has a strong desire to participate, concerns over potential future access persist. Moreover, the rise in anti-TNB legislation restricting access to facilities, teams, and activities has increased this anxiety for TNB persons (Dhanani & Totton, 2023).

Another common experience is the desire to align their physical abilities with their gender identity (Pérez-Samaniego et al., 2019). Elling-Marchartzki (2017) explained that TNB persons engaging in physical activity or sport often share a concern that others will perceive a disconnect between their displayed physical performances and their desired gender identity. This disconnect between congruent internal experience and external perception can be balanced with increased embodiment from participation. However, this is not always the case for many TNB people and athletes. For example, people assigned male at birth may have mixed feelings about their muscle mass or aerobic capacity during transition in competitions against women. While such features may help in sport competitions, it can also alienate them from their competitors and bring unfair scrutiny to their participation. Trans men may seek to increase muscle mass and strength to achieve a level of competition with their peers, though trans men who have achieved high levels of sporting success prior to transition have shown that such parity is closer than many in society may believe. Additionally, nonbinary people can often feel that the adherence to a gendered sport may devalue or negate their identity in the eyes of others regardless of their assigned gender (Murawsky, 2023).

However, there are also significant differences in the experiences of TNB persons in physical activity. One major source of difference is people's experience of physical activity as pretransition youth performing in their gender assigned at birth. Evidence by Elling-Machartzki (2017) indicated that TNB persons assigned male at birth often reported more negative memories of physical education classes in school and being less active in physical activities or organized sports as boys and young men. This may be due to the traditionally masculine cultural meaning assigned to athletics previously discussed in this chapter. People assigned male at birth who develop an awareness of their own gender identity at a young age may experience a dissonance between their identity and the cultural pressure put on them in spaces of physical education. According to Elling-Machartzki (2017), "Such narratives were more often told by trans women about their youth as boys. They commonly recalled negative memories of physical education classes in school and had not been very active in [physical activity and sport] as boys and young men" (p. 261). Elling-Marchartzki quoted from a trans woman who explained, "Before my transition, I never participated in sports. You need some kind of self-respect, which I absolutely didn't have" (p. 261). Such quotes illustrate the negative influences of social norms, sports, and peers on TNB experiences in physical activity.

On the other hand, TNB people assigned female at birth exhibited a heightened prevalence of positive recollections surrounding their early engagement in physical activities, particularly concerning embodiment and self-esteem. It is noteworthy that trans men frequently express a greater inclination for participating in sports during their childhood, particularly favoring "boys' sports" such as football, while harboring a strong disapproval towards activities typically associated with girls, including rhythmic gymnastics and sports that enforce gender-specific clothing regulations. These differences in experiences of physical activities pretransition effectively demonstrate the conventional role of sports in relation to the construction of masculine identity and differentiation from femininity as discussed previously (Elling-Machartzki, 2017). This illustrates the impact that cultural values and gender norms associated with physical activity can have on TNB people even pretransition and precognizance of their identity.

Following transition, trans women may face greater barriers to participation due to societal expectations about femininity as well as the beliefs that cisgender women are less physically capable and require protection (McClearen, 2022). Trans women encounter barriers to participation, such as exclusion based on discriminatory policies or practices specifically applied in women's sports related to perceived concerns about fairness and competitive advantage, as well as safety in contact sports (Cleland et al., 2022). Additionally, trans women may confront social stigma, prejudice, and discrimination within sports settings, which they report impact their overall well-being and enjoyment of the activities (Jones et al., 2017).

Trans men may face less of these societal expectations, but still experience barriers due to their gender identity or discrimination based on their perceived biological sex (Jones et al., 2017). Trans men have a range of experiences and feelings about sports and physical activity, just like any other group of people. However, Caudwell (2014) explained that there are some common experiences and concerns that trans men may face when it comes to sports and physical activity. Many trans men report feeling more comfortable participating in sports and physical activity after they begin hormone therapy and undergo physical changes that align with their gender identity. For example, trans men who take testosterone may experience an increase in muscle mass, which can help them feel more confident and capable in sports. On the other hand, some trans men may feel uncomfortable participating in sports and physical activity due to concerns about their appearance or being misgendered. Many sports have gender-segregated teams and facilities, which can be difficult for trans men who do not feel comfortable in either male or female spaces. Additionally, trans men may experience discrimination or harassment in sports and physical activity settings which can make it difficult for them to feel safe and included, which can lead to anxiety, fear, and avoidance of these activities (Caudwell, 2014).

To conclude, it is important to note the research (Elling & d'Escury, 2017; Jones et al., 2017) indicating that the experiences of TNB people in physical activity can vary widely depending on their individual circumstances, such as their level of physical ability, access to supportive communities, and personal preferences and interests. In summary, while trans men and women may share some common experiences in physical activity, it is important to recognize the unique challenges and opportunities faced by individuals of all gender identities and work towards creating safe, inclusive, and welcoming physical activity spaces for everyone.

INTERSECTIONALITY IN TRANS AND NONBINARY ENGAGEMENT IN PHYSICAL ACTIVITIES

In the realm of physical activity, sports, and physical education, Whiteness is still the dominant culture. Simon et al. (2022) noted that this becomes a barrier because the experiences of TNB people are deeply intertwined with intersectionality. Intersectionality plays a crucial role in shaping the unique challenges and barriers TNB people face. Herrick and Duncan (2018) found that past experiences with sport and physical education are largely dominated by instances of heterosexism, and that one's identity as a woman or as a person of color become further areas of discrimination in the sporting settings. They noted the complexity of experiences that emerged when intersecting and overlapping minority identities encountered systems of oppression (i.e., cissexism, dominant masculinity, etc.) in sporting settings. Harassment, bullying, and exclusion from sports and physical activity can be common.

For TNB people of color, the journey in physical activity and sport is often marked by a complex interplay of gender identity and racial or ethnic identity. The interlocking oppressions of racism and trans prejudice can exacerbate disparities in access to resources, acceptance, and representation. For example, Black and Hispanic TNB athletes frequently contend with not only transprejudice, but also systemic racism, which can manifest in reduced opportunities, increased scrutiny, and a lack of culturally competent support within sports settings. The case of CeCé Telfer, the first openly trans woman to win a National Collegiate Athletic Association track and field championship exemplifies this. Telfer's journey underscores the compounded difficulties of being a Black trans woman athlete, where she faced not only anti-TNB bias, but also racism (Brassil, 2021). The intersection of these multiple minoritized identities can lead to a heightened vulnerability to mental health struggles, as TNB people of color navigate a sports culture that historically prioritizes cisgender and White narratives. For instance, consider the story of Schuyler Bailar, the first openly trans NCAA Division I swimmer. Bailar's experience highlights not just the challenges faced by a TNB athlete, but also the nuances added by his identity as an Asian American (Freeman, 2024). His experiences shed light on the intersectional hurdles, including both transprejudice and racial stereotyping, that athletes like him must navigate.

The narrative shifts slightly when considering different racial and ethnic groups within TNB communities. Asian American and Indigenous TNB athletes often face unique cultural stigmas and stereotypes that can influence their sports experiences in distinct ways. In addition to transprejudice, Asian American TNB athletes may grapple with lowered expectations and stereotypes about being good at academics but not sports, while Indigenous TNB athletes might confront a lack of visibility and representation in mainstream sports culture. These varied experiences underscore the need for MHPs to adopt a nuanced and intersectional approach when addressing the needs of TNB people of color. See Chapter 6 for a more in-depth discussion of the experiences of TNB people of color.

CHALLENGES FOR TRANS AND NONBINARY PERSONS' ENGAGEMENT IN PHYSICAL ACTIVITIES

Physical activities are not only important for people's well-being but may also warrant particular focus for TNB persons. TNB youth face several barriers to physical activity, including social isolation, harassment, discrimination, and a lack of safe spaces to engage in physical activity. Gender-segregated sports and locker rooms can also be problematic for TNB youth who may not feel comfortable in either male or female spaces (Elling-Machartzki, 2017). Additionally, many TNB youth may experience body dysphoria or discomfort with their physical appearance, which can make engaging in physical activity a challenge. These barriers can prevent TNB youth from receiving the physical and mental health benefits of regular exercise and lead to a higher risk of health problems later in life as discussed previously. Finally, the hegemonic hypermasculinity common in competitive sporting cultures may contribute to a sense of isolation or disconnect from the social norms surrounding such activities, leading some TNB individuals to not engage in these activities. So, while competitive sports may be a bastion of social acceptance for some TNB athletes, it can also exacerbate feelings of alienation and isolation. These experiences are particularly foundational in adolescence as social acceptance and positive peer relationships are integral to TNB mental well-being (Tankersley et al., 2021).

For youth and adolescents, becoming or staying involved in physical activity is often difficult. Two studies have shown that TNB populations tend to have significantly less voluntary involvement in physical activities such as school sports or extracurricular activities than their cisgender peers (Aparicio-García et al., 2018; Bishop et al., 2020). Evidence indicates the disparity in physical activity may stem from TNB youth feeling unsafe or uncomfortable in environments that typically segregate along gender (Greenspan et al., 2019). Additionally, TNB youth may have received, witnessed, or feared discrimination and hostile behavior when using locker rooms or gender-segregated athletic facilities, especially considering the increasing amount of discriminatory legislation aimed at restricting TNB students' participation in school sports teams or their access to public spaces such as locker rooms and bathrooms (Kulick et al., 2019). Indeed, the *2019 National School Climate Survey* measuring the experiences of LGBTQ youth noted as a key finding that school administrators were "often preventing or discouraging students from participating in school sports because they were LGBTQ" (Kosciw et al., 2020, p. 39).

The gap in participation and barriers to access are particularly problematic for this age range as physical activity behaviors formed during adolescence significantly influence physical activity throughout adulthood. Evidence indicates that the amount of engagement in physical activity during adolescence is a significant predictor of physical activity levels later in adulthood (Huotari et al., 2011). Thus, preventing or discouraging TNB youth from engaging in physical activity is likely to have significant negative impacts on their wellness and lifespan.

To address these barriers, Williams et al. (2023) suggest MHPs talk with TNB youth about their current and past experiences in physical activity and engagement as a way to uncover insights that may impact their engagement or lack thereof. This conversation could open a dialogue about how gender identity development, transprejudice, and the binary nature of much physical activity and sporting settings influence participation. Importantly, this conversation can help TNB youth reengage with activities that were once enjoyable and healthy. If a TNB youth is not currently, nor in the past, engaged in physical activity, this can be a "change" conversation to help the youth adopt healthy and protective habits to manage stress. Williams et al. (2023) provide a matrix of activities and inquiries for MHPs to promote physical activity with clients and advocate for reducing barriers for TNB youth in community settings.

TNB adults also face several barriers to physical activity including discrimination, lack of access to appropriate facilities, and concerns about safety and visibility. For TNB people, discrimination can make it difficult to access traditional physical activity spaces. Many gyms, sports teams, and fitness classes may not be welcoming to TNB people or may not have policies in place to protect them from discrimination or harassment. TNB adults may also face a lack of access to appropriate facilities, such as locker rooms and restrooms. Many gyms and fitness centers have gender-segregated locker rooms, which can be uncomfortable or unsafe for TNB individuals. TNB adults may avoid physical activity due to concerns about accessing facilities.

Safety and visibility are also major concerns for TNB adults who want to engage in physical activity. TNB individuals may be at a higher risk of harassment or violence, both in public spaces and in physical activity environments. Additionally, many TNB people may not feel comfortable being visible while engaging in physical activity due to concerns about their appearance or being misgendered. The idea of embodiment of one's gender becomes much more salient when participating in physical activity. TNB people have to reconcile outward perception of others and the internal experience of their body being used in a physical space. Some TNB athletes competing in their gender assigned at birth struggle with feeling like their bodies cannot conform to their internal experience of gender because of their participation in athletics. Some athletes may feel pressure to delay transitioning until after their careers are completed and must find ways to cope with their gender dysphoria. For nonathletes, the barriers often prevent TNB adults from receiving the physical and mental health benefits of regular exercise and can lead to a higher risk of health problems later in life. It is essential to create safe and inclusive spaces for TNB individuals to engage in physical activity, including policies that protect against discrimination and harassment, gender-neutral facilities, and supportive staff and trainers.

PROMOTING TRANS- AND NONBINARY-AFFIRMING PHYSICAL ACTIVITY SPACES

For MHPs, being a sound advocate for TNB people to participate in physical activity and sport extends beyond the office. Being an advocate for TNB people requires the creation of inclusive physical activity spaces for TNB clients through intentional efforts to promote safety, comfort, and respect for all participants. It also requires that MHPs work with TNB clients to find the types of activities that they resonate with. MHPs also have a duty to support TNB clients as they go through the learning process of finding physical activities that they don't resonate with and how their relationship with their body changes. Making safety plans for going into new spaces to do physical activity and planning check-ins to go over how different activities feel to do are just the foundation of what it looks like to help these clients. In terms of advocacy, here are some examples of physical activity spaces that can be more inclusive for TNB people:

- **All-gender facilities:** Providing all-gender locker rooms, restrooms, and changing areas can create a more welcoming environment for TNB people who may not feel comfortable in gender-segregated spaces.
- **Inclusive policies:** Establishing policies that protect against discrimination and harassment based on gender identity and expression can help ensure that TNB people feel safe and welcome in physical activity spaces.
- **Diverse programming:** Offering a variety of physical activity programs that are accessible and appropriate for individuals of all gender identities and abilities can help create a more inclusive environment.
- **Training for staff and coaches:** Providing training for staff and coaches on how to create a welcoming, affirming, and inclusive environment for TNB individuals can help ensure that they feel supported and respected in physical activity spaces. This also includes providing training on how TNB communities benefit from physical activity.

- **Challenge myths:** Challenging transprejudicial and transmisogynisitc myths and misconceptions about participation in physical activity and sport for TNB individuals, while emphasizing the importance of the physical and mental health benefits that go along with inclusive spaces that promote physical activity, can help TNB people feel welcome and understood in physical activity spaces. This advocacy can be done in personal interactions, public forums, social media, and community gatherings.
- **Partnering with LGBTQ+ organizations:** Partnering with LGBTQ+ organizations and community groups can help promote awareness and create a more inclusive environment for TNB people in physical activity spaces.

By implementing these strategies, physical activity spaces can become more welcoming and inclusive for TNB communities, helping to ensure that everyone can enjoy the physical and mental health benefits of regular exercise.

CHAPTER SUMMARY

The politicization of TNB participation in competitive sports has stoked anti-TNB attitudes that have further reduced TNB participation in broad forms of physical activity. The experiences of TNB individuals in physical activities can be marked by discrimination, harassment, and fear, making it challenging for them to engage in these activities. Such experiences occur against the backdrop of gendered stereotypes that have historically shaped sports culture and continue to influence contemporary sporting spaces. Yet physical activity is vital for everyone's health, and it can be particularly important for TNB individuals who may face health disparities. Physical activities also play a role in connecting one's sense of self to their physical body while offering a platform for individuals to express their gender identity while generating positive embodied experiences that contribute to self-awareness and pride in one's identity. Further efforts should not only focus on TNB-affirming policies in competitive sport but also include ways to make physical activity spaces more inclusive for TNB communities, implementing all-gender facilities, inclusive physical education policies, diverse programming at physical activity spaces, and partnerships with TNB organizations to promote safety, comfort, and respect in these spaces.

REFERENCES

Aparicio-García, M. E., Díaz-Ramiro, E. M., Rubio-Valdehita, S., López-Núñez, M. I., & García-Nieto, I. (2018). Health and well-being of cisgender, transgender and non-binary young people. *International Journal of Environmental Research and Public Health, 15*(10), 2133. https://doi.org/10.3390/ijerph15102133

Barnes, K. (2023). *Fair play: How sports shape the gender debate*. St. Martin's Press.

Bishop, A., Overcash, F., McGuire, J., & Reicks, M. (2020). Diet and physical activity behaviors among adolescent transgender students: School survey results. *The Journal of Adolescent Health, 66*(4), 484–490. https://doi.org/10.1016/j.jadohealth.2019.10.026

Block, M. (2022, June 29). *Americans are deeply divided on transgender rights, a poll shows*. National Public Radio. https://www.npr.org/2022/06/29/1107484965/transgender-athletes-trans-rights-gender-transition-poll

Brassil, G. (2021, June 1). 'For my people': A transgender woman pursues an Olympic dream. New York Times. https://www.nytimes.com/2021/06/01/sports/olympics/cece-telfer-olympic-trials.html

Cahn, S. K. (2015). *Coming on strong: Gender and sexuality in women's sport*. University of Illinois Press.

Carson, V., Hunter, S., Kuzik, N., Wiebe, S. A., Spence, J. C., Friedman, A., Tremblay, M. S., Slater, L., & Hinkley, T. (2016). Systematic review of physical activity and cognitive development in early childhood. *Journal of Science and Medicine in Sport, 19*(7), 573–578. https://doi.org/10.1016/j.jsams.2015.07.011

Caudwell, J. (2014). [Transgender] young men: Gendered subjectivities and the physically active body. *Sport Education and Society, 19*(4), 398–414. https://doi.org/10.1080/13573322.2012.672320

Cleland, J., Cashmore, E., & Dixon, K. (2022). Why do sports fans support or oppose the inclusion of trans women in women's sports? An empirical study of fairness and gender identity. *Sport in Society, 25*(12), 2381–2396. https://doi.org/10.1080/17430437.2021.1942456

Coleman, E., Radix, A. E., Bouman, W. P., Brown, G. R., de Vries, A. L. C., Deutsch, M. B., Ettner, R., Fraser, L., Goodman, M., Green, J., Hancock, A. B., Johnson, T. W., Karasic, D. H., Knudson, G. A., Leibowitz, S. F., Meyer-Bahlburg, H. F. L., Monstrey, S. J., Motmans, J., Nahata, L., . . . Arcelus, J. (2022). Standards of care for the health of transgender and gender diverse people, version 8. *International Journal of Transgender Health, 23*(Suppl. 1), S1–S259. https://doi.org/10.1080/26895269.2022.2100644

Cooky, C., & Dworkin, S. L. (2013). Policing the boundaries of sex: A critical examination of gender verification and the Caster Semenya controversy. *Journal of Sex Research, 50*(2), 103–111. https://doi.org/10.1080/00224499.2012.725488

Dhanani, L. Y., & Totton, R. R. (2023). Have you heard the news? The effects of exposure to news about recent transgender legislation on transgender youth and young adults. *Sexuality Research & Social Policy, 20*(4), 1–15. https://doi.org/10.1007/s13178-023-00810-6

Durwood, L., McLaughlin, K. A., & Olson, K. R. (2017). Mental health and self-worth in socially transitioned transgender youth. *Journal of the American Academy of Child & Adolescent Psychiatry, 56*(2), 116–123. e112. https://doi.org/10.1016/j.jaac.2016.10.016

Eime, R. M., Young, J. A., Harvey, J. T., Charity, M. J., & Payne, W. R. (2013). A systematic review of the psychological and social benefits of participation in sport for children and adolescents: Informing development of a conceptual model of health through sport. *The International Journal of Behavioral Nutrition and Physical Activity, 10*(1), 98. https://doi.org/10.1186/1479-5868-10-98

Elling, A., & d'Escury, K. C. (2017). Between stigmatization and empowerment: Meanings of physical activity and sport in the lives of transgender people. In E. Anderson & A. Travers (Eds.), *Transgender athletes in competitive sport* (pp. 54–67). Routledge. https://doi.org/10.4324/9781315304274-6

Elling-Machartzki, A. (2017). Extraordinary body-self narratives: Sport and physical activity in the lives of transgender people. *Leisure Studies, 36*(2), 256–268. https://doi.org/10.1080/02614367.2015.1128474

Fausto-Sterling, A. (2021). A dynamic systems framework for gender/sex development: From sensory input in infancy to subjective certainty in toddlerhood. *Frontiers in Human Neuroscience, 15*, 613789. https://doi.org/10.3389/fnhum.2021.613789

Freeman, M. (2024, March 29). Schuyler Bailar is fighting for trans representation in swimming. *USA Today.* https://www.usatoday.com/story/sports/2024/03/29/schuyler-bailar-trans-swimmer-athlete-harvard/72295645007/

Gleaves, J. (2017). Sport as meaningful narratives. *Journal of the Philosophy of Sport, 44*(1), 29–43. https://doi.org/10.1080/00948705.2017.1280407

Gleaves, J., & Lehrbach, T. (2016). Beyond fairness: The ethics of inclusion for transgender and intersex athletes. *Journal of the Philosophy of Sport, 43*(2), 311–326. https://doi.org/10.1080/00948705.2016.1157485

Greenspan, S. B., Griffith, C., & Watson, R. J. (2019). LGBTQ+ youth's experiences and engagement in physical activity: A comprehensive content analysis. *Adolescent Research Review, 4*(2), 169–185. https://doi.org/10.1007/s40894-019-00110-4

Guttmann, A. (1994). *Games and empires: Modern sports and cultural imperialism.* Columbia University Press. https://doi.org/10.7312/gutt91262

Haas, A. P., Rodgers, P. L., & Herman, J. (2014). *Suicide attempts among transgender and gender non-conforming adults: Findings of the national transgender discrimination survey.* American Foundation for Suicide Prevention.

Hargie, O. D., Mitchell, D. H., & Somerville, I. J. (2017). 'People have a knack of making you feel excluded if they catch on to your difference': Transgender experiences of exclusion in sport. *International Review for the Sociology of Sport, 52*(2), 223–239. https://doi.org/10.1177/1012690215583283

Harris, S., Jedlicka, S., Pielke Jr, R., & Ryan, H. (2023). The politics of exclusion: Analyzing US state responses to interscholastic transgender athletes. *International Journal of Sport Policy and Politics,* 1–22. https://doi.org/10.1080/19406940.2023.2242878

Harrow, S. (2016). *British sporting literature and culture in the long eighteenth century.* Routledge. https://doi.org/10.4324/9781315570303

Herrick, S. S. C., & Duncan, L. R. (2018). A qualitative exploration of LGBTQ+ and intersecting identities within physical activity contexts. *Journal of Sport & Exercise Psychology, 40*(6), 325–335. https://doi.org/10.1123/jsep.2018-0090

Hillman, C. H., Erickson, K. I., & Kramer, A. F. (2008). Be smart, exercise your heart: Exercise effects on brain and cognition. *Nature Reviews Neuroscience, 9*(1), 58–65. https://doi.org/10.1038/nrn2298

Huotari, P., Nupponen, H., Mikkelsson, L., Laakso, L., & Kujala, U. (2011). Adolescent physical fitness and activity as predictors of adulthood activity. *Journal of Sports Sciences, 29*(11), 1135–1141. https://doi.org/10.1080/02640414.2011.585166

Ivy, V. (2021). If "ifs" and "buts" were candy and nuts: The failure of arguments against trans and intersex women's full and equal inclusion in women's sport. *Feminist*

Philosophy Quarterly, 7(2). Advance online publication. https://doi.org/10.5206/fpq/2021.2.10726

Ivy, V. (2023). Trans women are women, and sport is a human right. *Journal of Olympic Studies, 4*(2), 3–19. Advance online publication. https://doi.org/10.5406/26396025.4.2.02

James, S. E., Herman, J. L., Rankin, S., Keisling, M., Mottet, L., & Anafi, M. A. (2016). *Executive summary of the report of the 2015 U.S. Transgender Survey*. National Center for Transgender Equality.

Jones, B. A., Arcelus, J., Bouman, W. P., & Haycraft, E. (2017). Sport and transgender people: A systematic review of the literature relating to sport participation and competitive sport policies. *Sports Medicine, 47*(4), 701–716. https://doi.org/10.1007/s40279-016-0621-y

Jones, B. A., Haycraft, E., Bouman, W. P., & Arcelus, J. (2018). The levels and predictors of physical activity engagement within the treatment-seeking transgender population: A matched control study. *Journal of Physical Activity & Health, 15*(2), 99–107. https://doi.org/10.1123/jpah.2017-0298

Karkazis, K., & Jordan-Young, R. (2020). Sensing race as a ghost variable in science, technology, and medicine. *Science, Technology & Human Values, 45*(5), 763–778. https://doi.org/10.1177/0162243920939306

Katzmarzyk, P. T., Powell, K. E., Jakicic, J. M., Troiano, R. P., Piercy, K., Tennant, B., Committee, P. A. G. A. (2019). Sedentary behavior and health: Update from the 2018 physical activity guidelines advisory committee. *Medicine and Science in Sports and Exercise, 51*(6), 1227–1241. https://doi.org/10.1249/MSS.0000000000001935

Kosciw, J. G., Clark, C. M., Truong, N. L., & Zongrone, A. D. (2020). *The 2019 national school climate survey: The experiences of lesbian, gay, bisexual, transgender, and queer youth in our nation's schools. A report from GLSEN*. ERIC.

Kulick, A., Wernick, L. J., Espinoza, M. A. V., Newman, T. J., & Dessel, A. B. (2019). Three strikes and you're out: Culture, facilities, and participation among LGBTQ youth in sports. *Sport Education and Society, 24*(9), 939–953. https://doi.org/10.1080/13573322.2018.1532406

Kurtzleben, D. (2021, 11 March 2021). *Political dispute over transgender rights focuses on youth sports*. National Public Radio. https://www.npr.org/2021/03/11/974782774/political-dispute-over-transgender-rights-focuses-on-youth-sports

Langer, S. (2019). *Theorizing transgender identity for clinical practice: A new model for understanding gender*. Jessica Kingsley Publishers.

McClearen, J. (2022). "If you let me play": Girls' empowerment and transgender exclusion in sports. *Feminist Media Studies, 23*(4), 1361–1375. https://doi.org/10.1080/14680777.2022.2041697

Merleau-Ponty, M. (2004). *Maurice Merleau-Ponty: Basic writings*. Psychology Press.

Moon, I. (2019). 'Boying' the boy and 'girling' the girl: From affective interpellation to trans-emotionality. *Sexualities, 22*(1–2), 65–79. https://doi.org/10.1177/1363460717740260

Mücke, M., Ludyga, S., Colledge, F., & Gerber, M. (2018). Influence of regular physical activity and fitness on stress reactivity as measured with the trier social stress test protocol: A systematic review. *Sports Medicine, 48*(11), 2607–2622. https://doi.org/10.1007/s40279-018-0979-0

Murawsky, S. (2023). The struggle with transnormativity: Non-binary identity work, embodiment desires, and experience with gender dysphoria. *Social Science & Medicine (1982), 327*, 115953–115953. https://doi.org/10.1016/j.socscimed.2023.115953

Olson, K. R., Durwood, L., DeMeules, M., & McLaughlin, K. A. (2016). Mental health of transgender children who are supported in their identities. *Pediatrics, 137*(3), e20153223–e20153223. https://doi.org/10.1542/peds.2015-3223

Pérez-Samaniego, V., Fuentes-Miguel, J., Pereira-García, S., López-Cañada, E., & Devís-Devís, J. (2019). Experiences of trans persons in physical activity and sport: A qualitative meta-synthesis. *Sport Management Review, 22*(4), 439–451. https://doi.org/10.1016/j.smr.2018.08.002

Pieper, L. P. (2014). Sex testing and the maintenance of western femininity in international sport. *The International Journal of the History of Sport, 31*(13), 1557–1576. https://doi.org/10.1080/09523367.2014.927184

Pieper, L. P. (2016). *Sex testing: Gender policing in women's sports*. University of Illinois Press. https://doi.org/10.5406/illinois/9780252040221.001.0001

Reisner, S. L., Bradford, J., Hopwood, R., Gonzalez, A., Makadon, H., Todisco, D., Cavanaugh, T., VanDerwarker, R., Grasso, C., Zaslow, S., Boswell, S. L., & Mayer, K. (2015). Comprehensive transgender healthcare: The gender affirming clinical and public health model of Fenway Health. *Journal of Urban Health, 92*(3), 584–592. https://doi.org/10.1007/s11524-015-9947-2

Schultz, J. (2014). *Qualifying times: Points of change in us women's sport*. University of Illinois Press. https://doi.org/10.5406/illinois/9780252038167.001.0001

Schultz, J. (2018). *Women's sports: What everyone needs to know*. Oxford University Press.

Simon, M., Lee, J., Evans, M., Sucre, S., & Azzarito, L. (2022). A call for social justice researchers: Intersectionality as a framework for the study of human movement and education. *Kinesiology Review, 11*(2), 149–157. https://doi.org/10.1123/kr.2021-0009

Singh, A., Uijtdewilligen, L., Twisk, J. W., van Mechelen, W., & Chinapaw, M. J. (2012). Physical activity and performance at school: A systematic review of the literature including a methodological quality assessment. *Archives of Pediatrics & Adolescent Medicine, 166*(1), 49–55. https://doi.org/10.1001/archpediatrics.2011.716

Storr, R., Nicholas, L., Robinson, K., & Davies, C. (2022). 'Game to play?': Barriers and facilitators to sexuality and gender diverse young people's participation in sport and physical activity. *Sport Education and Society, 27*(5), 604–617. https://doi.org/10.1080/13573322.2021.1897561

Streed, C. G., Jr., Beach, L. B., Caceres, B. A., Dowshen, N. L., Moreau, K. L., Mukherjee, M., Poteat, T., Radix, A., Reisner, S. L., & Singh, V. (2021). Assessing and addressing cardiovascular health in people who are transgender and gender diverse: A scientific statement from the American Heart Association. *Circulation, 144*(6), e136–e148. https://doi.org/10.1161/CIR.0000000000001003

Taha-Thomure, R., Milne, A. S., Kavanagh, E. J., & Stirling, A. E. (2022). Gender-based violence against trans* individuals: A netnography of Mary Gregory's experience in powerlifting. *Frontiers in Psychology, 13*, 854452–854452. https://doi.org/10.3389/fpsyg.2022.854452

Tankersley, A. P., Grafsky, E. L., Dike, J., & Jones, R. T. (2021). Risk and resilience factors for mental health among transgender and gender nonconforming (TGNC) youth: A systematic review. *Clinical Child and Family Psychology Review, 24*(2), 183–206. https://doi.org/10.1007/s10567-021-00344-6

Thorpe, H., Nelson, M., Scovel, S., & Veale, J. (2023). Journalists on a journey: Towards responsible media on transgender participation in sport. *Journalism Studies, 24*(9), 1–19. https://doi.org/10.1080/1461670X.2023.2206920

Torres, C. R., Lopez Frias, F. J., & Patiño, M. J. M. (2022). Beyond physiology: Embodied experience, embodied advantage, and the inclusion of transgender athletes in competitive sport. *Sport, Ethics and Philosophy, 16*(1), 33–49. https://doi.org/10.1080/17511321.2020.1856915

Veale, J. F., Watson, R. J., Peter, T., & Saewyc, E. M. (2017). Mental health disparities among Canadian transgender youth. *The Journal of Adolescent Health, 60*(1), 44–49. https://doi.org/10.1016/j.jadohealth.2016.09.014

Williams, C. R., McKenna, J. L., Artessa, L., & Moore, L. B. M. (2023). Team effort: A call for mental health clinicians to support sports access for transgender and gender diverse youth. *Journal of the American Academy of Child & Adolescent Psychiatry, 62*(8), 837–839. https://doi.org/10.1016/j.jaac.2023.01.022

Young, I. M. (1980). Throwing like a girl: A phenomenology of feminine body comportment motility and spatiality. *Human Studies, 3*(1), 137–156. https://doi.org/10.1007/BF02331805

Young, I. M. (2002). Lived body vs gender: Reflections on social structure and subjectivity. *Ratio, 15*(4), 410–428. https://doi.org/10.1111/1467-9329.00200

Zelle, A., & Arms, T. (2015). Psychosocial effects of health disparities of lesbian, gay, bisexual, and transgender older adults. *Journal of Psychosocial Nursing and Mental Health Services, 53*(7), 25–30. https://doi.org/10.3928/02793695-20150623-04

Index

A

Academic advocacy, 63–64
Acceptance
  benefits of, 196
  caretaker and sibling, 245–246
  religious, 356
  TNB families and, 196
  TNB older adults and, 272, 283
Accessibility and physical activity, 381, 385
ACF (advocacy coalition framework), 69
ACLU (American Civil Liberties Union), 49
Activism
  client, 148–149
  effects of, 149
  history of, 25
  Indigenous, 358
  public, 272
Adoption, 134–135, 198
Adversity, 27
  navigating, 147
  responding to, 283–284
Advocacy
  agenda-setting and, 67
  client, 41
  communication and, 68
  community, 152
  crisis hotlines and, 332
  cultural competency and, 151
  defining, 57
  effective, 58–59
  empowerment and, 60
  evidence-based models for, 67–71
  framing and, 67–68, 70
  health care, 44–47
  institutional, 61–62, 150–151, 277–278
  interdisciplinary collaborative care (ICC) and, 66
  interpersonal, 150
  intersectionality and, 65
  legislative, 58, 62–63, 65
  levels of, 60, 64–65, 152
  media, 62
  networking and, 69
  professional, 62
  public engagement and, 68
  research interpretation and, 70
  sports, 386–387
  stakeholder engagement and, 70
  sustainable, 63
  TNB adolescents and, 255–256
Advocacy coalition framework (ACF), 69
AFAB (assigned female at birth), 23
Affirmation
  defining, 4
  therapeutic, 147
  trauma-informed care (TIC) and, 300
Age
  gender-affirming surgery and, 44
  gender transition and, 241
  health care access and, 42
  identity disclosure and, 196–197
Agenda-setting and advocacy, 67
Agender, 22, 164, 169
AMAB (assigned male at birth), 23
American Civil Liberties Union (ACLU), 49
American Indian Gay and Lesbian
    Conference, 358

American Psychological Association (APA) Guidelines for Psychological Practice With Transgender and Gender Nonconforming People, 20
Americn Counseling Association (ACA) Advocacy Competencies, 60–63
Anticrossdressing laws, 168
Anti-TNB attitudes
  history of, 106–107
  religion and, 351–352
  rise of, 51, 374
  sports and, 373
  TNB older adults and, 278–279
  trauma and, 297
Anti-TNB legislation
  anxiety and, 51, 58
  bad science and, 122–123
  escalation of, 150, 255
  historical, 168
  mental health providers (MHPs) and, 224
  mutual aid and, 202–203
  name changes and, 224
  negative effects of, 51
  resisting, 189
  sports and, 20–21, 374–375, 385
  suicidality and, 319–320, 323
  TNB adolescents and, 304–305
  TNB youth and, 212–214, 246
  trauma and, 304–305
Anxiety
  anti-TNB legislation and, 51, 58
  compound stress and, 119
  nonbinary (NB) individuals and, 169
  TNB individuals and, 7
APA Policy Statement on Affirming Evidence-Based Inclusive Care for Transgender, Gender Diverse, and Nonbinary Individuals, Addressing Misinformation, and the Role of Psychological Practice and Science, 51
APA Presidential Task Force on Evidence-Based Practice, 33
Ashley, Florence, 22
Assigned female at birth (AFAB), 23
Assigned male at birth (AMAB), 23
Association for Behavioral and Cognitive Therapies, 120
Asylum seekers, 48–49
Athletes
  female POC, 377
  gender diversity in, 121–122
  media coverage of TNB, 374

Autism
  emotional dysregulation and, 253
  gender-affirming hormone therapy (GAHT) and, 253
  gender dysphoria and, 118–119
  suicidality and, 319
  TNB individuals and, 245
  trans women and, 118
Autonomy
  health care, 32–33
  suicidality and, 331
  TNB youth and, 213
Awachie, Tochukwu, 25

B

Baby boomers, 270
Bad science
  anti-TNB legislation and, 122–123
  consequences of, 105–107
  history of, 105–106
  social media and, 107–108
  sports and, 121
Bailar, Schuyler, 384
Barlow, David, 120
Bassi, Aléx, 24
Bathroom bills, 48
Behavioral Risk Factor Surveillance System, 115
Biases
  anti-TNB, 19
  evaluating, 111
  experimental, 108–110
  health care, 134
  research, 112
  spiritual, 363, 366
Biden administration, 6
Bigender, 164
Binary normativity
  defining, 171
  effects of, 172
  religion and, 354–355
  resisting, 166, 177
Birth-assigned sex
  gender transition and, 242–243
  physical activity and, 382
  social dysphoria and, 243
Bissu, 167
Blockers. *See* Medical puberty blockade
Body dysphoria
  physical activity and, 385
  spirituality and, 351
Boi, 23, 164

Book bans, 213
Broaching behavior, 36, 143, 228
The Brown Boi Project, 23
Buddhism, 356
Butch, 165
Bvlbancha Collective, 141

C

Caregivers
 communal, 190
 emotional strain on, 219
 emotional support for, 220
 name changes and, 223–224
 trust and, 216
Care planning, 280–281
Chest binding, 253
Child custody evaluations, 88
Cisheteronormativity
 mental health providers (MHPs) and, 189–190
 TNB parents and, 192–193
 trauma and, 295
Cisnormativity, 104, 171
Cissexism, 104–110
Cis–trans binary, 168–169
Clustered communities, 39
Cognitive behavioral therapy (CBT), 144, 147
Collaboration
 autonomy through, 331
 client–provider, 35
 interdisciplinary, 66–67, 80–82
 medical, 94
 trauma-informed care (TIC) and, 310
The Collaborative Assessment and Management of Suicidality, 331
Colonialism
 gender binary and, 24, 167
 Indigenous communities and, 24, 137, 355–356
 spirituality and, 350–351, 355–356
Communication
 advocacy and, 68
 appropriate modes of, 95
 educating providers through, 95–96
 interdisciplinary collaborative care (ICC) and, 78, 81–82
 mental health providers (MHPs) and, 81
 TNB parents and, 196
Community
 advocacy and, 152
 building, 203
 clustered, 39
 kinship networks and, 149
 mental health providers (MHPs) and, 203
 nonbinary (NB) individuals and, 176
 online, 176–177
 resilience and, 148
 strengthening connection in, 149
Compound stress
 anxiety and, 119
 racism and, 134
 TNB adolescents and, 304
Compression of morbidity, 276
Conception, 198
Concern points, 331–332
Confidentiality
 challenges to, 39
 informed consent and, 40–41
 TNB youth and, 248–249
Consent. *See also* Informed consent
 interdisciplinary collaborative care (ICC) and, 85
 protocols for, 41
 TNB mental health clients and, 85
Continuing education, 83–84
Convenience samples, 113
Conversion therapy. *See also* Gender identity change efforts (GICE)
 criticisms of, 120
 popularity of, 120
 suicidality and, 324
Convoy Model of Social Relations, 283
Coparenting, 194–195
Correctional environments
 discrimination and, 48
 gender identity in, 7
 TNB-affirming care in, 86–87
 vulnerability and, 48
Cotransition, 195, 195–196
Counseling
 faith-based, 86
 pride and, 180–181
 spirituality and, 86, 362–363
Crisis hotlines
 advocacy and, 332
 benefits of, 151
 need for, 325
Crisis management
 interventions in, 324–326
 mental health providers (MHPs) and, 64
 preparations for, 333
 suicidality and, 328–330

Critical consciousness
    building, 27
    liberation and, 137–138
    mental health providers (MHPs) and, 149
Critical race theory, 6, 27
The Cultural Assessment for Risk of Suicide (CARS), 328
Cultural competency, 36
    advocacy and, 151
    cultural humility vs., 25
    developing, 147
    language and, 36
Cultural heritage
    estrangement from, 217
    nonbinary (NB) identity and, 179
    spiritual practices and, 346
    TNB identity and, 82–83
Cultural humility
    benefits of, 22, 25–26
    cultural competency vs., 25
    theoretical frameworks for, 27
The Cultural Theory and Model of Suicide, 328

D

Data analysis, 117
Data warehouses, 116–117
DBT, 66, 144. *See* Dialectical behavior therapy (DBT)
Deadname, 23, 224
Decolonial psychotherapy, 146–147
Demi, 164
Desisting, 222
Detransitioning, 260–261
    misconceptions about, 123, 222
    motivations for, 223
    TNB adolescents and, 260–261
    TNB youth and, 222–223
Developmental stages
    affirming care throughout, 238
    gender identity throughout, 213
    gender transition and, 217, 241–242
Diagnosis
    autism, 118, 245
    ethical considerations for, 32–33
    gender dysphoria, 32–33, 52, 96
    influences in, 34
    mental health providers (MHPs) and, 78, 137
    TNB-affirming care and, 151
    utility of, 46

Diagnostic and Statistical Manual of Mental Disorders (DSM-5-TR), 32, 46, 296
Diagnostic and Statistical Manual of Mental Disorders (DSM-III), 45
Diagnostic misclassification vs. dysphoria, 46
Dialectical behavior therapy (DBT), 66, 144
Disclosure
    intimacy and, 259
    nonverbal, 180
    situational, 180
    therapeutic alliance and, 38
    TNB parents and, 195
    unplanned, 226
Discrimination
    correctional environments and, 48
    identity-based, 48
    mental health providers (MHPs) and, 35
    minority stressors and, 190
    nonbinary (NB) individuals and, 170
Disordered eating, 169, 172, 258
Dissociation, 304
    TNB adolescents and, 258
Distal minority stressors, 307, 321
    discrimination, 170
    invalidation, 170
    misgendering, 170
    proximal vs., 35
    rejection, 170
    victimization, 170
Distraction
    coping through, 177
    gender dysphoria and, 256
    resilience and, 177
    suicide safety plans and, 329–330
Dobbs v. Jackson Women's Health Organization, 193
Documentation
    health care access and, 44–47
    identity, 43–44
    mental health provider (MHP), 43, 79, 88
    sufficient forms of, 46
Donald Trump, 6
DSM-5-TR. *See Diagnostic and Statistical Manual of Mental Disorders*
DSM-5-TR (Diagnostic and Statistical Manual of Mental Disorders), 32
DSM-III (Diagnostic and Statistical Manual of Mental Disorders), 45

E

Eating disorders, 169, 172, 258
Ecological theory, 146
Education
  continuing, 83–84
  mental health providers (MHPs) and, 47, 255–257
  sexual and reproductive health, 250–251
  social transition, 250–251
  sociopolitical, 149
  trauma-informed, 309
Educational burdening, 170–171
Educational settings
  alternative, 229
  interdisciplinary collaborative care (ICC) in, 84–86
  managing harmful, 229
  mental health providers (MHPs) and, 35–36, 229
Elections and TNB rights, 7
Embodiment
  gender euphoria and, 351
  gender roles and, 379–380
  goals for, 90, 254, 351
  physical activity and, 379–380
Emotional dysregulation
  autism and, 253
  hormone therapy (HT) and, 92
  minority stressors and, 143–144
Empathy
  facilitating, 241
  nonbinary (NB) identity and, 178
  TNB parents and, 198–199
Empowerment
  advocacy and, 60
  interdisciplinary collaborative care (ICC) and, 94
  mutual aid and, 203–204
  TNB POC, 149
  trauma and, 299
Enby, 164
End-of-life planning, 279
Environmental support, 245–246
Erikson's theory of psychological development, 278
Ethics
  mental health providers (MHPs) and, 46–48, 58, 256–258
  practical, 32–41
  professional codes of, 108–109
  responsibility to, 58

Ethnoracial Equity and Inclusion Work Group, 296
Evidence-based advocacy models, 67–71
  advocacy coalition framework (ACF), 69
  multiple streams framework (MSF), 67–68
  narrative policy framework (NPF), 68–69
  social determinants of health (SDOH) policy model, 71
  unified model of advocacy, 69–71
External distal stressors, 168–169, 307, 321

F

Factors in suicidality
  access to care, 324
  anti-TNB legislation, 319–320, 323
  conversion therapy, 324
  internalized transprejudice, 327
  medical discrimination, 326
  minority stress, 323, 326–328, 330
  perceived burdensomeness, 322
  social support, 323
  stigma, 325
  thwarted belongingness, 322
Family
  alternative structures of, 139–140
  connection to, 179
  identity disclosure and, 195–196
  mental health providers (MHPs) and, 41, 215, 218–219
  protective factors in, 196
  spirituality and, 86
  TNB youth and, 82–83
Family emergence, 199
Family planning, 197–198
  mental health providers (MHPs) and, 305
Family Resilience Framework, 283
Family support
  protective factors of, 136–137, 170
  resilience and, 136–137
  suicidality and, 323
  TNB adolescents and, 259–260
  TNB older adults and, 281
  TNB youth and, 213
Feed the Second Line, 141
Femme, 165
Fertility
  affirming care for, 94
  hormone therapy (HT) and, 92, 252
  preservation of, 251

Framing and advocacy, 67–68, 71
Free speech, 50

G

GAHT. *See* Gender-affirming hormone therapy (GAHT)
GAMST (gender-affirming medical and surgical treatment), 43, 46–47
Gatekeeping
  countering, 9–10
  health care, 10
  impact of, 275, 331
  interdisciplinary collaborative care (ICC) and, 90
Gays and Lesbians Living in a Transgender Society, 64
Gender-affirming care
  advocating for, 64–65, 68
  barriers to, 217
  embodiment in, 380
  evidence-based support for, 51
  name changes and, 223–224
  parents (of TNB individuals) and, 217–218
  regret rate for, 222–223
  role of mental health providers (MPHs) in, 90, 135, 151–152
  timing of, 213, 217–218
  TNB older adults and, 275–276
  TNB youth and, 212, 218, 255
Gender-affirming care bans
  escalation of, 255
  language and, 122
  TNB youth and, 44, 58, 201
Gender-affirming counseling
  assessments in, 246–248
  missteps in, 299–300
  spirituality in, 362–363
  TNB older adults and, 282–284
  TNB youth and, 214–217, 249
Gender-affirming hormone therapy (GAHT)
  autism and, 253
  cardiovascular effects of, 378
  emotional impacts of, 253
  medical puberty blockade and, 252
  neurodivergence and, 253
  puberty and, 243
  secondary sex characteristics and, 252–253
  TNB older adults and, 271
  TNB youth and, 240, 252–253

Gender-affirming medical and surgical treatment (GAMST), 43, 46–47
Gender-affirming surgery
  age and, 44
  letters and documentation for, 93–94
  managing expectations for, 94
  mental health providers (MHPs) and, 93–94, 254
  regret after, 123
  TNB adolescents and, 253–254
  TNB older adults and, 271
  types of, 254–255
Gender-based sport participation, 121–122
Gender binary, 9
  colonialism and, 24, 167
  Indigenous communities and, 167–168, 358
  navigating, 47–48
  origin, 167
  racism and, 167–168
Gender diversity
  antiquated use of, 20
  athlete, 121–122
  expected, 214
  history of, 167–168
  TNB scientific research and, 104
  voices of, 104
Gender dysphoria, 46
  autism and, 118–119
  definition of, 175
  diagnosing, 32–33, 52, 96
  diagnostic misclassification vs., 46
  distraction and, 256
  external causes of, 46, 175
  gender euphoria vs., 175–176
  gender incongruence and, 256–257
  internalized, 212
  puberty and, 242–244
  rejections of, 145
  safety and, 301
  spirituality and, 361
  therapeutic assessments of, 145, 247
  TNB adolescents and, 256–257
  TNB parents and, 198
  TNB youth and, 211–212
Gender essentialism, 104–105, 113
Gender euphoria
  definition of, 175, 240
  embodiment and, 351
  gender dysphoria vs., 175–176
Gender expression, 33, 106, 165

Gender fluidity
  definition of, 164
  expressions of, 22–23
  navigating, 218
Genderflux, 164
Gender history
  disclosing, 226–227
  documenting, 91
  TNB youth and, 214
Gender identity
  correctional environments and, 7
  culture-specific, 22
  disclosure of, 38
  gender modality vs., 169
  history of, 167
  Indigenous communities and, 24, 167
  legal documents and, 7, 43
  measures of, 222
  mental health providers (MHPs) and, 38
  neurodivergence and, 304
  nonbinary, 164
  parenting and, 193
  physical activity and, 381–382
  pronouns and, 22
  pronouns vs., 165
  public restrooms and, 7
  sexual orientation and, 21–22
  sexual orientation vs., 33
  spectrum of, 33
  statements of, 215
  TNB youth and, 8, 214
Gender identity change efforts (GICE), 49–50, 240
Gender incongruence
  gender dysphoria and, 256–257
  influential factors of, 241
  TNB adolescents and, 239
Genderless, 164
Gender modality, 22, 124, 169
  gender identity vs., 169
Gender nonconforming, 5, 20, 164–165
Gender norms
  athletic, 382
  breaking, 243
  cultural, 82
Gender Outlaw: On Men, Women, and the Rest of Us, 21
Gender presentation, 250
Gender privilege, 36–37
Genderqueer, 164
  identity development as, 135
  use of, 5, 23

The Gender Quest Workbook, 250
Gender roles
  challenging, 70
  embodiment and, 379–380
  essentialist view of, 104
  sports and, 376–377
  TNB adolescents and, 242–243
Gender-supportive environments, 218–219
Gender transition
  age and, 241
  birth-assigned sex and, 242–243
  developmental stages and, 217, 241–242
  nonbinary, 174
  sexual orientation and, 242–243
  TNB parents and, 198–199
Gender vs. sex, 21
General Social Survey, 115
Generational trauma
  healing, 146–147
  impact of, 297
  TNB older adults and, 275
Gerontology, 136, 270
GICE (gender identity change efforts), 49–50, 240
GLAAD LGBTQ+ Glossary of Terms, 20
Graduate training programs, 47, 65, 125
Grief, 352
  TNB older adults and, 278
Guidelines for Psychological Practice With Transgender and Gender Nonconforming People, 35

H

Harassment
  health impact of, 378
  sports and, 383–384
  trauma and, 304–305
Harm reduction, 139
Harry Benjamin International Gender Dysphoria Association, 9
Health care
  advocacy in, 44–47
  autonomy in, 32–33
  barriers to, 325–326
  bias in, 134
  collaboration in, 94
  documentation and, 44–47
  telehealth and, 80
  TNB older adults and, 273, 276
  TNB POC youth and, 244
  veterans and, 202

Health coalitions, 65
Health outcomes
  interdisciplinary collaborative care (ICC) and, 81
  physical activity and, 378–379
  racism and, 134–135
Hijra, 24, 357
Hinduism, 357
Historical memory, 6
Homelessness, 42
Homicide, 42
Homophobia and racism, 106
Hormone levels, 122
Hormone therapy (HT)
  emotional dysregulation and, 92
  fertility and, 92, 252
  informed consent and, 91–92
  Standard of Care models for, 91–92
House of Tulip, 141
Houses, 140
Hughes, Charles, 106

I

ICD-11. See *International Statistical Classification of Diseases and Related Health Problems (ICD-11)*
Identity disclosure
  age and, 196–197
  considerations for, 259
  family and, 195–196
  parenting and, 195–197
  TNB adolescents and, 259
  TNB older adults and, 271–272
  unplanned, 226
Incarceration, 42, 244
Indigenous communities
  colonialism and, 24, 137, 355–356
  gender binary and, 167–168, 358
  gender identity and, 24, 167
  lifemaps and, 365
  spirituality and, 357–359
  Western culture and, 358–359
Indigiqueer, 350
Infertility, 252
Informed consent
  confidentiality and, 40–41
  definition of, 40–41
  hormone therapy (HT) and, 91–92
  therapeutic assessment and, 47
Institutional advocacy, 61–62, 150–151, 277–278

Insurance coverage
  ban on, 51
  mental health providers (MHPs) and, 47, 96
  TNB-affirming care and, 96–97
Interdisciplinary collaborative care (ICC), 77
  advocacy and, 66
  benefits of, 34, 84
  case study in, 82–83
  client involvement in, 94
  communication and, 78, 81–82
  consent and, 85
  decentralized systems of, 79, 97
  educational settings and, 84–86
  empowerment and, 94
  gatekeeping and, 90
  health outcomes of, 81
  models of, 66, 97–98
  referral networks and, 79, 97
  release of information in, 80, 85
  TNB mental health clients and, 80–82
  TNB youth and, 92
  treatment planning and, 81
Intergenerational relationships, 282
Interjurisdictional practice, 51
Internalized stigma, 321
International Statistical Classification of Diseases and Related Health Problems (ICD-11), 32, 51, 296
Interpersonal advocacy, 150
Interpersonal-Psychological Theory of Suicide (IPTS), 322
Intersectionality, 6
  advocacy and, 65
  defining, 36
  parenting and, 190–191
  physical activity and, 383–384
  pride and, 147
  theory of, 36
  therapeutic, 143
  TNB older adults and, 273–275, 283–284
  TNB POC youth and, 228
  TNB scientific research and, 191–192
Intersex traits, 22, 303
Intimacy
  disclosure and, 259
  TNB aging and, 278–279
  trauma and, 305
Intrapersonal relationships, 150
Invalidation, 170

IPTS (Interpersonal-Psychological Theory of Suicide), 322
Iridescent Life Course Perspective, 282

J

JAMA Psychiatry, 120
Journal Article Reporting Standards (JARS), 110–111
Joy and flourishing, 8

K

Kinship networks
  alternative, 138–140
  community connection and, 149
  resilience and, 137
Knowledge ownership, 124

L

Language
  accessible, 40
  cultural competency and, 36
  evolution of, 20–21
  gender-affirming, 23, 96
  gender-affirming care bans and, 122
  gendered, 36–37
  Indigenous, 358
  masculinity and, 164
  modeling affirming, 274
  TNB-affirming care and, 25
  TNB scientific research and, 124
Legal documents
  gender identity and, 7, 43
  gender marker change on, 43–44, 88–89
Legislation
  advocacy and, 58, 62–63, 65
  anti-TNB, 6–7, 19, 104
  bathroom bills in, 48
  engaging with, 65
  storytelling in, 68–69
  TNB parents and, 193
Letters and documentation
  gender-affirming surgery and, 93–94
  protocol for writing, 93
  utility of, 46
LGBTQIA+ community, 20
Liberation
  critical consciousness and, 137–138
  defining, 137
  mutual aid and, 137–138
  oppressive ideologies and, 146
  psychology of, 6, 27
Life expectancy, 23, 278
Lifemaps and Indigenous communities, 365
Lifespan developmental theory, 200
  TNB aging and, 270

M

Māhū, 24, 167
Manualized therapies, 144
Masculinity
  language and, 164
  privilege in, 37
  sports and, 121, 376
Masculinization, 253
Media
  advocacy and, 62
  representation in, 19, 257
  TNB athletes in, 374
Medical discrimination, 170, 273, 326
Medical puberty blockade. *See* Puberty suppression
Medical transition
  nonbinary (NB) individuals and, 173–174
  social vs., 221
  TNB older adults and, 271
  TNB youth and, 229–230
Medicare, 96
  TNB older adults and, 277
Menstrual suppression, 253
Mental health provider (MHP) competencies. *See also* ACA Advocacy Competencies; Multicultural and Social Justice Counseling Competencies
  awareness of systemic oppression, 364–365
  interdisciplinary practice, 34
  liberation psychology, 137
  self-awareness, 364–365
  spirituality, 360–361
Mental health providers (MHPs). *See* Documentation, mental health provider (MHP); gender-affirming care
  allied, 84
  anti-TNB legislation and, 224
  cisheteronormativity and, 189–190
  communication and, 81
  community connection and, 203, 255–256

Mental health providers (*continued*)
  crisis management and, 64
  critical consciousness and, 149
  diagnosis and, 78, 137
  discrimination and, 35
  educational settings and, 35–36, 229
  education and, 47, 255–257
  ethics and, 46–48, 58, 256–258
  family and, 41, 215, 218–219
  family mediation, 241
  family planning and, 305
  gender-affirming surgery and, 93–94, 254
  gender identity and, 38
  historical role of, 45, 90
  insurance coverage and, 47, 96
  interdisciplinary roles of, 85–86
  managing emotions as, 220
  mutual aid and, 138, 202–203
  parents (of TNB individuals) and, 218–221, 247–250
  racial awareness in, 144
  spirituality and, 86
  suicidality and, 327
  terminology and, 25–26, 36–38
  TNB adolescents and, 238–239
  TNB identities of, 38
Mental health providers (MHPs) as gatekeepers, 59, 151
  history of, 45, 90
Meta-analyses, 111
Microaggressions
  assessment of, 307–308
  interpersonal, 323
  misgendering and, 170
  nonbinary (NB) individuals and, 170
  racialized, 134–135
Millstone Act, 122
Minority stress model, 4, 35, 176
  assessing risk and resilience with, 307
  suicidality and, 320–321, 328
Minority stressors
  definition of, 190
  discrimination and, 190
  effects of, 169, 213
  emotional dysregulation and, 143–144
  multiple, 321
  reducing, 240
  TNB adolescents and, 239
  TNB youth and, 213–214, 220
  types of, 239

Misgendering
  microaggressions and, 170
  pronouns and, 165
  responding to, 150
Misinformation, 229
Misrepresentation, 105–107
Morbidity, compression of, 276
Mortality, 278
Multicultural and Social Justice Counseling Competencies, 26
Multicultural and Social Justice Cultural Competencies, 150
Multigender, 164
Multiple streams framework (MSF), 67–68
Mutual aid
  anti-TNB legislation and, 202–203
  defining, 138
  empowerment and, 203–204
  history of, 138, 203
  liberation and, 137–138
  mental health providers (MHPs) and, 138, 202–203
  social media and, 202–203
  TNB families and, 202–203
  TNB scientific research and, 138
  types of, 141, 203–204

N

Name changes, 44
  anti-TNB legislation and, 224
  caregivers and, 223–224
  gender-affirming care and, 223–224
  TNB youth and, 223
Narrative policy framework (NPF), 68–69
National Center for Transgender Equality, 66, 88
National Health Interview Survey, 115
National Institutes of Health, 114
NC Public Facilities Privacy & Security Act (HB2), 48
Neopronouns, 165
Networking and advocacy, 69
Neurodivergence
  gender-affirming hormone therapy (GAHT) and, 253
  gender identity and, 304
  TNB youth and, 220, 245
Neuroscience, 113–114
Neutrois, 164
1993 Archives of Sexual Behavior, 107
Nonbinary gender identification marker, 44

Nonbinary (NB) identity
    cultural heritage and, 179
    definition of, 164
    empathy and, 178
    strengths of, 178–181
    trans vs., 168, 172
    victimization and, 170, 173
Nonbinary (NB) individuals
    anxiety and, 169
    community connection in, 176
    discrimination and, 170
    educational burdening of, 170
    medical transition and, 173–174
    mental health in, 169
    microaggressions and, 170
    misconceptions about, 171–173
    parenting and, 191
    proximal minority stressors and, 168
    psychological stress and, 169
    resilience and, 176–178
    social support and, 170
    stereotypes of, 172

O

Oedipal complex, 107
Older Americans Act, 276–277
Online communities, 177
Oppressive ideologies
    evading, 136, 137
    liberation and, 146
    TNB scientific research and, 104
Overdiagnosis, 171

P

Parenting
    definition of, 192
    gender identity and, 193
    identity disclosure and, 195–197
    intersectionality and, 190–191
    nonbinary (NB) individuals and, 191
    TNB joy and, 201
    TNB scientific research and, 191–192
Parents (of TNB individuals)
    counseling for, 219–220, 249–250
    gender-affirming care and, 217–218
    harassment of, 250
    managing expectations of, 220
    mental health providers (MHPs) and, 218–221, 247–250

pronouns and, 225–226
reactions from, 216
therapeutic alliance and, 260
TNB-affirming care and, 200–201
Passing, 24, 259
Paternalism, 59
Pathologization
    behavioral, 144
    gender identity, 45–46, 50
    rejection of, 120
PCC. *See* Person-centered care (PCC)
P&ENM (polyamorous and ethically nonmonamous) parenting, 191–192
Personal identity
    developing, 135
    pride in, 147–148
    social transition and, 221–222
Person-centered care (PCC), 275
    models of, 282–284
PFLAG National Glossary, 20
Phalloplasty, 254
Physical activity. *See also* Sports
    accessibility and, 381, 385
    advocacy in, 386–387
    birth-assigned sex and, 382
    body dysphoria and, 385
    embodiment through, 379–380
    gender-affirming practices in, 387–388
    gender identity and, 381–382
    health outcomes and, 378–379
    intersectionality in, 383–384
    TNB adolescents and, 385–386
    TNB POC experiences with, 384–385
    TNB-specific benefits of, 380–381
Pioneer Network, 275
Policy advocacy coalitions, 69
Policy change frameworks, 67–68
Political negotiation, 69
Polyamorous and ethically nonmonogamous (P&ENM) parenting, 191–192
Polycule, 194
Positionality statements, 112
Posttraumatic stress disorder (PTSD), 296–297
    assessing, 306–307
Power dynamics
    interlocking, 65–66
    relationships and, 38
    religious, 351
    therapeutic, 302

Preferred Reporting Items for Systematic
    Reviews and Meta-Analyses
    (PRISMA), 111
Pregnancy, 198
Pride
    counseling and, 180–181
    cultivating, 147
    generation of, 270
    identity, 136, 147–149
    intersectionality and, 147
    resilience and, 177
    TNB POC communities and, 136, 146
Primary care, 89
    interdisciplinary, 94–96
Professional ethics codes, 108–109
Pronouns, 165–166
    changing, 166
    correcting, 225
    gender identity and, 22
    gender identity vs., 165
    gender-neutral, 165
    misgendering and, 165
    neo-, 165
    parents (of TNB individuals) and, 225–226
    privacy concerns with, 166
    sharing, 166
    singular, 225–226
    they/them, 165–166
    TNB youth and, 224–225
    using multiple, 165
Proximal minority stressors. *See
    also* Minority stress
    distal vs., 173
    examples of, 307
    nonbinary (NB) individuals and, 168
Psychological stress, 50
    nonbinary (NB) individuals and, 169
    TNB POC rates of, 134
Psychopathia Sexualis, 106
PSYPACT, 80
PTSD. *See* Posttraumatic stress disorder (PTSD)
Puberty
    gender-affirming hormone therapy
        (GAHT) and, 243
    gender dysphoria and, 242–244
    social transition and, 221
    Tanner Stage 2 of, 221
    TNB adolescents and, 239
Puberty suppression
    gender-affirming hormone therapy
        (GAHT) and, 252
    mental health outcomes of, 242
    suicidality and, 212, 240, 324
    TNB adolescents and, 242
    TNB youth and, 92, 242
Public accommodations, 42, 47–48
Public engagement, 68
Public engagement and advocacy, 68
Public restrooms
    access to, 63, 170, 386
    gender identity and, 7
    privacy concerns in, 48
Public spaces
    gendered experiences in, 380
    safety in, 42, 386
    TNB families and, 204

Q

Qualitative research, 112–113
Quantitative research, 113
Queen, 24
Queer, 23
Queer time, 200–201

R

Racism
    compound stress and, 134
    effects of, 42
    gender binary and, 167–168
    health outcomes and, 134–135
    homophobia and, 106
    sports and, 384
    TNB mental health clients and, 27
    TNB POC youth and, 227–228
Rapid Onset Gender Dysphoria (ROGD),
    119–120
Referral networks
    gatekeeping, 10
    interdisciplinary collaborative care (ICC)
        and, 79, 97
    TNB-affirming care, 51
Refugees, 48–49
Rejection
    behavioral responses to, 174
    existential, 352
    expectations of, 321
    gender-related, 170
    religious, 348–349, 359
Relationships
    child–parent, 88, 198–199
    counselor–caregiver, 216–217
    intergenerational, 282
    intrapersonal, 150
    multiple and dual, 38–40, 191

power dynamics and, 38
social, 136
Release of information (ROI), 39, 41, 80
Religion
  anti-TNB attitudes and, 351–352
  binary normativity in, 354–355
  defining, 346
  Eastern, 355–356
  oversimplification of, 353–354
  psychological harm from, 348–349
  role of the body in, 351
  spirituality vs., 347
  suicidality and, 319
  TNB POC communities and, 350
  TNB scientific research and, 348–350
  Western culture and, 349, 353
Reminiscent therapy (RT), 280
Renaming and TNB parents, 194
Reproductive health and TNB older adults, 278–279
Research, bias in, 112
Research interpretation and advocacy, 70
Resilience
  assessing for, 179
  community and, 148
  cultivating, 4, 148
  defining, 136, 148
  distraction and, 177
  factors of, 136
  family support and, 136–137
  kinship networks and, 137
  nonbinary (NB) individuals and, 176–178
  points of therapeutic intervention for, 148
  pride and, 177
  resistance through, 136–137, 148–149
Resilience theory, 4, 27
Retransition. *See* Detransition
Retraumatization, 81
Reyna, 24
Richards, Renée, 122, 374
ROGD (Rapid Onset Gender Dysphoria), 119–120
ROI. *See* Release of information (ROI)
RT (reminiscent therapy), 280

S

Sacred, 346
Safety
  assessment of, 298
  gender dysphoria and, 301
  school, 229

social support and, 301–302
trauma-informed care (TIC) and, 300–301, 309
travel, 195
validating concerns for, 47–48
SAPCs (Social Aid and Pleasure Clubs), 141
SDOH (social determinants of health) policy model, 71
Secondary data sources, 115–118
Secondary sex characteristics
  development of, 238
  diversity in, 121
  gender-affirming hormone therapy (GAHT) and, 252–253
Self-harm, 257–258
Sex. *See also* Secondary sex characteristics
  birth-assigned, 242–243
  definition of, 21
  gender vs., 21
  religious definition of, 351–353
Sex and Gender: The Transsexual Experiment, 106
Sexual orientation
  defining, 21
  gender identity and, 21–22
  gender identity vs., 33
  gender transition and, 242–243
Sexual Orientation and Gender Identity Module, 115
Sexual orientation change efforts (SOCE), 50
Social acceptance
  advocating for, 69
  alternative sources of, 138–139
  sports and, 385
Social aid and pleasure clubs (SAPCs), 141
Social determinants of health (SDOH) policy model, 71
Social dysphoria and birth-assigned sex, 243
Social media
  bad science on, 107–108
  influence of, 119, 249
  mutual aid and, 202–203
  representation on, 177
Social rejection, 212
Social support
  nonbinary (NB) individuals and, 170
  safety and, 301–302
  suicidality and, 323–324, 329
  TNB older adults and, 281–282
  trauma and, 301–302
  trauma-informed care (TIC) and, 310

Social transition
  assessing readiness for, 226
  benefits of, 221–222, 227
  definition of, 221
  medical vs., 221
  personal identity and, 221–222
  puberty and, 221
  risks of, 227
  steps of, 250
  TNB POC youth and, 227–228
Sociological frameworks, 308
Soul wound, 297
Spirituality
  affirming, 360–361
  bias in, 363, 366
  body dysphoria and, 351
  clinical assessment of, 362–363, 366
  colonialism and, 350–351, 355–356
  counseling and, 86, 362–363
  defining, 346
  family and, 86
  gender-affirming counseling and, 362–363
  gender dysphoria and, 361
  Indigenous communities and, 357–359
  mental health providers (MHPs) and, 86, 360–361
  reclaiming, 359
  rejection from, 348
  religion vs., 347
  suicidality and, 359
  treatment planning and, 362
  well-being and, 148, 347–348
Spiritual practices
  benefits of, 346
  cultural heritage and, 346
  denial of access to, 352
  negative outcomes of, 348–349
  strategies for integrating, 365–366
  therapeutic application of, 347, 363–364
  therapeutic assessment and, 361–363
Sports. *See also* Physical activity
  advocacy in, 386–387
  anti-TNB attitudes and, 373
  anti-TNB legislation and, 20–21, 374–375, 385
  bad science and, 121
  cultural history of, 375–376
  gender diversity and, 121–122
  gender roles in, 376–377
  harassment and, 383–384
  masculinity and, 121, 376

  racism and, 384
  social acceptance and, 385
  testosterone and, 122, 383
  TNB exclusion from, 121–122, 373–374
  TNB students and, 385
  trans men and, 383–384
  trans women and, 382–383
  violence and, 386
  visibility and, 386
  vulnerability and, 384
Stakeholder engagement and advocacy, 70
Standard of Care (SOC) model for hormone therapy, 91–92
Standards of Care for the Health of Transgender and Gender Diverse People, 378
Standards of Care, Version 8, 214
Stealth, 259
Stigma
  identities and, 33
  internalized, 321
Stoller, Robert, 106
Strength-based counseling, 179–180
Stress. *See* Compound stress; external distal stressors; minority stress model; minority stressors
Stud, 23
Substance use, 7
Suicidality. *See also* Factors in suicidality
  anti-TNB legislation and, 319–320, 323
  autism and, 319
  autonomy and, 331
  conversion therapy and, 324
  crisis management and, 328–330
  facilitating disclosure of, 327, 330–331
  family support and, 323
  mental health providers (MPHs) and, 327
  minority stress model and, 320–321, 328
  protective factors from, 323–324, 327–329, 331
  puberty suppression and, 212, 240, 324
  religion and, 319
  social support and, 323–324, 329
  spirituality and, 359
  therapeutic interventions for, 257–258, 331–332, 333
  TNB individuals and, 7, 317
  TNB older adults and, 279
  TNB POC communities and, 318
  veterans and, 319, 330

Suicide safety plans, 327–329
    client autonomy in, 331
    distraction and, 329–330
    effectiveness of, 328
    engagement with, 331
    steps of, 329–330
    TNB-affirming, 329–330
Symbolic politics, 68
Systemic authority, 137

T

Telehealth
    health care access and, 80
    interstate, 51, 202
    veterans and, 80
Telfer, CeCé, 384
Terminology
    changes in, 22
    cultural competence through, 36
    gender expansive, 218
    medicalized, 20
    mental health providers (MHPs) and, 25–26, 36–38
    problematic, 24
    resources for learning, 20
    TNB POC, 23
The Terms Paradox, 21
Testosterone
    naturally occurring, 377
    side effects of, 253
    sports and, 122, 383
Theories
    critical race, 27
    ecological, 146
    intersectionality, 27, 36, 65–66
    liberation psychology, 27
    resilience, 27
Therapeutic age of consent, 40
Therapeutic alliance
    disclosure and, 38
    parents (of TNB individuals) and, 260
    TNB POC communities and, 143
    TNB youth and, 216, 249
    trauma and, 302
    trust and, 309
Therapeutic assessment
    gender dysphoria and, 145, 247
    informed consent and, 47
    instruments of, 248–249
    intersectional, 214
    parent sessions in, 247

spiritual practices and, 361–363
    steps of, 247
    systems perspective in, 247
    TNB youth and, 214, 248–249
Therapeutic interventions
    anti-oppressive, 145
    goals of, 221
    individualized, 221
    outdated, 45
Therapy
    affirmation in, 147
Thick trust capital, 139–140
    vulnerability and, 139
Thomas, Lia, 373–374
303 Creative LLC v. Elenis, 193
TIC. *See* Trauma-informed care (TIC)
Time-of-transitioning, 241–242, 271–272
Title IX, 6, 64
TNB adolescents
    advocacy and, 255–256
    anti-TNB legislation and, 304–305
    compound stress in, 304
    detransitioning and, 260–261
    dissociation and, 258
    family support and, 259–260
    gender-affirming surgery and, 253–254
    gender dysphoria and, 256–257
    gender incongruence and, 239
    gender roles and, 242–243
    identity disclosure and, 259
    mental health providers (MHPs) and, 238–239
    minority stressors and, 239
    nonsurgical services for, 255
    physical activity and, 385–386
    puberty and, 239
    puberty suppression and, 242
    strengths of, 240
    unique experience of, 238–239
TNB-affirming care
    age limitations in, 44
    autonomy in, 32–33
    challenges to, 95
    clinical care guidelines for, 43
    competency in, 27, 95
    contentious attitudes towards, 43
    correctional environments and, 86–87
    criminalization of, 51
    definition of, 4–5
    diagnosis and, 151
    empirical support for, 33
    ethical issues within, 32–41

TNB-affirming care (*continued*)
  evidence-based practices in, 33
  growth in, 25–28
  historical models of, 90–91
  history of, 45
  improvements in, 90
  insurance and, 96–97
  interdisciplinary, 10, 47
  language and, 25
  parents (of TNB individuals) and, 200–201
  positive outcomes of, 45–46, 51
  reducing barriers to, 151
  referral networks in, 51
  scrutiny of, 50–51
  sociopolitical context around, 50–51
  suicide safety plans in, 329–330
  training opportunities in, 97
  trauma-informed, 49
TNB aging
  intimacy and, 278–279
  lifespan developmental theory and, 270
  medical violence in, 306
TNB communities
  anxiety in, 7
  familiarity with, 19
  generational differences in, 24
  health disparities in, 379–380
  homelessness in, 42
  homicide rates in, 42
  incarceration rates in, 42
  organizers in, 12
  overdiagnosis in, 171
  persecution of, 48
  physical activity in, 379–380
  substance use in, 7
  surgical intervention rates in, 43
  trauma rates in, 295
TNB families
  acceptance and, 196
  communication in, 196
  continuity in, 196
  counseling for, 204
  empathy in, 198–199
  health care access for, 197
  lifespan development in, 200
  mutual aid and, 202–203
  protective factors in, 196–197
  public spaces and, 204
TNB identity
  benefits of, 240
  cultural heritage and, 82–83

  disclosure of, 195–197
  essentializing, 114
  medicalization of, 105–106
  mental health provider (MHP), 38
  misrepresentation of, 105–106
  models of, 300
  pathologization of, 171
  pride in, 240
TNB individuals
  additional stressors of, 35
  advocating for, 41
  anxiety and, 7
  autism and, 245
  incarcerated, 42
  life expectancy of, 278
  population size of, 269
  suicidality and, 7, 317
  tropes of, 9
TNB joy
  centering, 302, 320
  parenting and, 201
  TNB scientific research and, 12
TNB leadership, 125
TNB mental health clients
  consent and, 85
  identities of, 8–9
  interdisciplinary collaborative care (ICC) and, 80–82
  racism and, 27
  relationships among, 39
  social identities of, 42
TNB older adults
  acceptance and, 272, 283
  advocating for, 274
  anti-TNB attitudes and, 278–279
  concerns of, 271–272
  family support and, 281
  gender-affirming care and, 275–276
  gender-affirming counseling and, 282–284
  gender-affirming hormone therapy (GAHT) and, 271
  gender-affirming surgery and, 271
  generational trauma and, 275
  grief and, 278
  health care and, 273, 276
  identity disclosure and, 271–272
  intersectionality and, 273–275, 283–284
  medical transition and, 271
  Medicare and, 277
  POC, 273
  reproductive health and, 278–279

social support and, 281–282
suicidality in, 279
supportive roles of, 269
time-of-transitioning in, 271–272
trauma-informed care (TIC) and, 275
victimization of, 275–276
visibility and, 270
TNB parents
  cisheteronormativity and, 192–193
  communication and, 196
  disclosure and, 195
  empathy and, 198–199
  family protective factors in, 196
  gender dysphoria and, 198
  gender transition and, 198–199
  legislation and, 193
  renaming and, 194
  transitioning, 198–199
  uplifting, 192
  visibility and, 190
TNB POC-affirming counseling
  broaching behavior in, 143
  diagnostic conceptualization in, 144
  goals of, 145
  liberatory approaches to, 143–149
  oppressive constructs in, 143
  treatment planning and, 145–147
TNB POC communities
  compounded inequities in, 134–136
  counseling approaches in, 143
  physical activity in, 191–192
  pride and, 136, 146
  psychological stress in, 134
  religion in, 350
  suicidality in, 318
  supportive interventions for, 146
  terminology in, 23
  therapeutic alliance and, 143
  TNB scientific research and, 135
  trauma in, 295
  violence and, 134–135
TNB POC youth
  harassment rates in, 244
  health care access and, 244
  intersectionality and, 228
  mental health outcomes of, 244
  racism and, 227–228
  resilience factors for, 245
  social transition and, 227–228
TNB scientific research
  bias in, 112
  crisis intervention in, 324–325

deficit-based approaches to, 135
evaluating, 111
gender diversity and, 104
history of, 106
intersectionality in, 191–192
language and, 124
misrepresentations of findings in, 108
mutual aid and, 138
oppressive ideologies and, 104
overgeneralizations of, 107–108
parenting and, 191–192
process-oriented approach to, 104, 124
qualitative, 112–113
quantitative, 113
recommendations for, 123–125
recruiting for, 113, 124
religion and, 348–350
sampling in, 114, 116
study design in, 191
TNB joy and, 12
TNB POC communities and, 135
trauma and, 296
underfunding of, 105
TNB students
  nonbinary, 168
  sports and, 385
  supporting, 36, 58
  threats to, 224
TNB youth
  anti-TNB legislation and, 212–214, 246
  autonomy in, 213
  confidentiality and, 248–249
  detransitioning and, 222–223
  family and, 82–83
  family support and, 213
  gender-affirming care and, 212, 218, 255
  gender-affirming care bans and, 44, 58, 201
  gender-affirming counseling and, 214–217, 249
  gender-affirming hormone therapy (GAHT) and, 240, 252–253
  gender dysphoria in, 211–212
  gender history and, 214
  gender identity and, 8, 214
  improving quality of life for, 240
  interdisciplinary collaborative care (ICC) and, 92
  medical transition and, 229–230
  mental health outcomes for, 212
  minority stressors and, 213–214, 220
  name changes and, 223

TNB youth (*continued*)
  needs of, 211–212
  neurodivergence and, 220, 245
  pronoun usage and, 224–225
  puberty suppression and, 92, 242
  social transitions in, 221, 226–227
  supporting, 40, 85–86
  therapeutic alliance and, 216, 249
  therapeutic assessment and, 214
  therapeutic relationships for, 216
  victimization and, 303–304
Tokenism, 112–113
Tolerance, 357
Top surgery. *See* Masculinization
Trans, 5, 168
Trans feminine, 165
Transgender resilience intervention model (TRIM), 176
Transgenero, 24
Trans Hub Language, 20
Trans Lifeline, 332
Trans Lifeline Glossary, 20
Trans masculine, 165
Transmedicalism, 117
Trans men in sports, 383–384
Trans Metlife Survey, 350
Transprejudice
  effects of, 240
  internalized, 307
  racialized, 227
  resisting, 3, 199
  trauma and, 297
Transsexualism, 45
Trans women
  autism in, 118
  caregiving in, 190
  dysphoria in, 243
  sports and, 382–383
  violence and, 42, 295
Trauma
  anti-TNB attitudes and, 297
  anti-TNB legislation and, 304–305
  assessment of, 306–308
  cisheteronormativity and, 295
  coping with, 304–305
  developmental impact of, 303–304
  empowerment and, 299
  examples of TNB, 294–295
  harassment and, 304–305
  healing from, 296–302
  intergenerational, 297
  intersectional sources of, 306

  intersex experience with, 303
  intimacy and, 305
  long-term effects of, 296
  multiple definitions of, 293
  social support and, 301–302
  sociopolitical influences on, 297
  therapeutic alliance and, 302
  TNB scientific research and, 296
  transprejudice and, 297
Trauma-informed care (TIC)
  affirmation in, 300
  collaboration in, 310
  defining, 298
  principles of, 309
  safety in, 300–301, 309
  social support and, 310
  TNB older adults and, 275
The Trauma Recovery Model for Transgender, Nonbinary and Gender Expansive People of Color, 299
Travel, 89, 195
Treatment planning
  interdisciplinary collaborative care (ICC) and, 81
  spirituality and, 362
  TNB POC-affirming counseling and, 145–147
  TNB POC considerations in, 145–147
  trauma-informed, 306
TRIM (transgender resilience intervention model), 176
Trust
  caregivers and, 216
  cultivating, 138–139
  therapeutic alliance and, 309
2019 National School Climate Survey, 385
Two-Spirit individuals, 24, 167, 358–359

U

Unified model of advocacy, 69–71
United States Transgender Survey (USTS), 116
United States v. Skrmetti, 7
USTS (United States Transgender Survey), 116

V

Veterans
  health care and, 202
  suicidality and, 319, 330
  telehealth and, 80

Victimization
  nonbinary (NB) identity and, 170, 173
  TNB older adults and, 275–276
  TNB youth and, 303–304
Violence
  anti-TNB, 301, 302
  LGBTQ+ affiliated, 42
  sports and, 386
  surgical, 303
  TNB POC communities and, 134–135
  trans women and, 42, 295
Visibility
  effects of, 8
  sports and, 386
  TNB older adults and, 270
  TNB parents and, 190
Von Krafft-Ebing, Dr. Richer Freiherr, 106
Voting rights, 153, 212
Vulnerability
  correctional environments and, 48
  sports and, 384
  thick trust capital and, 139

W

Watchful waiting, 217

Well-being
  spirituality and, 148, 347–348
  TNB youth, 215
Western culture
  centering of, 349–350
  Indigenous communities and, 358–359
  religion and, 349, 353
World Professional Association for Transgender Health Standards of Care, 43–45, 253–254
World Professional Association for Transgender Health (WPATH), 66, 229
WPATH Global Education Initiative, 97
WPATH Standards of Care Version 8, 96
WPATH (World Professional Association for Transgender Health), 66, 229

Y

Youth Risk Behavior Surveillance System, 116

Z

Zulu parade, 141

About the Editors

Anneliese Singh, PhD, LPC, is a professor in the School of Social Work with a joint appointment in the Department of Psychology and serves as the associate provost for academic excellence and opportunity at Tulane University. Their research explores racial healing, racial trauma, and trans and queer liberation, with special attention to people of color and young people. Dr. Singh has written extensively on multicultural and social justice competency development in the helping professions, and equity and justice efforts in higher education. Dr. Singh is the author of *The Racial Healing Handbook: Practical Activities to Help You Challenge Privilege, Confront Systemic Racism, and Engage in Collective Healing* and *The Queer and Trans Resilience Workbook*. Dr. Singh founded the Trans Resilience Project to translate their LGBTQ+ research findings into school and community-based change efforts, including National Institutes of Health–funded work with trans and nonbinary people in Project AFFIRM and the Transgender Inclusion Empowerment Support project. Anneliese is a licensed counseling psychologist and professional counselor, and they are a fellow of the American Counseling Association and American Psychological Association. Anneliese's TEDx Talks have explored gender liberation. She is a South Asian, mixed race, genderqueer femme who has worked with trans and nonbinary communities as a community organizer and scholar–activist for over 30 years. Anneliese passionately believes in and strives to live by the ideals of Dr. King's beloved community, as well as Audre Lorde's reminder that "without community, there is no liberation." Dr. Singh is @anneliesesingh on Instagram and LinkedIn.

Rafe McCullough, PhD, LPC, LMHC, NCC, is an associate professor of Professional Mental Health Counseling in the Department of Counseling, Therapy, and School Psychology at Lewis & Clark College in Portland, Oregon. Dr. McCullough has counseling specializations in both clinical mental health and professional school counseling. His writing, research, and interests center on multicultural and social justice counseling and advocacy, disability and disability justice, clinical practice with youth and young adults, supporting trans educators, and affirming clinical practices for queer and trans clients. For over 25 years, Dr. McCullough has been involved in sustained advocacy and deep engagement within trans communities, supporting and fighting for trans people's rights to exist and to live full lives, especially trans and nonbinary youth. Dr. McCullough is a licensed professional counselor and a licensed school counselor, currently providing services to trans and nonbinary young adults, the youth, and their families. For him, this work is profoundly personal, and he is fiercely passionate about care for trans and nonbinary communities. He believes in the power of joy, wonder, curiosity, and humor to help his cherished community face and navigate the challenges ahead.